2599

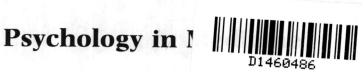

Psychology in M

For Charnwood, Church Row and Cothall,
which provided asylum.

A medical man likes to make psychological observations

George Eliot, *Middlemarch* (1871)

...more than half of practical medicine is psychology...

John Ryle, *The Natural History of Disease* (1936)

Psychology in Medicine

I.C. McMANUS MA, MD, PhD

Senior Lecturer in Psychology, St Mary's Hospital Medical School,
Imperial College of Science, Technology and Medicine, London, UK,
and University College London, UK

Consulting Editor

PETER RICHARDS MA, MD, PhD, FRCP

Professor of Medicine and Dean, St Mary's Hospital Medical School,
Imperial College of Science, Technology and Medicine, London, UK

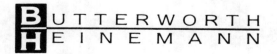

Butterworth-Heinemann Ltd
Linacre House, Jordan Hill, Oxford OX2 8DP

 PART OF REED INTERNATIONAL BOOKS

OXFORD   LONDON   BOSTON
MUNICH   NEW DELHI   SINGAPORE   SYDNEY
TOKYO   TORONTO   WELLINGTON

First published 1992

© Butterworth-Heinemann Ltd 1992

British Library Cataloguing in Publication Data
McManus, I. C.
  Psychology in Medicine
  I. Title
  150
ISBN 0 7506 0496 4

CV
WLM100

Typeset by Lasertext Ltd., Stretford, Manchester
Printed and bound in Malta by Interprint Limited

Contents

Preface

In his *Provincial Letters*, Pascal apologized for writing such a long letter, but he didn't have time to write a short one; but brevity in writing is not easy, as the young Ruskin recognized when he wrote to his father 'I would write a short, pithy, laconic, sensible, concentrated, and serious letter if I could...'. I was asked to write a short book, and like many before me I thought it would be easier than writing a long one and found that it is not. This book is perhaps still too long, and that is a heinous crime in writing for medical students, for their curriculum is horribly overloaded. Those words they do read have to seem relevant, readable, interesting, and to communicate the excitement and interest of the subject. Whether this book does that it is not for n e to say, but it is more likely to do so than in its lengthier first draft.

Although aimed principally at medical students, I hope that this book may also find another target. Many doctors qualified before psychology established itself as an accepted part of the medical curriculum. Some will now wish to discover what psychology is about; maybe out of curiosity or perhaps because while studying some other medical phenomenon they have come across those nebulous 'psychological factors', which are so frequently invoked as explanation, and accompanied by much arm-waving — and they wish to know what psychology has to offer. I hope that this small book will provide a quick answer to their questions.

In carrying out any task we all have role-models. The *cognoscenti* of textbook style might be interested to know that I have tried, although certainly with less success, to write a book that combines features from the best three textbooks that I know: McKeown and Lowe's *Textbook of Social Medicine*, Roitt's *Essential Immunology*, and Cavalli-Sforza and Bodmer's *The Genetics of Human Populations*. They showed me that textbooks can be well-written, well-illustrated, present ideas as well as facts, and be enjoyable.

The original idea for this book came from Peter Richards, and his patience and commitment have been supported by Richard Barling and then Susan Devlin from Butterworth-Heinemann; I hope it was worth waiting for. Needless to say the book started out as a series of lecture notes, which have been developed, polished and refined; my thanks to a decade of students at St Mary's on whom I have honed the material presented here. The book could not have been written without those who provided a place of refuge from the London bustle; my grateful thanks to my parents, to David and Wilhemina Lockwood, and to Geraldine McNeill all of whom kept me fed, watered and warm while I spent the days writing. The final stages of the book could not have been completed without Jack Van Horn's enthusiasm and commitment. Finally, as always, my thanks to Diana Lockwood for providing support throughout the project.

Chris McManus
London, 1991

1

Introduction

- Psychology is a young science, with its own special methods and theories for measuring and understanding phenomena.
- Preclinical teaching should not principally provide factual material, which is only forgotten, but a broader conceptual understanding.
- Psychology is often perceived as a 'difficult' subject, partly because of the multiple theories, which work over different time scales, and partly because of a supposed absence of 'facts'.
- The method of study known as SURFACE LEARNING, with its emphasis upon rote-learning, will not work well in studying the behavioural sciences. Instead DEEP LEARNING, with its emphasis upon ideas and principles, is required.
- Psychology is not taught only to help you understand other people, but also to help you understand yourself, and your relation to other people.

Psychology, along with sociology, is a newish entrant to the already crowded preclinical curriculum. The General Medical Council first recommended the inclusion of behavioural sciences in the medical curriculum in 1957, the advice was reinforced by the Royal Commission on Medical Education ('The Todd Report') of 1968, and during the 1970s most medical schools appointed special teachers in both psychology and sociology. It is surprising therefore that psychology and sociology are sometimes still controversial, with students and staff arguing their legitimate place within the medical curriculum. Rather than being seen as akin to the traditional preclinical sciences of anatomy, physiology and biochemistry, they are instead viewed as mere commonsense dressed up in complicated words. Such a view is however rapidly disappearing as it is accepted that an understanding of behaviour is central to the treatment of disease and the promotion of health. In 1991 the British government issued a consultative document entitled *The Health of the Nation*, which recognized this explicitly:

'...there is considerable emphasis in this document on the need for people to change their behaviour – whether on smoking, alcohol consumption, exercise, diet, avoidance of accidents [or]...sexual behaviour. The reason is simple. We live in an age where many of these main causes of premature death and unnecessary disease are related to how we live our lives.'

Psychology, and its place in the training of medical students, is frequently misunderstood. Few would dispute the place of anatomy, or other preclinical subjects, although often their purpose is not properly comprehended. A detailed knowledge of anatomy is not relevant to the daily practice of most doctors, or even to most surgeons except in their particular area of specialisation. Neither are medical students taught anatomy so that a quarter of a century hence they will recall, instantly and without hesitation that the musculo-phrenic and superior epigastric arteries are branches of the internal thoracic artery, or that teres major, teres minor, the humerus and the long head of triceps are the defining features of the quadrilateral space. As a matter of empirical fact, most students will forget such information soon after being examined in it. Nevertheless the careful and systematic study of anatomy does leave a residue within the student; an awareness of the three-dimensional inter-relations of body components, a conceptual grasp of the relations and functions of muscle, artery, vein and nerve. Without detailed study, this anatomical awareness would not be possible. The dividends on this investment of time are paid throughout the doctor's career whenever the structure of the body is considered, be it in carrying out a lumbar puncture, contemplating the fate of a peanut inhaled by a child, or viewing a tomographic scan. Anatomy is not medicine, but is a basis of medicine: clinical skills are built upon such foundations. Additionally, anatomy is taught well or badly according to the extent to which its eventual applications are considered.

Psychology is likewise basic to medicine. It does not intend to provide specific skills of daily use in the actual practice of medicine. Rather its purpose is to make you aware that human beings have a psychological dimension to them (as well as chemical, cellular, physiological, anatomical and social dimensions), and in particular that illness inevitably has a host of psychological aspects. As a doctor whose role is to treat the *whole* patient (rather than being a mere technician concerned solely with one detailed topic), you must necessarily understand the broad principles underlying thought and behaviour. The specific details are not of enormous importance (and indeed, as in all sciences, will evolve so that ideas once thought to be correct may be seen as erroneous or even laughable by future generations). What does matter is understanding the approach of the subject, its own especial flavour. Most medical students have already been trained in the physical sciences (such as chemistry) and in biological sciences (such as biology and physiology). Each subject has its own 'logic', an approach that recognizes the inherent problems specific to its own subject matter, and allows scientifically valid conclusions to be reached. The logic of chemistry cannot simply be transplanted into the physiology laboratory for many reasons; an important one is that physiological phenomena are inherently more variable than chemical processes. Likewise the logic of psychology often differs from other preclinical sciences.

Psychology attempts to teach a number of things. First and foremost it tries to convince the student that although in some ways psychological phenomena are inherently different from other biological phenomena, they are not necessarily beyond scientific analysis. On the contrary, psychology has evolved its own special techniques and methods for studying what might otherwise seem to be scientifically intractable problems concerned with such subjective phenomena as feelings, moods, interests and perceptions. These methods and theories provide a set of conceptual tools that can be applied to a whole range of situations. These concepts could be taught by considering many different situations (such as the psychology of political opinion, social behaviour in rats, or perception in pigeons). However, in the present context, the subject is better taught with examples, wherever possible, which are relevant to medical practice, because that way the future application of the ideas will be obvious. Nevertheless, it must be remembered that the specific information is not the core of the subject; instead it is the underlying general principles and ideas. Therefore, although this book discusses in some detail the problems of bereavement, and does not mention the problems of being diagnosed as diabetic, this does not mean that only the former is 'important'. Each may well be important in your future practice, and each shares certain features. The central feature of each is *loss*, with all that implies; loss of a friend or relative in one case, of a way of life and of a sense of one's own well-being in the other. By understanding how loss affects the bereaved you will also gain insights into the role of loss in the newly diagnosed diabetic. This book is short and I have therefore chosen the topics using two criteria: to illustrate important psychological principles or to discuss important practical problems that will be met in practice; and, preferably, both. Nevertheless, the book does not pretend to be comprehensive; there are many larger books and journals in libraries for those wishing to develop their new conceptual tools on more substantial material.

The other important approach of this book, and it is one in which I especially hope that it differs from many other introductory textbooks, is its emphasis upon *evidence*. Psychology is an empirical science and as such is based on data. Most illustrations in this book are not theoretical or generalized abstractions from data, but show actual experimental results. The underlying message is that psychology is done by measuring things which at first sight may seem almost immeasurable. Often these measures are straightforward and easy to apply, requiring apparatus only as complicated as a pencil, paper and stopwatch. As such psychology is ideal for student research projects, as well as for complicated research programmes. As always in science, though, the difficult part is not simply collecting data but collecting the *right* data, and interpreting them as a convincing answer to a specific research problem; then others can repeat the study, extend the results, and advance the theory further.

Psychology in medical schools has a reputation as a 'difficult' subject. Why is this? Students often say there are many technical terms; the implication is that these are unnecessary, being more easily stated in ordinary language. However, all sciences have their technical terms (anatomy perhaps being the most extensive), and their purpose is to make important but subtle differences between concepts. Psychology is no exception. Everyday language is a deceptive friend and must be extended if it is to describe the subtleties of thought and mind. Another complaint is that psychologists cannot make up their minds, and insist on giving several different theories to describe a single process. More annoyingly, the psychologists apparently insist on students knowing *all* of the theories, although it would surely seem obvious that only one can actually be correct, and hence *that* is the one to be learnt. The problem here is more subtle, being partly connected with the nature of psychology, and partly with the nature of students.

Psychology works on many different time scales, from simple learning processes lasting a few minutes, to social phenomena over days, weeks, and months, and to developmental processes literally encompassing the entire life-span. Different levels of explanation are needed to account for processes from all of these points of view (in the same way as a building needs plans, elevations and sections if it is to be described properly). In other cases there are indeed rival theories, each with evidence in its favour, but none of which can account for all that needs to be explained. Final judgement must therefore be reserved at present. Students must use their critical powers to assess the relative merits of the rival theories, determine how well they fit the data, and consider how future data may allow one to accept a particular theory and to reject another. Understandably the response of students to such uncertainty is often to feel confused.

The sense of confusion engendered by the behavioural sciences is partly a function of previous education. Science as taught in school is typically cut and dried. Facts are facts, and there is little problem. Preclinically this is also true of many of the subjects, and reflects their later stage of development as sciences. To use an astronomical metaphor, topographical anatomy, the oldest of the preclinical sciences, is like a long burnt out star, a white dwarf, a dense but hardly illuminating mass. The mature sciences of biochemistry and physiology are like our own sun, seemingly fixed and immutable, producing a deceptively clear, even light; deceptive because at the sun's centre considerable heat and energy are being generated from the controversies of researchers, although those phenomena are hardly discernible to the student. Psychology and sociology are akin to young, new star systems, distantly perceived through ever more powerful telescopes. Appearing on the scene only recently, the turmoil at their heart is apparent even from afar, and as yet their light is neither strong nor predictable. It is controversy, in the form of disparate theories, that fuels the reactions behind them, and which illuminates the world around them. Overall there is a sense of excitement in anticipating the eventual evolution of what will probably be new star systems, albeit ones whose final form is far from clear.

A further problem for students is in the way that they study the basic social sciences, which is influenced by the knowledge that they need to pass the essential exams at the end of the preclinical course. Two major approaches to learning have been identified by educational psychologists. SURFACE LEARNING is the mere rote-learning of material, which is passively absorbed in its totality, seemingly without any obvious intervention of mind or brain, later to be spewed forth onto the exam paper, and subsequently to be forgotten forever. It is an efficient method if the quantities are relatively small, and the exam is similar in structure to the material taught. It is however educationally unedifying for student and teacher alike. By contrast, DEEP LEARNING is the understanding of principles and ideas, so that novel problems can be approached, and controversies critically evaluated. It is what most teachers would say is the purpose of a university education, although many students fail ever to see this, as often as not because of the limited nature of their teaching. Deep learning is hard work, requiring extensive thought, but is very efficient in the long term because only one idea needs to be learned, rather than many specific instances. Much teaching in medical schools regrettably encourages a mindless surface learning approach (and some cynics say that is why they are often called medical *schools* rather than universities). For some subjects, surface learning can work well. It does *not* work well for psychology or sociology (or for that matter, for physiology, with its emphasis upon systems theory, or for statistics, which are other subjects often felt to be 'difficult'). The prescription for success is simply stated: psychology is about the mind, and the mind will not be understood without the application of hard work from another mind, your own.

Psychology and sociology have a further role as basic medical sciences that is nothing to do with a cold, calculating and rigorous application of scientific principles to other people in other situations, but is instead to do with helping you to understand yourself. While reading, thinking and learning about processes such as 'perception', 'memory', 'thinking' or 'learning', you will inevitably realize that you yourself are simultaneously carrying out those tasks. Psychology is not a soulless knowledge about a remote organism; instead it concerns you yourself and all you do, and it can help develop a self-awareness, an insight, which would be difficult to attain otherwise. Similarly when learning about social psychology there will be an awareness that you are also part of a social world in which you have certain motives and drives. And on a more sober note, you also are mortal, will inevitably become ill, be treated as a patient and eventually die, as will those around you. These processes are inexorable, and are a part of the human condition. Denial of them in yourself or in others will help neither you nor your patients in your future professional career; and of course denial is itself also a psychological process that will be studied. Part of the role of psychology in a preclinical course is to remind you that medicine is not just about enzymes, electrodes, scalpels and drugs but is about people, other human beings like yourself who react to events and have similar problems and views of the world. Psychology is not only a science, it is a human science, and it is in a broad sense part of the humanities. Theories of education have sometimes been likened to a jug or spectacles. The jug model regards students as a vessel into which facts are poured until full. The spectacle model says that education provides a pair of glasses through which the student can see the world differently and more clearly. Psychology's role is unashamedly that of extending your vision, both outwards and inwards.

Basic processes

2

Perception and sensation

- The passive, almost instantaneous and automatic process of SENSATION must be distinguished from the active, slower, interpretation of the sensory world found in PERCEPTION.
- Even simple sensory judgements involve a decision process, which can be understood by SIGNAL DETECTION THEORY.
- Differences in decision making can be interpreted in terms of SENSITIVITY, the true differences in effectiveness of the sensory apparatus, and CRITERION, a willingness to produce FALSE ALARMS or MISSES.
- Perception uses prior expectations and likelihoods, coupled with the information present in a stimulus, to produce the most likely interpretation of a stimulus.
- ILLUSIONS result when errors arise in the processing of sensory images. Psychology exploits errors in order to understand how systems function.

Although similar in ordinary usage, perception and sensation have distinct meanings; the difference between seeing and 'seeing'. Look at Figure 2.1. Although the areas of black and white are easily made out, you will not see anything else in the figure because it has intentionally been printed upside down. Turn the book round and look again. Initially there are still only unconnected black and white patches. Suddenly though you will begin to make out a picture. Have a few hints: there is a black and white dog to the right of centre, nose to the left, sniffing the ground, with a tree behind, and the ground strewn with leaves. By now you should have seen it. If not, then keep looking. It is not a hoax; indeed it is a genuine photograph. Perhaps ask a friend if you still cannot work it out. The aim of this demonstration is that suddenly you should have 'seen' the meaningless black and white patches as a complex picture. The 'Aha!' phenomenon, at which you may have worked quite hard, is PERCEPTION, whereas the instantaneous, easy, seemingly trivial process of being aware of the black and white patches is the process of SENSATION.

Perception is an *active* process that we work at, often for a long time, and whose success depends both upon our present state, previous experience and knowledge, and expectations, which is why a hint

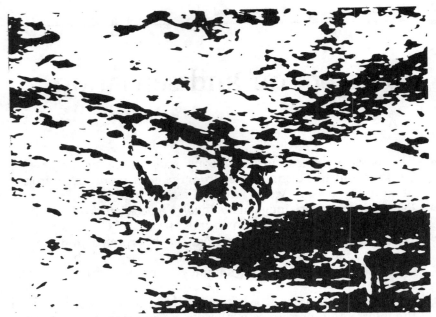

Fig. 2.1 This figure has intentionally been printed upside down. Before turning the book around, read the beginning of Chapter 2. Photograph by R C James.

helps so much with Figure 2.1. Sensation, however, is the *passive* process of transducing physical events from the world into neural activity in the brain, so that we are aware of them; sensation is unaffected by knowledge, experience or expectations. Sensation and perception are clearly distinguished when we try to build machines that can do them. Optical sensing devices that produce a voltage in proportion to light intensity have been known for many years and form the basis of television cameras; such a device could easily differentiate the black and white areas in Figure 2.1. However computers that can scan the output from a camera and print 'Dog, park, autumn', do not exist and their construction provides many problems, not merely technical, but reflecting our far deeper inability to program knowledge and experience. The uses of such a device would be enormous; an example would be automatically examining photomicrographs of cervical smears to detect malignant change, a task which presently is tedious, time-consuming, error-prone and involves large numbers of highly trained staff.

Although sensation is apparently totally passive, this is only true when the sensory system is considered in isolation. Any real judgement about sensation always actually involves higher psychological processing. Consider an actual study.

A doctor, D, palpated the abdomen of 65 patients with his hand and used tactile sensations to decide whether the spleen was enlarged.

	Doctor's judgement					
Doctor D		Normal	Enlarged	Total	Detection rate	False alarm rate	Overall success rate

Doctor D		Normal	Enlarged	Total	Detection rate	False alarm rate	Overall success rate
	Normal	43	5	48			
Actual size					12/17 = 0.61	5/48 = 0.10	(43 + 12)/65 = 0.85
	Enlarged	5	12	17 / 65			
Doctor E		Normal	Enlarged	Total	Detection rate	False alarm rate	Overall success rate
	Normal	27	21	48			
Actual size					16/17 = 0.94	21/48 = 0.44	(27 + 16)/65 = 0.66
	Enlarged	1	16	17 / 65			
Doctor F		Normal	Enlarged	Total	Detection rate	False alarm rate	Overall success rate
	Normal	35	13	48			
Actual size					8/17 = 0.47	13/48 = 0.27	(35 + 8)/65 = 0.66
	Enlarged	9	8	17 / 65			

Fig. 2.2 Doctors' clinical judgements (based on palpation of the abdomen) of whether or not the spleen is enlarged or normal; the judgements are compared with an objective assessment of true spleen size obtained by technetium scintigraphy. Doctor D is an actual physician (data reported by Sullivan S and Williams R (1976), Reliability of clinical techniques for detecting splenic enlargement, *Br Med J*, **2**, 1043–4), whereas doctors E and F are hypothetical individuals to illustrate the principles of signal detection theory.

Spleen size was also determined objectively by technetium scintigraphy. Figure 2.2 shows that in the 48 patients with a normal spleen, the doctor regarded the spleen as enlarged in five cases (10.4%), and in the 17 patients with an enlarged spleen the doctor recorded an enlarged spleen in 12 cases (70.6%). Therefore in a typical study of ability to carry out physical examinations, doctor D is moderately accurate, being correct in 55 of 65 patients (84.6%).

Now consider two other hypothetical doctors, E and F, who might also have done the study. Dr E is only correct in 42 (64.6%) of the patients, as is Dr F. Are then Drs E and F less sensitive than Dr D? Not necessarily. Drs E and F may be less *sensitive* (perhaps having poorer technique, or less sensitive fingers), but it might also be that Drs E and F differ in the *caution* that they use, and hence achieve a lower overall success rate. Consider the most cautious doctor imaginable, who worries so much about erroneously saying a spleen is enlarged that all patients are described as 'normal'. Although this decision is actually correct in 48 patients who truly had normal spleens, such data can say nothing about true ability to distinguish normal from abnormal, only about clinical and professional priorities.

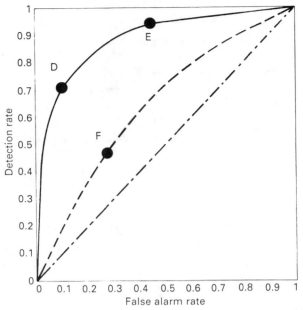

Fig. 2.3 The receiver operating curves (ROC) for the three individuals of Figure 2.2. The curved lines indicate lines of equal sensitivity (d'), so that Drs D and E are of equal true sensitivity. The straight, diagonal line indicates 'chance' or random responding in which the subject is completely unable to carry out the task (i.e. $d' = 0$). Increasing threshold or criterion (*beta*) is indicated by distances along the dashed curves from the bottom left-hand corner, so that Dr D is more cautious than Dr E, whereas Drs D and F are of similar degrees of caution.

Caution (or CRITERION) and SENSITIVITY can be distinguished from a subject's complete pattern of responses. Figure 2.2 shows the four response types that occur in each subject: two combinations are correct (enlarged spleen reported as enlarged, and normal spleen reported as normal) and two types are incorrect; FALSE POSITIVES (normal spleen reported as enlarged), and false negatives or MISSES (enlarged spleen reported as normal). These responses are summarized as the DETECTION RATE, the proportion of enlarged spleens detected in those patients with enlarged spleens, and the FALSE ALARM RATE, the proportion of enlarged spleens reported in patients with normal spleens.

Figure 2.2 shows that Dr D has a moderate detection rate (71%) and a low false alarm rate (10%), whereas Dr E has a high detection rate (94%) and a very high false alarm rate (44%). Dr D is good at reassuring normal subjects, whereas Dr E is good at detecting disease in the abnormal. Dr F has both a low detection rate (47%) and a moderately high false alarm rate (27%). Figure 2.3 shows the data plotted on a RECEIVER OPERATING CURVE (ROC). The X-axis shows the false alarm rate and the Y-axis the 'hit-rate', the proportion of detections in patients with enlarged spleens. For such curves, subjects with similar criteria lie on lines running perpendicular to the diagonal, and subjects with similar sensitivities lie on the lines parallel to the diagonal. We can now better describe Drs D, E and F. Drs D and E are actually equally sensitive but Dr D is more cautious than Dr E. Dr F however, is less sensitive than Drs D and E. In the psychological literature this is known as a SIGNAL DETECTION EXPERIMENT, and the sensitivity and criterion are, for historical reasons, conventionally represented by d' and beta respectively. Figure 2.4 and its caption gives the mathematical background for understanding d' and *beta*.

Both d' and *beta* may differ in different subjects, and can also change within a single subject. Decreased attention or concentration can reduce d', as may various drugs, whereas experience and learning can increase d'. Altering a task's rewards, costs and demands can alter *beta*: if the cost of failure (e.g. the patient dying of malaria, undiagnosed because the spleen was wrongly said to be normal) is greater than the cost of a false alarm (e.g. the patient receives a few weeks' drug treatment) then the proportion of detections and the false alarm rate will both rise. Reversing the costs of detections and false alarms will decrease the detection and false alarm rates.

Signal detection theory also shows how patients may differ in interpreting symptoms such as pain. In Chapter 20 we will ask if some patients are genuinely more *sensitive* to pain, or if they *report* pain more often. Do analgesic drugs act by *reducing* pain or do they alter the reporting of pain?

Signal detection theory applies both to the simplest of sensory judgements, such as detecting faint flashes of light, and to complex judgements, such as whether a patient requires immediate surgery. In all such situations differences in *true ability* must be distinguished from differences in *response tendency*.

PERCEPTION makes *decisions* based on the raw sensory information that is presented to the brain. A PARTICULAR sensory event, such as a pattern of light, is *interpreted* as a more UNIVERSAL response such as 'dog'; we recognize not only a specific animal, but also an object typical of the class of animals called dogs. Interpretation often goes beyond the information given, so we see what we *expect* to see. This is shown in an experiment in which Bruner asked subjects to sort a pack of playing cards by suit. As well as the four standard suits the pack also contained cards with a heart printed in black or a spade printed in red: few subjects noticed these cards, but instead sorted them as the standard suits which they had *expected* to see.

For any particular stimulus we have several hypotheses, which change in likelihood as further evidence is given. Occasionally we cannot settle on a single hypothesis, resulting in ILLUSIONS such as the

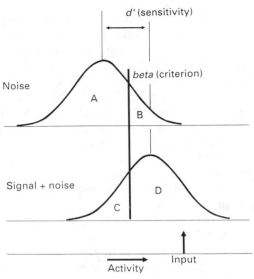

Fig. 2.4 Consider the activity occurring in a sensory nerve or in a central pathway. If no signal is present there will still be background or resting activity, or NOISE, varying from moment to moment, and probably distributed normally (see top distribution). When a true SIGNAL is present in addition to the background noise then the total activity will increase, and the overall distribution be shifted to the right (lower distribution). For any particular activity (e.g. 'Input', indicated at the bottom of the figure) the observer must decide if it results from a true signal or from background noise. The mathematically optimal strategy is to set a threshold, or criterion (*beta*), and say that all activity greater than this is signal and all activity less is noise. Thus since Input is greater than the criterion then it would be classified as a signal. Of course some actual signals (area C) will be reported as noise (misses), and some actual noise (B) will be reported as signals (false positives), although a majority of judgements (A + D) will be correctly assigned. As the observer shifts *beta* to left or right so the relative proportion of false positives to misses (B:C) will rise or fall; nevertheless *d'*, the true sensitivity of the observer, indicated by the differences in position of the peaks of the two distributions, remains the same. Only if the signal distribution shifts to the right (or if variabilities are reduced) does true sensitivity increase. The values plotted on the axes of the ROC curve are D/(D + C) on the ordinate and B/(A + B) on the abscissa.

NECKER CUBE (Fig. 2.5). After looking for a few moments you will see it reversing its perspective, so that it is seen from below rather than above; and a few seconds later it reverses back again. And indeed it never stops reversing. Perception continually works at the image, trying new hypotheses, but never reaching a definitive solution, because in this case there is insufficient evidence to distinguish them. The rate of reversal is proportional to intelligence, suggesting that in part intelligence is a continual searching for solutions to problems.

The Necker cube and the signal detection task illustrate an important feature of experimental approaches to psychology. Only when things

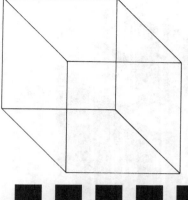

Fig. 2.5 The Necker cube, which can be seen either as a cube looked at from above and to the right, or as a cube looked at from below and to the left, the two interpretations continually and unpreventably alternating.

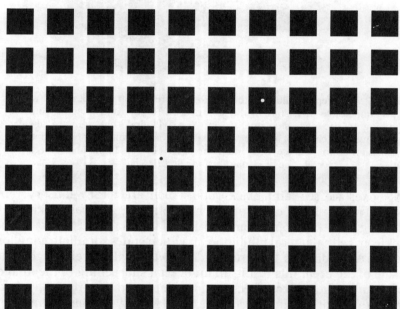

Fig. 2.6 A sensory illusion, the Hering Grid illusion. At the intersections can be seen a fuzzy grey spot, which is not truly present in the stimulus. The illusion is due to lateral inhibition in the ganglion cells of the retina. Note that the illusion is *not* an after-image. An after-image can be demonstrated in the figure by staring at the black dot for a minute or so, and then staring at the white spot. Superimposed on each black square should be seen a dark cross, which is an after-image resulting from the retinal activity arising from looking at the black dot. The after-image is due to fatigue of the cones in the retina.

go wrong, when we make *errors*, be they false positives, or the failure to see a set of lines as a single perception, do we gain insight into how the mind works. A perfect system tells us nothing about *how* it works.

Figures 2.6 and 2.7 shows several illusions coming from different sources. In the HERING GRID (Fig. 2.6) at the intersections between the

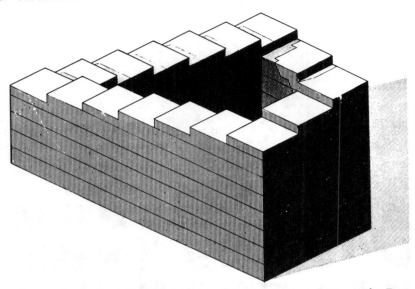

Fig. 2.7 A perceptual illusion, the Penrose figure. If you cannot see why Fig. 2.7 is impossible then start at the step nearest to you, and imagine yourself climbing to the next step and so on. You will find that you are always ascending, which is of course geometrically impossible. Reproduced with permission from Penrose L S and Penrose R (1958), Impossible objects: a special type of visual illusion, *Br J Psychol*, **49**, 31.

black boxes we see faint black dots, which are totally illusory. The dots are particularly clear at intersections we are *not* looking at, indicating that they come from non-foveal vision. This SENSORY ILLUSION arises from retinal lateral inhibition, in which cones stimulate ganglion cells corresponding to the area and *inhibit* ganglion cells slightly to the side of the area; this results in an overall sharpening of the image. Occasionally the process becomes visible, as in Figure 2.6, where ganglion cells at the intersection are so laterally inhibited that they apparently correspond to a darker area in the image. The workings of the sensory system are thus revealed to us by the illusion. Sensory illusions are distinguished from PERCEPTUAL ILLUSIONS, in which an error of *interpretation* is present, but the sensations are correct. However long we look at the Penrose figure (Fig. 2.7) we are unable to see it as a real three-dimensional figure, because the available information is conflicting.

Perception usually has to be learnt. As a demonstration, take a small electronic flash gun and ask a friend to hold it about six feet from you. Stare at the centre of the flash gun, and discharge it. You will get a strong AFTER-IMAGE, which is enhanced by blinking. Look at the palm of your hand and you will 'project' the after-image as a small purplish patch, shaped like the flash-gun aperture. Now look at a distant wall. The after-image looks larger. This is surprising because the after-image is fixed on your retina and cannot change its size. Context alters the apparent size. Distant objects in reality have smaller retinal images than those that are close. If an object known to be far away (the wall) produces the same retinal image as a closer object (your hand) then the only interpretation is that the more 'distant' object is also larger. This is known as Emmert's Law, and it is due to SIZE CONSTANCY: objects stay the same PHENOMENAL SIZE as they go further away, despite their retinal images shrinking. This constancy is apparently learnt, small children genuinely thinking that distant objects are indeed smaller.

Perception often makes assumptions about the way the world looks, for only then can it disambiguate otherwise indistinguishable hypotheses. Consider the problem of deciding whether a visual object is moving. When an image moves across our retina, two possibilities arise: it corresponds to an object moving in the world, or it corresponds to a motionless object viewed by a moving eye. There can be no *visual* information that distinguishes these hypotheses. There are two ways in which we might distinguish. We might have receptors in the eye-muscles, which tell us if our eyes are moving. Alternatively we might say, 'I have not told my eyes to move, therefore they cannot be moving, and therefore the moving image must correspond to a moving object'. Although it seems unlikely, the latter explanation is shown to be correct by a simple experiment.

Close your eyes and gently place your fingertip on the lower outer eyelid, and then carefully open your eye and push gently on the eyeball. The whole world seems to move. Of course the world is not actually moving, so why do you perceive it as such? Pushing the eye produces a moving visual image, but you have not told the eye to move, and hence it must be that the world is moving; and so it appears to be. Generally the assumption works well, but occasionally it fails, and we then have an illusion of the world moving and gain insight into how the system works.

Sensation and perception are our only basis for a knowledge of the world. All information has arrived through those systems, and hence might be illusory or deceptive. As we encounter new stimuli we must ask whether they arise from outside or within our perceptual systems. Both we and our patients can be fooled by our perceptions, be it when we are examining an abdomen for an enlarged spleen, or looking at a chest X-ray or ultrasonogram, or when a patient is describing a pain or other symptom.

3

Learning

- In learning, an organism changes its future behaviour in response to the consequences of its previous behaviour, and forms novel associations between stimuli and responses.
- PAVLOVIAN OR CLASSICAL CONDITIONING involves a CONDITIONED STIMULUS producing a CONDITIONED RESPONSE, such as salivation, that normally would be produced as the result of an UNCONDITIONED REFLEX.
- SKINNERIAN OR OPERANT CONDITIONING involves an alteration in the rate of a behaviour, such as lever-pressing, due to REWARD or PUNISHMENT.
- Classical and operant conditioning seem to be separate processes, and differ procedurally, in the types of behaviour they apply to, and in their response to EXTINCTION.
- PUNISHMENT can decrease the frequency of an operant behaviour, and in the case of ONE-TRIAL AVERSIVE CONDITIONING after illness or poisoning can result in long-lasting behavioural change.
- Not all learning involves classical or operant conditioning. Other types include LATENT LEARNING, and MODELLING or IMITATION LEARNING.

Benefiting from experience requires an organism to change its behaviour in different circumstances; the process is LEARNING and the information stored is called MEMORY. Mainly for practical reasons, learning is usually studied in animals and memory in man, and despite different methodologies it is the same process being studied.

The first systematic studies of learning were the famous experiments of the Russian physiologist, Ivan Pavlov (1849–1936), who measured the amount of salivation in dogs in his laboratory. Dogs reflexly produce saliva when food is presented. More interestingly, Pavlov showed that if a bell is rung before food is presented then dogs will salivate to the sound of the bell alone. This is PAVLOVIAN or CLASSICAL CONDITIONING. In learning theory terms, the food is an UNCONDITIONED STIMULUS (US) that produces an UNCONDITIONED RESPONSE (UR) via a reflex. The bell is a CONDITIONED STIMULUS (CS) that eventually also produces salivation, the CONDITIONED RESPONSE (CR). Although the UR and CR appear to be identical, they are not precisely identical, and hence have different names. In classical conditioning, an animal acquires new behaviours (e.g. salivating to a bell), which are potentially adaptive.

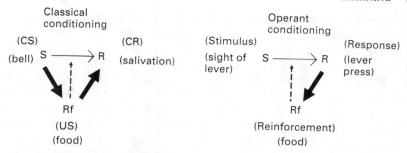

Fig. 3.1 The relations between the stimulus (S), the response (R), and the reinforcement (Rf) in classical and operant conditioning. Invariant links are indicated by heavy arrows, either being inbuilt reflexes (as in the case of the Rf-R link in classical conditioning) or being designed into the experiment as invariant (as in the S-Rf and Rf-R links in classical and operant conditioning respectively). Learned connections are indicated by light arrows. The influence of the reinforcer is shown by a dashed line, in strengthening a learned connection.

A different form of learning, described in the 1930s by the American psychologist B F Skinner (1904–1990), is called OPERANT, INSTRUMENTAL or SKINNERIAN CONDITIONING. At first it seems very different to classical conditioning. A hungry rat is placed in an experimental cage (a SKINNER BOX) that contains a lever, which the rat can push, and a trough in which a food pellet may appear. Eventually, perhaps by accident, the rat pushes the lever and a food pellet appears. Soon the rat is pushing the lever continuously to obtain food. In the terminology of operant conditioning, the lever press is a RESPONSE, the food is a REINFORCER. The response is REWARDED and hence increases in rate (to such an extent that a hungry rat may spend much of its day lever-pressing). The reinforcer acts because it satisfies a basic DRIVE (hunger in this case, but perhaps thirst, sleep, sex or warmth).

Much controversy has arisen as to whether classical and operant conditioning are the same fundamental process, or are separate (a 'two-process theory'). Most researchers now accept there are indeed two separate processes, which are differentiated in several ways. Firstly, there are procedural differences. Consider classical conditioning (Fig. 3.1). A stimulus, S, is *always* followed by a reinforcer (Rf) (indicated by the solid arrows). That reinforcer *always* causes a response (R). The reinforcer then causes a *direct* link to be set up between S and R, which gradually becomes stronger on each presentation of S and R. (Note that although this is classical conditioning, I have purposely used the language of operant conditioning to emphasize the similarities.) Figure 3.1 also shows operant conditioning. The animal sees the lever (S), and makes the response (R) of pushing it. This response *always* causes reinforcement to appear, in the form of food. The effect of the reinforcer is to strangthen the link between S and R so that in future the sight of the lever is more likely to make the animal press it. It should now be obvious that in both types of conditioning, new links are created between stimulus and response; this whole area is sometimes called s-r psychology. The difference is that in one case the experimenter controls the stimulus (i.e. the bell is always rung before food) and in the other it is the reinforcer that is controlled (i.e. food is always given when the lever is pressed). There is also an additional link in the case of classical conditioning, in that the reinforcer (the US) automatically causes a response (the UR) by a reflex, whereas in operant conditioning no such prior links exist. In addition, for operant conditioning to work organisms need to be able to monitor their own behaviours (i.e. in general they are voluntary actions), whereas no such feedback is necessary for classical conditioning to occur, which frequently involves involuntary autonomic responses.

A final difference between the two types of learning emerges when reinforcement is withdrawn. If the bell is rung but *no* food is subsequently presented then the salivation responses to the bell gradually die away, a process known as extinction. By contrast if, in operant conditioning, a press of the lever produces *no* food then the rat *increases* its rate of lever pressing, the extinction burst, and only then does the behaviour finally extinguish completely.

It has been necessary to describe these two types of learning in some detail because they underlie many behaviours, both human and animal, and can be used to explain a wide range of abnormal behaviours, from temper tantrums in children, to the development of phobias. Consider even the everyday observation of seeing somebody walk up to a lift, press the button and find the lift doesn't come; invariably they then press the button perhaps half a dozen more times, an extinction burst, before finally walking up the stairs. Rationally, there is little justification for such behaviour, because it is most unlikely that the switch itself is faulty.

In classical conditioning, the phenomenon of *secondary conditioning* is of great importance. Consider a dog trained to salivate to a bell. If we now turn on a light, and follow the light by the bell, but do not follow the bell by food on that occasion, the bell will produce its conditioned response of salivation, and eventually the animal will salivate to the light, even though the light and food have never themselves been presented. By such mechanisms, long complex chains of behaviour can be created.

Operant conditioning has developed a massive and complex terminology. A few terms are worth knowing. If instead of rewarding the animal for every response (continuous reinforcement) one rewards only after, say, *every* tenth lever press, this is called a fixed ratio (FR) schedule of reinforcement, and if one rewards only *on average* each tenth press, but sometimes after two and sometimes after forty presses, then this is variable-ratio (VR) reinforcement, which has the property

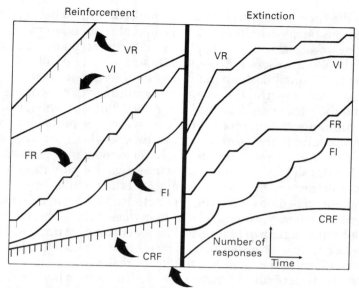

Fig. 3.2 Behaviour under different operant schedules (CRF Continuous reinforcement; FI Fixed interval; VI Variable interval; FR Fixed rate; VR Variable rate), both during reinforcement and during extinction. The CUMULATIVE RECORDS show time along the abscissa and responses on the ordinate, each lever press moving the pen upwards by a small fixed amount. Presentation of rewards is indicated by a downward tick on the record. Redrawn with permission from Walker S (1984), *Learning theory and behaviour modification*, London, Methuen, 54.

of being very resistant to extinction and of simulating many reward processes in the real world (for instance the gambler at the roulette table). If a reinforcer is given only after, say, *exactly* thirty seconds have passed since the previous reinforcer, then this is called a FIXED-INTERVAL (FI) reinforcement, and it produces its own characteristic pattern of responses, SCALLOPING, whereby the animal responds at a high rate just before the end of the critical time-interval (see Fig. 3.2). In contrast variable interval (VI) rewards, in which the animal is rewarded *on average* every 30 seconds, produce a steady sustained rate of responding (Fig. 3.2). In each type of reinforcement the animal can be considered to act in a way that maximizes its return for a minimum of effort. DISCRIMINATION LEARNING is when an animal learns to respond, say, to one lever when a blue light is on and to another lever when a red light is on. Such techniques can be used to ask subtle questions about, for instance, the colour perception of animals, particularly if combined with the phenomenon of STIMULUS GENERALIZATION, in which a stimulus like, but not identical to, the training stimulus is tested. We may ask whether a purple colour looks more like red or blue to a rat, by observing whether the rat trained as described above presses the 'blue' or the 'red' lever when presented with various purplish lights. Generalization also underlies the increasing range of objects to which phobic patients become sensitive, so that a phobia of spiders may generalize to a phobia of all insects, or perhaps to all small dark animals, and then to any animal.

A final but important variant on learning experiments is that although the reinforcers described so far (food, but also water, warmth, and in human societies, money) have increased the probability or the rate of responding, there are also PUNISHMENTS, which are aversive or unpleasant, and decrease the likelihood of responding; examples are mild electric shocks in animals, withdrawal of attention in the case of children, or fines or imprisonments for adults. Aversive, or punishment, schedules have the characteristic that the behaviour is reduced in frequency, so much so in many cases that it becomes very difficult for the organism to unlearn the association; extinction cannot readily occur as the response is never made and so the lack of a relationship with the action cannot be realized. ONE-TRIAL AVERSIVE CONDITIONING is particularly important in situations where a rat feels nauseous or ill after eating a particular food, and avoids that food in future. Such conditioning is probably responsible for many human food fads and preferences, and for CANCER ANOREXIA (see Chapter 26); if you eat strawberries for the first time at a party, and develop food poisoning within the next few hours (perhaps because of infected meat, or some other cause unrelated to strawberries) you may well develop a strong aversion to strawberries in the future. NEGATIVE REINFORCEMENT is technically not the same as punishment, being the *removal* of an *aversive* event, and therefore causing an *increase* in behaviour (since all reinforcers are defined as events that *increase* the rate of behaviour and all punishments as events that *decrease* the rate of behaviour; a negative reinforcer must therefore increase the rate of a behaviour and can only do this by removing something that is aversive). Therefore an animal being continually given electric shocks will work to press a lever to terminate the shocks, and the frequency of the lever-pressing behaviour is increased.

Thus far this chapter has emphasized classical and operant conditioning, the two forms of ASSOCIATIVE LEARNING. It might be objected that this emphasis is undue, and that there is no sense in which you might learn anatomy or psychology by schedules of reinforcement of reward for particular responses. That is indeed so, and there are other types of learning. However, the important thing about conditioning is that, so far as we can tell, it is the most primitive form of learning, occurring in all vertebrates and many invertebrates, and still being present and even frequent in man. It is the 'bottom-line'; it can always be used to modify behaviour, and frequently can be used to explain away apparently more complex and sophisticated behaviours. The most famous case is the horse, Clever Hans, who reputedly could

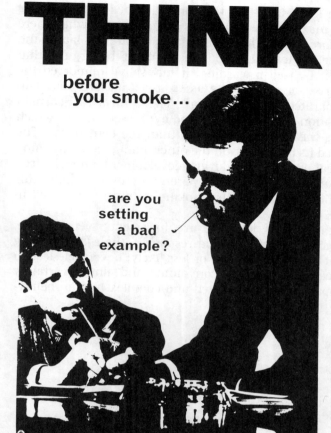

THINK

**before
you smoke...**

**are you
setting
a bad
example?**

Fig. 3.3 Child model-
ling parent smoking a
cigarette. Anti-smok-
ing advertisement pub-
lished by the Health
Education Council,
and reprinted with
permission.

solve arithmetic problems, tapping its hoof on the ground to count
out the answers, but in fact simply having been operantly conditioned
to respond to different expressions on the owner's face. In the mentally
subnormal and the mentally ill, conditioning becomes of great
importance, both in understanding and in treating abnormalities, and
in producing more socially acceptable behaviours, by such devices as
TOKEN ECONOMIES in which patients earn tokens for good behaviour, lose
them for antisocial behaviour, and can 'spend' them on rewards
(sweets or other reinforcers) — see Chapter 31.

Not all learning involves obvious, or direct, reinforcement. Edward
C Tolman (1886–1959) described the process known as *latent learning*.
A hungry, control rat learns to run through a complicated maze for
a food reward, and on each trial it runs faster and faster, as it learns
the route. A second non-hungry animal is placed in the maze without
food and is simply allowed to explore for a number of trials. Later it
is put into the maze when hungry and has to run though for food; it

learns the route in less trials than the control, showing that is was learning about the maze even when it was exploring, and when there was no direct reinforcement. The learning was apparently latent and only revealed later by testing, although it might be argued that because exploration is itself rewarding, it may have reinforced the learning. In MODELLING or IMITATION LEARNING, two rats are placed in adjacent cages separated by a glass wall. The control rat learns a complex discrimination task and is watched by the second rat, which when tested learns the task more quickly than the control rat. The test rat has modelled its behaviour on the other animal. Such learning is probably of great importance during development and children frequently model the actions of their parents or other adults; this occurs when a child imitates adults smoking by putting a pencil in its mouth (Fig. 3.3).

In summary, theories of learning are in essence very simple, involving the *association* of stimuli and responses, the *effects* making future behavioural associations more or less likely; nevertheless such simple processes can become very convoluted and almost certainly underlie many apparently sophisticated and complex human behaviours.

4

Memory

- Memory can be FRACTIONATED into several different types.
- ICONIC MEMORY is a buffer store lasting about half a second, and SHORT-TERM STORE is a limited capacity memory lasting about 15 seconds and holding 6 to 8 items.
- Recall from LONG-TERM STORE not only depends on the DEPTH OF PROCESSING during ENCODING, but is also affected by INTERFERENCE during retrieval.
- AMNESIA as a result of head injury can either be due to failure of encoding or consolidation (as in ANTEROGRADE AMNESIA or the RETROGRADE AMNESIA in the minutes before injury), or due to a deficit of retrieval (as in the longer-term RETROGRADE AMNESIA before injury).
- The memory deficit in KORSAKOFF'S SYNDROME is best explained as a deficit of retrieval rather than encoding, because learning does occur, albeit without conscious awareness.

Without memory we could have no conscious sense of past (or future) and would be consigned to a continuously changing but incomprehensible present, a situation in which some patients with brain lesions seem to find themselves. Memory is not a single process and much research has concerned the FRACTIONATION of memory to reveal the functional components. Different types of information are stored and retrieved differently. Most studies consider the idiosyncratic knowledge called EPISODIC MEMORY, the episodes of personal experience recalled in a specific context (what you had for breakfast today, or about your schooldays); SEMANTIC MEMORY is a more general knowledge about the world (that Bombay is south-west of Delhi, that Incan terns are black, or that the plural of mouse is mice), is independent of the context in which it was acquired (when did you learn that mice is the plural of mouse?), and which is similar to the semantic system of language (and can be damaged specifically in the condition of ANOMIC APHASIA — see Chapter 23). Semantic and episodic memory are both DECLARATIVE MEMORIES, capable of conscious recall, and are distinct from PROCEDURAL MEMORY, the knowledge of motor skills and conditioning, which are automatic and unconscious.

Consider what episodic memory must do. Fleeting experiences must be grasped, and held until placed in a more durable store than ephemeral electrical circuits (for memories can resist electroconvulsive shocks and general anaesthesia), and put where they can subsequently be found. Recall means finding the site of storage, extracting the memory, converting it to electrical events, and eventually outputting it. Failure at any stage means memory loss or AMNESIA for the event.

Many events are fleeting; indeed speech is so spread out in time that it has disappeared physically before the message is complete. To remember such events they must first be placed in a BUFFER STORE to await proper processing. This is best shown in the visual system. A very fast display is shown in a TACHISTOSCOPE. A subject looks at a screen with a central dot. The dot disappears, and a 3 × 3 array of letters appears for 50 milliseconds. The letters disappear and the subject has to name them; subjects are correct for four or five of the nine letters. Did the subject never see the remaining letters, or have they already been forgotten in the time it took to recall the other letters? Using a PROBE TECHNIQUE, we find that the letters were actually seen and then forgotten. After the letters are shown, a blank screen appears for t milliseconds, and then a high, medium or low pitched tone sound (the PROBE) indicates whether the top, middle or bottom row of letters should be reported. Subjects are 100% correct if the probe is presented immediately the stimuli have disappeared from the screen (Fig. 4.1). All the letters must therefore already be in memory, because the subject does not know which row is to be recalled until the stimuli have disappeared. The amount of forgetting depends upon t. The experiment shows the existence of ICONIC MEMORY, in which forgetting occurs by spontaneous decay, analogous to radioactive decay, with nothing able to prevent it. The half-life of iconic memory is about 450 milliseconds. Information still present after then survives because it has passed into the next stage. ECHOIC MEMORY is the auditory equivalent of iconic memory and has a similar half-life. Iconic memory is a mere copy of the sensory input but lasts longer than the input. However, sensory inputs need to be processed, or perceived, and information extracted. This requires a longer lasting buffer, a SHORT-TERM STORE or WORKING MEMORY, in which they are manipulated, processed, and kept while required.

Short-term store is easily demonstrated experimentally. A subject hears 15 one-syllable words read aloud, one per second, and then immediately recalls the words in any order. Words are recalled differently at different positions in the list (first, second, ... last), producing a SERIAL POSITION CURVE (Fig. 4.2), which has three portions: a PRIMACY EFFECT, words at the beginning being remembered well, a RECENCY EFFECT, words at the end being remembered well, and a flat portion in the middle, without a specific name, where words are remembered less well. If the experiment is repeated with the minor variation that there is a 30 second delay before recall starts in which the subject has to do a DISTRACTER TASK (e.g. counting aloud, backwards

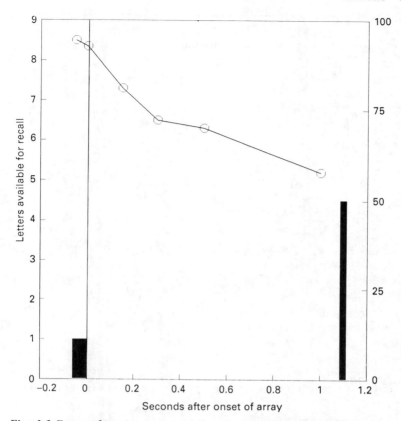

Fig. 4.1 Decay of iconic memory. A 3 × 3 array of letters was displayed for 50 milliseconds (shown by the small bar at the left). The dots show the numbers of letters available for recall when a probe was presented 0, 150, 300, 500 and 1000 milliseconds after the onset of the array. The bar at the right shows the number of letters recalled when the subjects are asked to recall the entire array. Adapted from Sperling G (1960), The information available in brief visual presentations, *Psychological Monographs*, **74**, (11).

in threes from a hundred), then the serial position curve shows no recency effect (Fig. 4.2). In the first experiment, the subject has been remembering some words by repeating them (REHEARSAL) in the same way that one remembers a telephone number for a minute or so. Rehearsal is disrupted in the second experiment and memory is impaired for the last few words. The recency effect is due to the short-term store, which is of LIMITED CAPACITY, and is disrupted by overwriting with other information (as in distraction). The information does not decay spontaneously but is disrupted by new information. It is like a juggler who can keep four balls in the air; if the action is interfered with, by using the hands for something else, then the balls are dropped and lost. Short-term store is important for processing language because

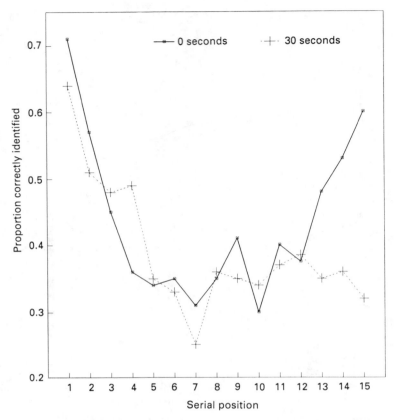

Fig. 4.2 The probability of a word being correctly recalled in a serial position experiment, according to its original position in the list. After reading out loud each of the 15 words, subjects carried out 0 or 30 seconds of a distracter task before recalling the words. Adapted from Glanzer M and Cunitz A R (1966), Two storage mechanisms in free recall, *Journal of Verbal Learning and Verbal Behaviour,* **5**, 351–60.

spoken words extend over time, and grammar requires words to be related to words spoken after a substantial delay (e.g. in '*the boy*, whose sister had long plaits and liked chasing kittens, *played* football', 'boy' must be held in working memory until 'played' appears).

If the recency effect reflects the short-term store, then the other parts of Figure 4.2 must be due to other, more durable memory, known as SECONDARY MEMORY, or LONG-TERM STORE whose properties can be explored by other variations of the serial position experiment. If words are read once every two seconds rather than once a second then memory is improved (Fig. 4.3), and if more items are read then performance on each item is worsened (Fig. 4.3). Greater resources improve recall, implying words are actively put in memory. This is confirmed if subjects are not told an experiment is on memory, but

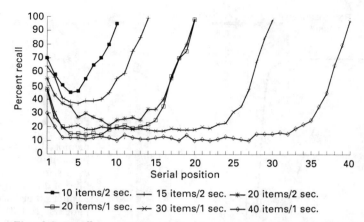

Fig. 4.3 Recall in a serial position experiment where lists are of different length, and items are presented either for one or two seconds. Words were read aloud and recall commenced immediately the list had finished. Adapted from Murdock B B (1962), The serial effect of free recall, *J Exp Psychol*, **64**, 482–8.

instead just to listen to words, and at the end are suddenly told to recall them; INCIDENTAL LEARNING is less good than INTENTIONAL LEARNiNG, showing that information is actively *put* into memory. Other experiments confirm that recall from long-term memory is principally dependent on the DEPTH OF PROCESSING at the time of learning.

The primacy effect is particularly interesting. Consider a subject who comes to the memory laboratory and carries out an experiment for the first time, obtaining a typical serial position curve like that in Figure 4.2. The experiment is then immediately repeated with different words and a similar curve obtained except that the primacy effect is diminished. And a third repetition gives a further diminution of the primacy effect. Why should this be? Think about the subject hearing the first word of the first experiment. They have a whole second to repeat the word to themself and they learn it well. The second word appears and now two words need remembering, so each is worked at less. This continues until fairly soon only the most recent three or four words can be rehearsed. Because first words are processed more they are remembered better. But that cannot explain why the primacy effect diminishes on each repetition (so-called PROACTIVE INTERFERENCE, in which previous learning disrupts future learning). The problem is not in LAYING DOWN or ENCODING the memory but in its RETRIEVAL. The first word of the first experiment is highly distinctive and is easily retrieved from memory. The first word of the second experiment is less distinctive, because already 15 other, potentially confusable, words are already in memory; and so on for the third list. Information must not only be actively put into memory but also must be retrieved, and INTERFERENCE between words prevents retrieval.

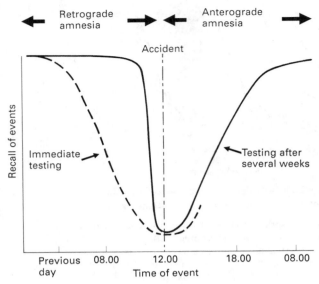

Fig. **4.4** A diagram-
matic summary of
memory loss, as shown
by failure to recall
events, in relation to the
time of the event before
or after an accident, for
patients tested either
immediately after or
several weeks after an
accident which occurred
at midday. See text for
further details.

Consider another experiment. Control subjects hear list A of ten
adjectives and when asked to recall are correct on 4.5 items. Other
subjects hear list A, but before recalling it, listen to another list B of
ten items, and only then are asked to recall list A. Success on list A
depends upon how similar B is to A. If B is 3-digit numbers, then on
average 3.7 items of A are remembered, and if B is nonsense syllables
then 2.6 items are recalled from A. Unrelated adjectives in B reduce
recall of A to 2.2 items, antonyms of the items in A reduce recall to
1.8 items, and if B consists of synonyms of A then only 1.3 items are
recalled. Since B is heard *after* A is learnt, any effects of B must be
upon retrieval rather than encoding (RETROACTIVE INTERFERENCE, in which
previous learning is disrupted by subsequent learning). Successful
memory therefore not only requires encoding, but also retrieval;
otherwise it is like a card index in which the cards are in random
order and although everything is there, nothing can be found.

Memory defects are common and illuminate underlying processes.
TRAUMATIC AMNESIA occurring after head injury is common, particularly
if unconsciousness is prolonged. A motorist may have an accident at
midday, just before lunch, be concussed for a few minutes, regain
consciousness, and be seen half an hour later in a hospital accident and
emergency department. Nothing about the accident and subsequent
events is remembered. Next morning there may still be no recall of
an ambulance or of the accident, but there are vague memories of
emergency treatment and clear memories of a hospital dinner the
previous night (Fig. 4.4). ANTEROGRADE or POST-TRAUMATIC AMNESIA (PTA)
is for events *after* the accident and is presumably due to concussion
disrupting cerebral functioning. Of greater interest is that even next

morning the patient may not remember events before the accident, such as getting up, having breakfast, and setting out on the journey. RETROGRADE AMNESIA (RA) extends backwards *before* the accident. Since memories of those events must have been encoded (normally people *can* remember the previous morning), RA must be a DEFICIT OF RETRIEVAL. That can be confirmed a month or two after the accident when the morning of the accident is remembered, showing that information had been present but not retrievable during the period of RA. The only exception is for the few minutes before the accident itself, memories of which never return, suggesting a failure of CONSOLIDATION, which is putting information into a durable form that can withstand concussion. That is confirmed in studies of patients receiving electro-convulsive shocks (ECS) to treat depression, to whom a word is said 10, 30 or 60 seconds before the shock; on regaining consciousness they recall words given 60 seconds before the shock but not words given 10 seconds before the shock, suggesting that consolidation takes about half a minute.

A rarer problem occurs in KORSAKOFF'S SYNDROME, the eventual outcome of WERNICKE'S ENCEPHALOPATHY, which occurs mainly in chronic alcoholism and is due to deficiency of vitamin B_6, thiamine. The predominant symptoms are a profound amnesia and CONFABULATION, a fabrication of plausible stories to conceal the memory deficit. The patient shows a complete inability to create new memories with nothing being recalled since the condition developed; a doctor or nurse is not recognized despite daily visiting for years. There is good recall of events from earlier in life, before the condition, and as a result they often believe that a different prime minister is in office, or even that a previous monarch is on the throne. If patients with Korsakoff's syndrome are tested on a serial position task then their results at first glance suggest that only the short-term store is present, showing just a recency effect (Fig. 4.5), and middle part completely missing, which has been interpreted as a pure deficiency of encoding in secondary memory. However Figure 4.5 shows some hints of a primacy effect in the amnesics and this suggests a different explanation involving recall deficits. If *some* items can be recalled from long-term store then there must be encoding and therefore other information might also have been stored but cannot be retrieved. That is supported by another experiment. Memory was tested indirectly by asking patients to name partial or fragmented stimuli (words or pictures; Fig. 4.6), the same objects or words being repeated with increasingly more intact forms until correct recognition occurred. To the subject this is not a memory experiment at all; however if the same words or objects are presented repeatedly then SAVINGS, needing successively less of a stimulus to make a correct response, demonstrate storage *and* retrieval of information. Korsakoff's patients never realize that they have seen the stimuli before but nonetheless they do show savings, and therefore

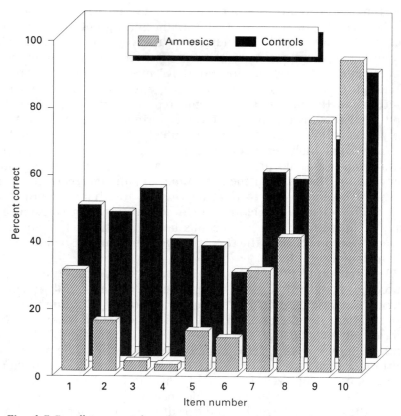

Fig. 4.5 Recall in a serial position experiment by amnesic patients with Korsakoff's syndrome, and by controls. Subjects were asked to remember a list of ten nouns which they read aloud from a card, one word being presented every three seconds. Adapted from Baddeley A D and Warrington E K (1970), Amnesia and the distinction between long- and short-term memory, *Journal of Verbal Learning and Verbal Behaviour*, **9**, 176–89.

must have adequate encoding and their deficit is one of retrieval, a deficit that is circumvented by providing 'hints' in the form of fragments. Such recognition without awareness in amnesia had first been described in CLAPAREDE'S PARADOX; the neurologist pricked the patient with a pin, left the room, returned a few minutes later and when the pin was produced the patient showed fear and moved away, but was unable to produce any conscious reason for the action.

An extremely rare form of amnesia was first described in a patient, now much investigated, called HM, who had severe, intractable epilepsy, particularly involving the temporal lobes. Since unilateral temporal lobectomy was known to benefit such patients, in 1953 it was decided to remove *both* temporal lobes. Postoperatively, HM had a profound anterograde amnesia, which still continues, along with

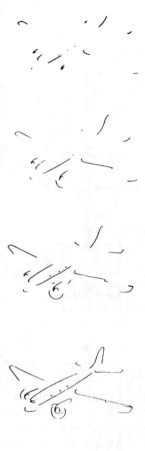

Fig. 4.6 Fragmented stimuli used to demonstrate savings in amnesic patients. Subjects are presented with progressively less fragmented versions of the stimulus until they can correctly recognize it. Reproduced with permission of authors and publishers from Warrington E K and Weiskrantz L (1968), New method of testing long-term retention with special reference to amnesic patients, *Nature*, **217**, 972–4; copyright 1968, MacMillan Magazines Ltd.

some retrograde amnesia, but no deficiency of short-term memory or of procedural memories (so that he can learn a complex motor task such as mirror-drawing, improving each day but never being aware of seeing the task before). Patients such as HM with the AMNESIC SYNDROME, which also occurs with encephalitis, cerebral anoxia and tumour, appear similar to Korsakoff's syndrome in their symptoms, although they do not confabulate. However careful testing suggests the two syndromes are different. When stimuli are presented very many times, both Korsakoff's and temporal lobe amnesics can remember at the same level as controls. Testing a day or a week later shows that Korsakoff's and controls have similar rates of forgetting,

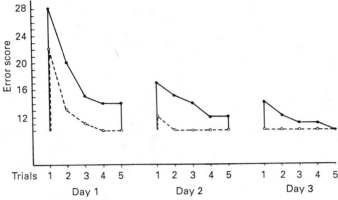

Fig. 4.7 Experiment using the fragmented stimuli of Figure 4.6,
which shows that amnesics (solid points) are capable of learning
to recognize the fragmented stimuli in Figure 4.6, albeit somewhat
more slowly than control subjects (open points). Reproduced with
permission of authors and publishers from Warrington E K and
Weiskrantz L (1968), New method of testing long-term retention
with special reference to amnesic patients, *Nature*, **217**, 972–4;
copyright 1968, MacMillan Magazines Ltd.

but that temporal lobe amnesics forget much more quickly, which
suggests different functional deficits.

This summary of memory deficits should not ignore the commonest
cause, ALZHEIMER'S DEMENTIA; diffuse cerebral damage particularly affects
the hippocampus and temporal lobes, and severe anterograde and
retrograde amnesia occur. The neurochemistry of Alzheimer's shows
a depletion of cholinergic neurones, which may be responsible for
memory loss. Cholinergic blockade can produce an amnesia, first
recognized by anaesthetists using hyoscine as a 'pre-med' with patients
often not even remembering being taken to theatre. The effect has
been confirmed experimentally. Attempts to improve memory in
demented patients by improving cholinergic transmission, either with
choline precursors or with cholinesterase inhibitors, have not as yet
been successful.

The neuro-anatomy of amnesia is confused. Korsakoff's syndrome
produces lesions of the mamillary bodies and the anterior thalamus,
whereas the critical lesion in the amnesic syndrome involves the
hippocampus. Since both are parts of the limbic system, it is suggested
that the circuit from hippocampus to mamillary bodies is involved in
retrieval. However, lesions of the fornix, which connects these areas,
do not always produce amnesia. More confusingly still, in animals,
lesions of hippocampus or mamillary bodies do not produce amnesia,
although recent work finds that damage to hippocampus *and* amygdala
results in amnesia in animals.

This account of memory deficits ends with an extremely rare syndrome which at first sight seems not to be a problem (and indeed seems advantageous), the HYPERMNESIC SYNDROME, in which patients are unable to forget. The Russian neuropsychologist A R Luria (1902–1977) described a patient, S, who automatically and uncontrollably used MNEMONICS (or memory strategies) to remember. In 1934, S was shown the following random formula:

$$N.\sqrt{d^2 \times \frac{85}{vx}} . \sqrt[3]{\frac{276^2 . 86x}{n^2v . \pi264}} n^2b = sv\frac{1624}{32^2} . r^2s.$$

He spent six or seven minutes remembering it, composing a short story to help, the beginning of which was:

> Neiman (N) came out and jabbed at the ground with his cane (.). He looked up at a tall tree which resembled the square-root sign ($\sqrt{}$) and thought to himself: 'No wonder the tree has withered and begun to expose its roots. After all, it was here when I built these two houses' (d^2) ['dom' is the Russian for house]...

This ran for a further hundred and fifty lines. Fifteen years later, in 1949, and completely unprompted, S recalled both the story and the formula perfectly. Such mnemonics can be helpful in normal memory since they organize and structure information (and many medical students have remembered the cranial nerves by recalling that 'On Old Olympus' Towering Tops A Finn And German Picked Some Hops' in which the initial letters correspond to the nerves, with the P standing for 'pneumogastric', the old name for the vagus nerve). Sadly, S derived little pleasure from his ability, which was automatic, and he found it to be a liability. The implication seems to be, as Freud had suggested, that it is necessary to forget in order to live happily.

This chapter has discussed the functional organization of memory but has hardly considered its structural organization. Where and how are memories stored? It is probably fair to say that at present we have little idea, but that a Nobel prize could await the person who unravels the mechanism. Several biochemical mechanisms have been suggested of which one of particular interest is LONG-TERM POTENTIATION. A brief, tetanic electrical stimulus (several seconds at 100 Hz) to the hippocampus results in an enhanced synaptic sensitivity, which can appear within ten minutes of stimulation, the mechanism being due to high intra-cellular calcium levels that irreversibly induce a protease whose action induces glutamate receptors and increases numbers of synaptic receptors. Blocking of glutamate transmission by 2-APV (2-amino-5-phophonovalerate) has since been shown to inhibit the learning of new material in rats. The cerebral localization of memory has been studied in 'model systems', and for low level tasks such as eye-lid conditioning, seems in part to be mediated by cerebellar mechanisms; a lesion to the middle cerebellar peduncle both abolishes and prevents re-acquisition of a conditioned eye-lid response on the contralateral side. The localization of higher memories, such as of visual discriminations, is far more diffuse, and studies of cerebral metabolism using isotopically-labelled 2-deoxyglucose during learning suggest that increased activity occurs throughout much of the cerebral cortex, limbic system, thalamus and cerebellum, although cingulate gyrus and hippocampus do seem to be especially involved. Such studies reinforce the suggestion that a specific memory for a specific event is not stored at a single cerebral location (as it might be in a computer), but rather is distributed throughout much of the brain, so that the entire integrated ensemble holds the memory (and hence memories in general are relatively resistant to localized cerebral damage). Recent analysis of such PARALLEL DISTRIBUTED PROCESSING (PDP) shows that it has many of the properties of memory, with an ability to learn complex events, based on only a few training trials, and without prior theoretical analysis, and that the memories so formed are like human memory in age and undergo 'graceful degradation', rather than sudden catastrophic failure.

5

Cognition

- Logic, the formal way in which logical problems are solved, and PSYCHO-LOGIC, the way in which these problems are solved by the human mind, are not the same.
- Logical SYLLOGISMS are typically solved by creating a mental image of the objects and then reading off the answer from the image.
- Scientific thought, which involves CREATIVITY, often shows the CONFIRMATORY BIAS typical of Baconian science, rather than attempting to disprove hypotheses as required by Popperian science.
- Estimates of probability are often erroneous due to the HEURISTICS of REPRESENTATIVENESS, taking a stereotypical example as statistically representative, and AVAILABILITY, items more available to consciousness being treated as more frequent.

Cognition, or 'thinking', is the general intellectual process of weighing evidence, making decisions and coming to conclusions, using imperfect evidence from the senses, experience or memory. Its general nature, the wide range of problems tackled, and the absence of conscious introspection (answers apparently just appearing in consciousness unbidden) make it both the centre of modern psychology, and also one of its most difficult areas of study. Here we will look at three aspects of a vast problem.

DEDUCTIVE LOGIC

Since people can solve logical problems it is assumed that they must use logic to solve them. That is not necessarily the case. My cat 'solves' complex three-dimensional problems when it catches a ball, although it knows little of Newton's laws or aerodynamics. Logic and PARA-LOGIC or PSYCHO-LOGIC (the ways logical problems are solved in our psyche) need not be the same. Consider a specific problem. You are given a simple SYLLOGISM, which states that 'If a patient's liver is enlarged then it is an abnormal liver'. You see a patient with a small liver. Can you assume it is normal? Many people will say 'yes', but that is an error. The rule does not say *only* large livers are abnormal.

Such errors of deduction are frequent, and yet usually we do not make serious errors of judgement. It seems that during a long chain of argument we make various guesses and assumptions. If we find a frank contradiction with earlier stages only then do we check and revise our earlier conclusions. If we decide our patient with a small liver has hepatic cirrhosis (i.e. an *abnormal* liver), then we will backtrack and spot our error, while if the liver is indeed normal then probably our error would stay undetected. Trial and error with continuous checking actually copes well with such problems.

Our problems with syllogisms suggest that deductive logic is not as straightforward psychologically as it might seem. Problem 1 below is an exercise in deductive logic for which 95% of students answer incorrectly. Try it yourself; the answer is at the end of the chapter.

Problem 1: Wason's THOG problem

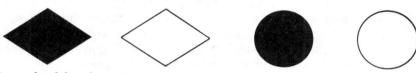

In each of the above designs there is a particular shape and a particular colour such that any of the four designs, which has one, and only one, of the features, is called a THOG.

The black diamond is called a THOG. What can you say, if anything, about whether each of the three remaining designs is a THOG? Indicate for each figure whether it definitely is a THOG, definitely is not a THOG, or whether there is insufficient information to decide. The correct answer, with an explanation, will be found at the end of the chapter.

Adapted with permission from Wason P C (1977), in Johnson-Laird P N and Wason P C, Eds, *Thinking: readings in cognitive science*, Cambridge, Cambridge University Press, 114–28.

If logic alone is not used to solve problems in deductive logic, then how are they done? One method builds a mental image on which the various items can be placed, so that eventually the answer can then simply be read off. For the problem 'Arthur is taller than Bill, Bill is taller than Charles. Is Arthur taller than Charles?' we make a picture of Arthur, place a shorter Bill alongside, and place a yet shorter Charles alongside Bill. It is then immediately obvious that Arthur is taller than Charles. The evidence for such a process is that problem solving depends on how information is presented and the ease of making a picture. Problems are more difficult when abstract rather than concrete (e.g. 'A > B' rather than 'Arthur is taller than Bill'), when terms are inconsistent with reality (e.g. 'Britain is larger than the United States'), if items are in a non-obvious order (e.g. 'B > C;

A > B), if negatives are used (e.g. 'Arthur is not shorter than Bill'), and if mixed relations are used (e.g. 'A > B; C < B'). Since none of these manipulations affect the pure logical task, they must therefore alter the way in which we approach the tasks *psychologically*, with the implication that logical problems are not solved purely by the application of logic.

INDUCTIVE LOGIC

Inductive logic, a controversial topic in the philosophy of science, transcends specific evidence to produce a generalization. If I show you the numbers, '31,28,31,30,31' and ask what is next you might induce they are the days in each month, and hence that the next is 30, the number of days in June. Francis Bacon (1561–1626) suggested that science creates hypotheses ('they are days in the month') and confirms them by testing with the next member; if the prediction is correct we then accept the hypothesis as proven. That view of science is not now generally accepted, being replaced by the view of Sir Karl Popper (1902–) that hypotheses cannot be proved, only disproved. Although 30 might indeed be the correct next number, our hypothesis may still be wrong; the series might be '31,28,31,30, 31,30,31,28,31,30,31,30,31,28 . . .'. This differentiation of Baconian and Popperian science is seen also in the *psychology* of induction. People show a strong bias to prove theories, looking only for supportive evidence, and do not collect the awkward evidence that might disprove the theories. Problem 2 below gives an example of this CONFIRMATORY BIAS, which you can try for yourself.

Problem 2: The scientist and nature

This problem can only be tried out with the assistance of a friend. Sit the friend down and tell them that you are 'Nature' and that they are a 'Scientist' whose job is to understand the way in which Nature works. They should only tell you the rule for the working of Nature when they are fairly certain, in the same way that they would only publish a scientific paper when they are fairly certain of its correctness. The data for the 'experiments' consists of triplets of numbers synthesized by the Scientist, for which Nature then indicates whether they are valid or not. The actual rule with which Nature assesses the data is that valid sequences consist of numbers in ascending order of magnitude. To give the Scientist a start you tell them that the sequence '2, 4, 6' is a valid sequence. They then give you triplets of numbers until they announce the rule. Record the numbers they provide and the rules that they announce, until finally they announce the correct rule.

See the end of the chapter for three examples of the pattern being solved.

PROBABILITY

Assessments of risk in medicine involve probabilities. One in 20 of the population carry the gene for cystic fibrosis, 1 in 20 000 babies have phenylketonuria; three in a million young women on oral contraceptives suffer cerebrovascular complications per year. How well do people handle probability?

A problem. A medical officer of health surveys all families of six children in the area. In 72 families the children are born in the order Boy, Girl, Boy, Girl, Boy, Girl. In how many families are the children in the order Boy, Boy, Boy, Boy, Boy, Girl? Statistically unsophisticated people usually say much less than 72, although 72 is indeed the most likely figure. This error shows the error of REPRESENTATIVENESS; the first family is more typical of family composition, and is therefore assumed to be more common than the second, less typical family, although this is not actually the case. Problem 3 below gives another example for you to try.

Problem 3: Linda, the philosophy graduate

Here is a brief personality sketch. Read it and then carry out the task below.

Linda is 31 years old, single, out-spoken, and very intelligent. She studied philosophy at university. As a student she was deeply concerned with student politics, was involved in campaigns against racial and sexual discrimination, and took part in several demonstrations against nuclear power.

Below are eight statements. Please rank them according to their likelihood of describing Linda, using 1 for the most likely and 8 for the least likely.

a. Linda is a teacher in a primary school.
b. Linda works in a book shop and takes Yoga classes.
c. Linda is active in the feminist movement.
d. Linda is a psychiatric social worker.
e. Linda is a subscriber to New Statesman.
f. Linda is a bank clerk.
g. Linda sells insurance.
h. Linda is a bank clerk and is active in the feminist movement.

See the end of the chapter for an analysis of the problem.
Adapted with permission from Tversky A and Kahneman B (1982) in Kahneman B, Slovic P and Tversky A, (eds.) *Judgment under*

uncertainty, Cambridge, Cambridge University Press, 84–98.

Another problem. Consider all the six letter English words which begin with the letter R (i.e. R-----). Now think of six letter words with an R in the third position (i.e. --R---). Which is more frequent? Most people say words beginning with R, although that is not actually the case. My word-processor found 1051 words beginning with R, and 1734 with R in the third position. However, we cannot search our memory so systematically; it is easier to find words beginning with R than with R in third place, and since the former are more AVAILABLE to consciousness we then assume they are more common. Problem 4 below gives another example, and Figure 5.2 shows results from a formal study of it.

Problem 4: Bus stops and sub-committees

For the two following problems, do not carry out any formal mathematical calculations; instead *estimate*, as quickly as possible, approximate answers to the questions.
a)   A bus has 10 different stops between its Start and Finish. Consider a bus that makes exactly three stops on the route. How many different combinations of stops can it make? Alternatively consider a bus that makes exactly seven stops; how many combinations of stops can it make?
b)   Consider a group of 10 people who have to form a committee. How many different sub-committees can be formed with just two members? How many sub-committees can be formed with exactly eight members?

Answers will be found at the end of the chapter.

Adapted with permission from Tversky A and Kahneman B (1982) in Kahneman B, Slovic P and Tversky A, Eds, *Judgement under uncertainty*, Cambridge, Cambridge University Press, 163–78.

These errors, which arise from the inappropriate application of the empirically derived working rules, or HEURISTICS, of availability and representativeness, can seriously distort probability estimates. Clinicians think cases typical of a disease are more common, and that cases remembered most easily (because bigger, nastier, bloodier, etc.) are more typical. Similarly the public estimates disease incidences from the reporting of cases in newspapers and media (Fig. 5.1). Diseases *thought* to be more common are those receiving most media exposure, and hence most *available*, even though they may not actually be more common.

These examples show thinking often goes wrong. Deductive logic is not always used accurately or systematically, inductive logic confirms rather than disproves hypotheses, and estimates of probability made from experience are frequently inaccurate. Such findings have important implications for diagnosis, scientific research and epidemiology.

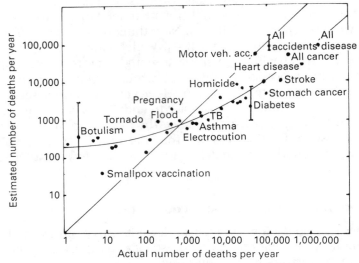

Fig. 5.1 Estimates made by American subjects of the numbers of deaths per year in the United States from a number of causes, compared with the actual number of deaths. The diagonal straight line indicates accurate estimates. The curved, fitted, line shows that, in general, rare causes of death are overestimated, and common causes underestimated. Causes of death that are overestimated relative to the general pattern (the curved line) are those which typically are reported more frequently in the media (road accidents, flood, tornado, botulism), whereas those under the curved line are typically under-reported by the media (stomach cancer, diabetes, electrocution, smallpox vaccination). Reproduced with permission from Slovic P, Fischoff B, and Lichtenstein S (1982), in Kahneman B, Slovic P and Tversky A, Eds, *Judgment under uncertainty*, Cambridge, Cambridge University Press.

Answer to problem 1: Wason's THOG problem

The white circle is definitely a THOG and the other two figures are definitely *not* THOGs. In many studies of medical students and other students, the most common response is to say that the white circle is definitely not a THOG and that the status of the other two figures cannot be determined.

The problem is difficult because of the phrase 'one, and only one, of these features'. In logic this is called an 'exclusive-OR', the whole being true only if *one* of the items is true, and false if both are true; it differs therefore from the more common use of 'or', the 'inclusive-OR', in which the whole is true if either *or both* components is true.

The key components of the figures are their shape and colour. The black diamond is a THOG and hence the defining characteristics of 'THOGness' must be either 'black and circle' or 'white and diamond', for then the black diamond would only have one characteristic, and therefore be a THOG. However, we do not know which pair of characteristics is correct. Assume that it is 'black and circle'. The white circle is then also a THOG (having only one characteristic, a circle) and the other two figures are not THOGs, having either none or two characteristics. However, the defining characteristics may be 'white and diamond'. If so then the white circle is still a THOG (because now it has the single feature of being white), and the other two figures still have none or two characteristics, and hence are not THOGs. Therefore without knowing the precise characteristics of being a THOG, formal deductive logic can nevertheless tell us the status of all the other figures.

The difficulty of this problem, especially when carried out only in our heads, and its straightforward demonstration by a simple written argument, shows that formal logic is not necessarily the manner in which psychological processes solve such problems.

Answer to problem 2: the scientist and nature

The usual error in this study is that subjects propose hypotheses which they have not attempted to falsify, but only to confirm, and hence the hypotheses are usually too narrow, encompassing only the limited range of data that have already been seen to be valid. As an example, below are shown three protocols of actual subjects tested by Wason. Words printed in italics are the 'final rules' produced by subjects, whereas words in roman type are working hypotheses spoken aloud by subjects. Subjects 4 and 6 show typical errors, whereas subject 2 forms working hypotheses which are then tested explicitly by falsification.

The demonstration shows clearly that repeated confirmations cannot prove a hypothesis, whereas a single falsification is sufficient to disprove it. In addition it also shows how scientific thought does not consist solely of formal, logical deduction, but that it is also has a large component of CREATIVITY or LATERAL THINKING, which can itself be explored scientifically using tasks such as this.

Subject 2. Female, aged 21.
    '3 6 9: three goes into the second figure twice and into the third figure three times; 2 4 8: perhaps the figures have to have a lowest common denominator; 2 4 10: same reason; 2 5 10: the second number does not have to be divided by the first one; 10 6 4: the highest number must be last; 4 6 10: the first number must be the lowest; 2 3 5: it is only the order that counts; 4 5 6: same reason; 1 7 13: same reason.
    The rule is that the figures must be in numerical order; (16 minutes).

Subject 4. Female, aged 19.
    '8 10 12: two added each time; 14 16 18: even numbers in order

of magnitude; 20 22 24: same reason; 1 3 5: two added to preceding number.
The rule is that by starting with any number two is added each time to form the next number. 2 6 10: middle number is the arithmetic mean of the other two; 1 50 99: same reason.
The rule is that the middle number is the arithmetic mean of the other two. 3 10 17; same number, seven, added each time; 0 3 6: three added each time.
The rule is that the difference between two numbers next to each one is the same. 12 8 4: the same number is subtracted each time to form the next number.
The rule is adding a number, always the same one to form the next number. 1 4 9: any three numbers in order of magnitude.
The rule is any three numbers in order of magnitude.' (17 minutes).

Subject 6. Male, aged 23.
'8 10 12: step interval of two; 7 9 11: with numbers not divisible by two; 1 3 5: to see if rule may apply to numbers starting at two and upwards; 3 5 1: the numbers do not necessarily have to be in ascending or descending order; 5 3 1: could be in descending order.
The rule is that the three numbers must be in ascending order separated by intervals of two. 11 13 15: must have one number below ten in the series; 1 6 11: ascending series with regular step interval.
The rule is that the three numbers must be in ascending series and separated by regular step intervals.
The rule is that the first number can be arbitrarily chosen; the second number must be greater than the first and can be arbitrarily chosen; the third number is larger than the second by the same amount as the second is larger than the first. 1 3 13: any three numbers in ascending order.
The rule is that the three numbers need have no relationship with each other, except that the second is larger than the first and the third larger than the second.' (38 minutes).

Answers reprinted with permission of the author from Wason P C (1968), 'On the failure to eliminate hypotheses – a second look' in Wason P C and Johnson-Laird P H, *Thinking and Reasoning*, Harmondsworth, Penguin.

Answer to problem 3: Linda, the philosophy graduate

Only three of the statements, c, f and h are of interest, the rest being FILLERS, to obscure the true subject of the study. In a large group of subjects in a similar study, statement c, 'Linda is active in the feminist movement', was rated as second most likely, and statement f, 'Linda is a bank clerk' was rated as sixth most likely. Statement h, that 'Linda is a bank clerk and is active in the feminist movement' was

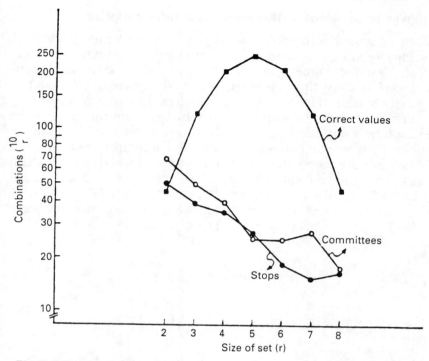

Fig. 5.2 Estimates of the number of combinations of items from 10 in the bus-stop and sub-committee problems described in problem 4. Each subject was asked to estimate the number of combinations of *r* items (between 2 and 8). Estimated values are compared with the correct values derived from probability theory. Reproduced with permission from Tversky A and Kahneman D (1982), in Kahneman B, Slovic P and Tversky A, Eds, *Judgment under uncertainty*, Cambridge, Cambridge University Press, 163–78.

rated as fourth most likely. Your results will show the same effect if item h is rated as more likely than the lower of c and f.

There must be some probability (P_c) that statement c is true, and similarly there is also a probability (P_f) that statement f is true. Since these probabilities must be less than one, then the probability that they are *both* true ($P_c \times P_f$) must be lower than the probability that either alone is true. But statement h, that 'Linda is a bank clerk and active in the feminist movement', is typically rated as *more* likely than one of its components.

The error arises due to a failure of the representative heuristic. The statements are regarded as typical of a particular sort of person, of a stereotype, and hence that stereotype is regarded as representative, so that the conjunction of the statements is accepted as more likely than its components.

Answer to problem 4: Bus stops and sub-committees

When presented with these problems, which are formally identical, statistically unsophisticated subjects, or even subjects who are sophisticated but under time pressure, will say that there are more patterns of three bus stops than of seven, and more committees of size two than of size eight (Fig. 5.2). In each problem the two answers should be identical (as can be seen intuitively by inverting the problem, by asking how many ways three stops can be *omitted* from the route, or how many ways can two people be *excluded* from the sub-committee).

The error occurs because of a failure of the availability heuristic. It is easier to think of combinations of three bus stops (1, 2 & 3; 1, 2 & 4; 1, 2 & 5; etc.) than of seven bus stops (1,2,3,4,5,6 & 7; 1,2,3,4,5,6 & 8; 1,2,3,4,5,6 & 9; etc.), and since the former are therefore more *available* to awareness they are judged as being more frequent.

6

Language

- Man is the only animal who has a language that shows arbitrary symbols which can be combined in an infinite number of ways. In chimpanzees, evidence for true language is very controversial.
- The basic unit of speech is the PHONEME, of which there are different sets in different languages.
- Phoneme perception, which shows CATEGORICAL PERCEPTION, is probably carried out by special cells in the temporal cortex.
- Infants are born with mechanisms for identifying phonemes from all human languages, but these mechanisms disappear if not exposed to appropriate speech inputs.
- Prosodic features such as INTONATION CONTOUR are important both in conveying stress and emphasis, and in regulating the interactions in conversations.
- NON-VERBAL COMMUNICATION, indicated by the eyes or by other body movements, is important in indicating emotion and in regulating interaction.

Language is fundamental to human society and perhaps even to human intellect. The brain and mind solve almost overwhelming problems in understanding spoken and written language, problems which can probably only be fully appreciated by those trying to program computers to extract meaning from spoken speech, in which, at present, success is far distant.

If language is defined as communication by ARBITRARY SYMBOLS, from which potentially *infinite* different statements can be produced, then it is probably unique to man. The dance of bees is not a language because the symbols are non-arbitrary and limited in scope. Bird song does have arbitrary symbols, but their scope is limited. The only possible exception is in chimpanzees, in which recent experiments have suggested that true language might exist. Nineteenth century attempts to make apes talk failed because the larynx and mouth are not physically suited to producing human sounds, and as a result modern researchers have either used deaf-and-dumb sign language or plastic cut-out symbols. Thus the monkey Sarah was taught the meaning of several hundred plastic symbols, which could be combined in grammatically formed sentences of some subtlety, understanding statements equivalent to 'If Sarah take banana then Mary no give Sarah chocolate', 'What colour is banana?' and a meta-linguistic statement, asking about the language itself, 'What colour is symbol for banana?'. Whether this behaviour is truly language is still not entirely clear, some psychologists arguing that the results could be explained merely in terms of conditioning (see, the 'Clever Hans' effect, described in Chapter 3).

Language can be sub-divided into several divisions; SYNTAX, to do with grammar (why 'the dog bit the man' and 'the man was bitten by the dog' are different), SEMANTICS, to do with meanings of words, PHONETICS to do with sounds in spoken speech, and PROSODICS, concerned with intonation patterns (which means that the words 'How do you do?' can be spoken with perhaps a dozen or more inflections of meaning). In this chapter, we shall be concerned principally with phonetics and prosodics. Syntax, particularly, is a technically complex area and is best omitted in an introductory account.

Speech sounds begin in the larynx, which rapidly 'chops' the expired air to produce a sound rich in harmonics, which then resonates in the tuned cavities of the mouth, pharynx and nose, their resonant frequencies being changed by moving the tongue, lips and soft palate. A SPEECH SPECTROGRAM (e.g. Fig. 6.1) shows that speech contains a series of bands of energy centred at different frequencies or FORMANTS, the lowest of which is called the FUNDAMENTAL or F1, and higher ones F2, F3, etc. In Figure 6.1, it is not obvious where many speech sounds stop and others start; the clarity and separation of words in spoken speech are generated by the brain, and are not present in the acoustic input. Speech components that are essential for producing particular sounds can be discovered by means of a SPEECH SYNTHESIZER, which produces a particular formant pattern, and subjects then say whether they hear it as a particular speech sound. Vowels are the continuous, relatively steady patterns of formants whereas consonants are transitory sounds. A consonant cannot be sounded on its own but must be sounded before or after a vowel; if the separate sound components of a consonant are sounded on their own they do not produce speech, but instead produce click-like noises. The formants comprising consonants are not fixed in their transitions, but depend upon the vowel following them (e.g. the /d/ sound in /di/ and /da/ in Figure 6.2).

The basic unit of spoken speech is the PHONEME, of which there are 44 in spoken English, and 120 or more in the languages of the world, some being common to most languages, others being present in only a few. In English, the phonemes broadly correspond with the letters, but are more extensive, so that 'ŋ' refers to the 'ng' sound at the end of 'thing', and /ə/ (called 'schwa/') is the 'er' sound at the beginning of 'about'. Phonemes which are different in one language need not be different in another, so that, for instance, the 'p' sound in 'up'

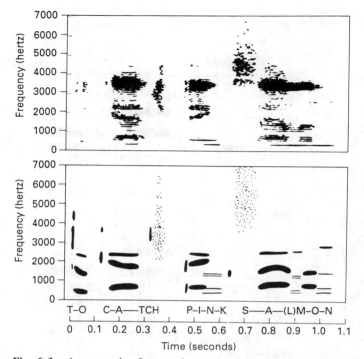

Fig. 6.1 An example of a speech spectrogram, in which time is shown on the abscissa, frequency on the ordinate, and amplitude is shown by the darkness of the record. The subject is saying the phrase 'To catch pink salmon'. The top box shows the actual spectrogram, and the lower box shows a diagrammatic representation, which can be put through the inverse process, using a SPEECH SYNTHESIZER or PATTERN PLAYBACK, to produce sounds which a normal listener will hear as the phrase 'To catch pink salmon'. Vowels (e.g. /ae/ in 'catch', or /i/ in 'pink') are seen to be extended continuous sounds made up of three formants. Consonants are transitory sounds preceding or following vowels, or are continuous noises (e.g. /s/ in 'salmon'). Reproduced from *Language and Speech*, p.66, by George A Miller. Copyright 1981 by W H Freeman and Company; reprinted with permission.

and 'lips' (technically aspirated and unaspirated respectively) are indistinguishable /p/ phonemes in English, but are separate phonemes in Hindi. The physical sounds making a phoneme may differ from occasion to occasion, but psychologically all are the same phoneme, in the same way that the letter A can be written differently by different people but is always the same letter. An analogy is with chemistry, phonemes being akin to atoms; chemistry depends only on which type of atom is involved, even though some of those atoms may have subtle physical differences in the form of isotopes. Thus $C^{12}O_2$ and $C^{14}O_2$ are chemically identical, although physically different. Just as

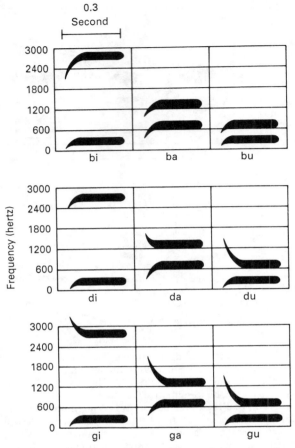

Fig. 6.2 Synthetic stimuli producing the consonants /b/, /d/ and /g/ before the vowels /i/, /a/ and /u/. The shape of the consonant depends upon the vowel following, e.g. the second (higher) formant of /d/ rises before /i/ and falls before /a/ and /u/. Reproduced from *Language and Speech*, p.66, by George A Miller. Copyright 1981 by W H Freeman and Company; reprinted with permission.

atoms are composed of smaller, sub-atomic particles, so phonemes are also composed of smaller units called FEATURES. These features, of which there are 13 in English, distinguish the phonemes. Thus, the stop consonants /b/, /d/, /g/, /p/, /t/, and /k/ differ in only two features: the PLACE OF ARTICULATION of the tongue, which is against the lips in the labial sounds, /b/ and /p/, against the teeth in the dental sounds /d/ and /t/, and against the soft palate in the velar sounds /g/ and /k/; and the onset of VOICING, the vibration of the larynx, which occurs after RELEASE of the consonant in the UNVOICED consonants /p/,

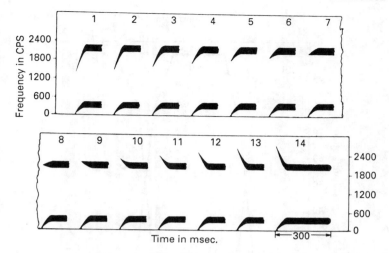

Fig. 6.3 *a*) A series of spectrographic patterns which at some points on the continuum are typical of naturally produced /bĕ/ (number 1), /dĕ/ (number 7), and /gĕ/ (number 14). From Lieberman A *et al.* (1957), The discrimination of speech sounds within and across phoneme boundaries, *J Exp Psychol*, **54**, 358–68.

/t/ and /k/, and before release in the VOICED consonants /b/, /d/ and /g/. Try speaking the sounds 'pat', 'tat', 'cat', 'bat', 'dat' and 'gat' and identifying where your tongue is placed and, by using your hand to feel the vibrations of your larynx, whether the sounds are voiced or unvoiced.

Perhaps the most exciting thing about phoneme perception is that it shows a fundamental difference from other forms of perception. If I play a sine-wave sound that gradually increases in frequency from 1300 Hz to 2900 Hz, you will hear a sound of gradually increasing pitch. By contrast, if I play the range of sounds shown in Figure 6.3a in which the initial frequency of the second formant shifts from 1300 to 2900 Hz you will not hear a continuously changing sound from /bĕ/ through intermediate values to /dĕ/ and then through more intermediate values to /gĕ/ but instead you will clearly hear each sound as *either* /bĕ/, *or* /dĕ/ *or* /gĕ/, with a very sudden changeover between the phoneme categories (shown in Fig. 6.3b). This CATEGORICAL PERCEPTION, in which all sounds are forced into pigeon-holes, without intermediate values, is almost entirely restricted to speech. There is good evidence that cells with such properties are located in the temporal lobe of the cortex, and that they can be ADAPTED by FATIGUE, in which repeatedly listening to the sound /bæ/ shifts the boundary between /bæ/ and /dæ/ (Fig. 6.3c). Damage to the temporal lobe can result in the deficit known as SPECIFIC WORD DEAFNESS or AUDITORY APHASIA in which a patient can hear and discriminate almost any sounds except speech sounds (see Chapter 23 for other types of aphasia).

Labelling data

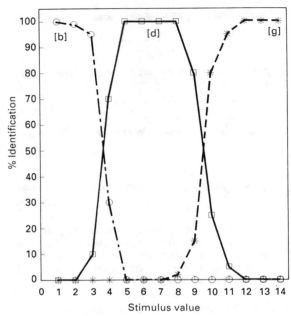

Fig. 6.3 *b*) Intermediate stimuli between /bě/, /dě/ and /gě/ are only actually heard as one of the three sounds, with no sense of blending between the possibilities. The ordinate shows the proportion of times that each sound in (a) was heard as /bě/, /dě/ or /gě/. Note the sudden and rapid changeovers. Adapted from Lieberman A *et al.* (1957), The discrimination of speech sounds within and across phoneme boundaries, *J Exp Psychol*, **54**, 358–68.

If phonemes have specific neural detectors, and languages differ in their phonemes, then how is it that an English speaker has the appropriate detectors for English phonemes? Two mechanisms might exist; listening to a language could induce appropriate detectors, or else *all* detectors may be present at birth and unused ones atrophy and disappear. The latter seems to be the case. By using either conditioning techniques or evoked potential methods, it can be shown that neonates can distinguish phonemes from birth onwards. Furthermore, they can also distinguish phonemes in languages other than their own, but the ability to make such distinctions disappears during the first year of life (Figures 6.4a and b). Such mechanisms may explain why second language learners can typically be distinguished from native speakers unless they have acquired their second language in the first years of life.

The correct use of spoken language requires not only that the words are enunciated correctly, but also that the overall INTONATION CONTOUR is appropriate. The fundamental pitch, or first formant, rises and falls continuously during speech, rising, for instance, at the end of a

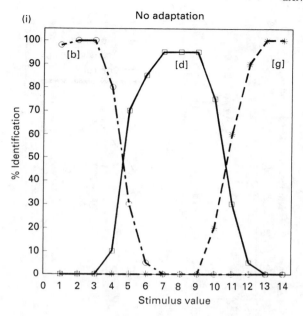

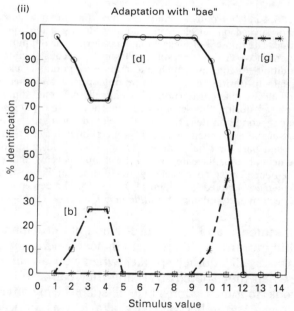

Fig. 6.3 *c*) The identification of a range of sounds between /b/ and /g/ by a single subject, *i*. before adaptation, and *ii*. after adaptation by listening to the sound /bæ/ 180 times during a 2 minute period, and then a further 1 minute of adaptation before testing on each stimulus. Note that the /d/-/g/ boundary is unchanged but that the /b/-/d/ boundary is disrupted, implying fatigue of a process detecting /b/ sounds. Adapted from Cooper W E and Blumstein S E (1974), A 'labial' feature analyzer in speech perception, *Perception and Psychophysics*, **15**, 591–600.

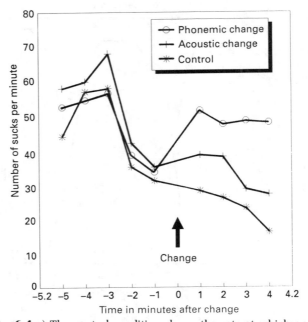

Fig. 6.4 *a*) The control condition shows the rate at which an infant sucked on an electronic dummy during a ten minute period. The number of sucks diminishes during the ten minutes (HABITUATION). A similar result applies in the 'acoustic change' condition (middle) in which one auditory stimulus is played repeatedly during the first five minute period and then an acoustically different (but not phonemically different) stimulus is played during the second five minutes. In the 'phonemic change' condition (left) the stimulus played during the second part of the experiment was a different phoneme from that in the first part, and habituation did not occur, indicating that the neonate must be categorizing the stimuli as being different, and hence must be perceiving the distinction between the phonemes. Adapted from Eimas P D (1985), The perception of speech in early infancy, *Scientific American*, **252**(1), 34–40.

questioning sentence and falling at the end of an emphatic sentence (and in writing we use '?', '!' and '.' to indicate such processes). These PROSODIC FEATURES tell another speaker when you are about to finish and hence when they should start, and they can also indicate when you will brook no interruptions. Like all such social conventions they can go wrong. A number of years ago it was noticed that Mrs Thatcher, who was then Prime Minister, was continually being interrupted by television interviewers. A careful analysis of the intonation contours (Fig. 6.5) revealed that at such 'disputed endings', Mrs Thatcher's voice pitch fell very quickly (normally a sign of an ending), and she looked directly at the interviewer (also a sign of an ending — see Fig. 6.6), but that her final pitch was not very

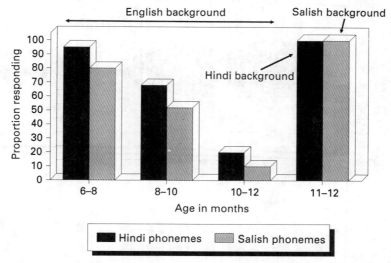

Fig. 6.4 *b*) Left three columns: The proportion of American infants at three different ages responding to a phonemic distinction that is either present only in Hindi (solid bars), or only in Salish (an American Indian tongue) (shaded bars). In native American infants the ability to perceive the distinction is present at 6 months but has disappeared by the age of 12 months. Rightmost column: the proportion of native Hindi or Salish infants who could make the Hindi or Salish distinction, respectively, remains at 100% at 12 months of age. Adapted from Eimas P D (1985), The perception of speech in early infancy, *Scientific American*, **252**(1), 34–40.

low (normally a sign of continuing to speak); the interviewers misinterpreted this combination of cues, thought that Mrs Thatcher must be finishing, and started to speak themselves, only to find that she in fact was continuing, having thought she had indicated that intention by keeping her final pitch high.

The use of direct eye-gaze to indicate the end of a speaking turn is only one of a whole set of NON-VERBAL COMMUNICATIONS presented by the eyes, which in most primates are surrounded by EYE-RINGS to make them more conspicuous — the eye-brows in man. So important are the eyes that when looking at faces we spend much of our time scanning them particularly. The eyes can convey direct information about emotional states (e.g. Fig. 6.7). They can also allow an inference about whether the truth is being told. Whilst deceiving, most people do not usually look the other person directly in the eye. An exception, in which direct eye-contact is maintained while lying, occurs in those individuals of the personality type known as HIGH MACHIAVELLIAN, after the Italian political theorist Niccoló Machiavelli (1469–1527), who refined deception as a political tool. The disconcerting effect of sun-glasses upon interaction is in large part due to the abolition of eye-contact.

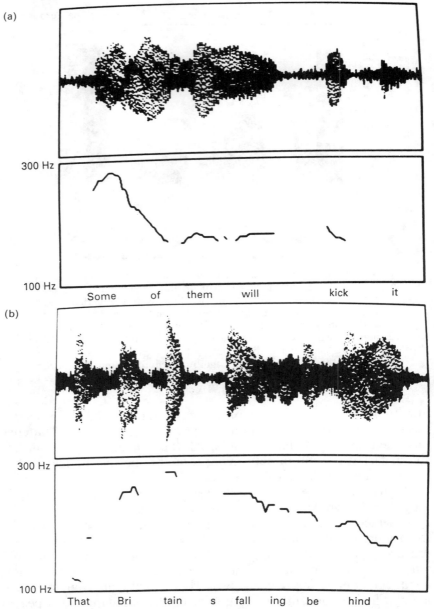

Fig. 6.5 The speech signals and the pitch of the fundamental frequency during two phrases spoken by Mrs Thatcher during television interviews. *a)* a FINAL UTTERANCE indicating the end of a bout of speaking, and for which the pitch falls quickly, and to a low level, and *b)* a MEDIAL UTTERANCE, with slower fall in pitch, and higher final pitch indicating an intention to continue speaking.

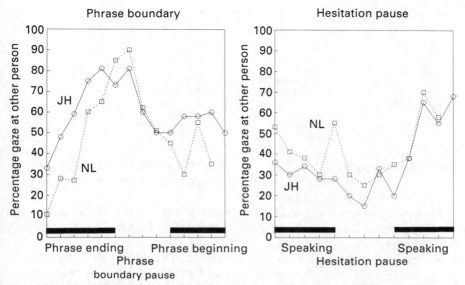

Fig. 6.6 The proportion of occasions on which two speakers are looking the other person directly in the eye during a total of 48 PHRASE BOUNDARIES (left), at which times a change of speaker can occur, and during 43 HESITATION PAUSES (right), in which the speaker intends to carry on speaking. Two different speakers, JH and NL, are indicated by separate lines. Redrawn with permission from Kendon A (1967), Some functions of gaze-direction in social interaction, *Acta Psychol Scand*, **26**, 22–63.

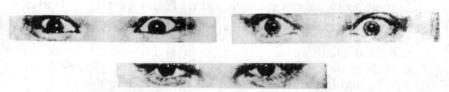

Fig. 6.7 The eyes are a direct source of information about emotional states. Reproduced with permission of author and publishers from Nummenmaa T (1964), *The language of the face*, Jyvaskala, University of Jyvaskala Studies in Education, Psychology and Social Research, Number 9.

In summary, spoken language is of crucial importance in human social communication, and as such special brain mechanisms have developed for its perception and production (see also Chapter 23), and these have been supplemented both by non-phonemic vocal mechanisms such as intonation, which conveys information about emotion and turn-taking, and by non-verbal mechanisms such as eye-gaze, for emphasizing linguistic features.

7

Intelligence

- Measurement of intelligence, using the methods of PSYCHOMETRICS, is in principle similar to the measurement of any other physical or biological quantity.
- Intelligence tests should be both RELIABLE and VALID. Tests can show CRITERION VALIDITY, FACE VALIDITY, CONSTRUCT VALIDITY and INTERNAL CONSISTENCY.
- Individuals differ in their intelligence. Attribution of these differences to genetic or environmental factors can only be relative to a particular time and population. Probably 40–50% of variance is genetic and 50–60% environmental in western populations.
- Genetic influences on IQ are best demonstrated in the children of monozygotic twins, where the confounding effects of differential treatment of twins by their parents can be taken into account.
- Monozygotic twins are less intelligent than dizygotic twins because of their postnatal environment rather than their prenatal environment.
- Children from small families and those born early in their family are relatively more intelligent. These environmental effects can be explained by Zajonc's CONFLUENCE MODEL, which considers the total intellectual environment to which the child is exposed.

Previous chapters have implied that individuals are all rather similar; and indeed they do have similar basic processes of perception, learning, memory, cognition, language, etc, and have similar brain structures. However people also *differ* psychologically, in their intelligence, personality, and in how they view the world. How do we measure differences in intellectual ability (PSYCHOMETRICS) and where do they come from?

INTELLIGENCE can either mean COMPETENCE, the highest intellectual activity of which a person is *capable* (but might not ever perform), or PERFORMANCE, almost tautologically defined as 'that which is measured by intelligence tests'). When in 1905 Binet and Simon described the first intelligence test, their intention was totally pragmatic:

'Our aim is, when a child is put before us, to take the measurement of his intellectual powers, in order to establish whether he is normal or if he is retarded.... we shall not seek in any way to establish or to prepare a prognosis and we leave the question of whether his backwardness is curable or not, capable of improvement or not, entirely unanswered'.

Doctors are mostly interested in intelligence as *performance*, when assessments are required for placing a backward child in an appropriate educational institution, in diagnosing reading or school difficulties, assessing head injury or brain disease in adults, or in research projects. Sometimes competence can be assessed: a child not doing well at school who has a high IQ is under-achieving, and hence competence is above performance.

Any form of measurement (be it of length, size, liver function or IQ) requires assumptions. For any form of measure, these assumptions can be assessed. To show the similarities I will compare a biochemical measurement (of liver function) with the psychological measurement of intelligence.

Measurement starts with an intuitive idea of how different items should be ordered. Liver function should be worse in an advanced cirrhotic than in mild hepatitis which in turn should be worse than for a normal individual. If a biochemical test did not put groups in that order it would be rejected. CRITERION VALIDITY is therefore the ability to predict a well-known and understood characteristic. Similarly an IQ test should, on average, put research scientists above bank clerks, and road sweepers above the congenitally idiot. This criterion is *necessary* for a measure, but it is *not sufficient*.

Patients with severe liver disease might also have impaired exercise tolerance, but it would not be a reasonable *measure* of liver failure because it has no obvious relation to liver metabolism *per se*. CONSTRUCT VALIDITY requires a plausible theoretical explanation for a test doing what it claims to do. Knowledge of Mozart's symphonies, or income, would probably show criterion validity as IQ tests, but would not show construct validity. Construct validity requires a definition, and for intelligence it is typically:

'The general ability to process abstract quantities, independent of cultural or education background, of memory, or of particular knowledge.'

IQ tests are therefore constructed to assess *only* intellectual ability, avoiding specific cultural knowledge, so that as far as possible they are CULTURE-FREE (although results from minority cultures must be interpreted carefully).

A patient will feel a blood test could reasonably assess liver function, but would be surprised if electrodes were put on their head. FACE VALIDITY means that those taking or use the test *feel* it is measuring what it should measure; and they have CONTENT VALIDITY when they measure *all* relevant aspects (so an intelligence test will assess verbal, spatial and other intellectual abilities, since all are included within the broad term 'intelligence').

A dozen different tests of liver function should all show broadly similar results; they should be correlated, or show INTERNAL CONSISTENCY. If the items of an IQ test are ordered from most difficult to easiest then a person answering any item should also answer correctly all easier items. A consequence is that if two scores are calculated, from the odd and even numbered items, then the scores should correlate highly (SPLIT-HALF RELIABILITY). Similarly if the same person is tested again after a few weeks both scores should be similar (TEST-RETEST RELIABILITY). Good tests should be reliable *and* valid (although tests may be highly reliable and yet have little validity).

Returning to liver failure it might be objected that there can be no such thing as 'liver failure' in the abstract. Perhaps there should be two separate measures, one of parenchymal liver failure, due to hepatocyte damage, and a second due to extrinsic damage of the biliary system, and each could have its own specific tests. And indeed abnormal levels of SGOT, SGPT or glutamine transaminase imply parenchymal damage, and abnormal alkaline phosphatase or 5-NT levels assess biliary tract damage. There then will be greater correlations between the items within one group than between items in different groups. The same applies to intelligence; items assessing verbal ability correlate more closely with other verbal items than with those measuring spatial ability. On this basis, Thurstone and Guilford suggested that there is no single, unitary intelligence, but only specific intelligences, each independent in some sense. Returning to liver failure it can be argued that whilst liver failure may have different causes, all that matters to the patient is the overall degree of failure, particularly as each may cause the other anyway. Therefore, it may be better to measure overall failure, and also to create a second measure of 'relatively parenchymal' versus 'relatively biliary'. A similar argument applies to intelligence. Since verbal, spatial and arithmetic sub-tests all intercorrelate, Burt, Spearman and others argued for measures of GENERAL INTELLIGENCE (G) and of COGNITIVE STYLE ('relatively verbal' versus 'relatively spatial'). The important thing about such controversies is that they are pseudo-controversies. Intelligence and liver failure are multidimensional concepts; the best single number to describe them is, in a real sense, arbitrary, depending on the purpose of our measure. Similarly, a rectangle can be described by its height and breadth, or by its area and perimeter; both are equivalent and contain equal information; area is better if you are a surveyor, and height and width if you are a carpenter. With liver failure, an overall measure is required to assess overall fitness for work, whereas deciding whether or not to operate requires a specific measure of the extent of extrinsic damage. With intelligence, different measures are needed for asking if a person is suitable for a sheltered workshop or if they have a specific reading defect.

Given that we can measure intellectual performance, how and why do individuals differ? Intelligence levels are normally distributed, with a mean of 100 and standard deviation of 15. This is hardly interesting as the tests are constructed to have such properties. Five per cent of the population therefore have an IQ above 125, and 5% below 75; and 0.1% above 143 and 0.1% below 57. To be more practical, an IQ of about 100 is needed to gain GCSE grades A or B, 110 to obtain A-levels and 120 to enter university; medical students have an average IQ of 125. Arguably an IQ of 70–75 is sufficient for independent existence in a technological society.

Many intelligence tests are in common use. Some, like RAVEN'S PROGRESSIVE MATRICES, cover the entire range of ability and are completely non-verbal. Tests in clinical use are the WAIS (WECHSLER ADULT INTELLIGENCE SCALE), the WISC (WECHSLER INTELLIGENCE SCALE FOR CHILDREN) and the WPPSI (WECHSLER PRE-SCHOOL AND PRIMARY SCALE OF INTELLIGENCE), which measure specific abilities as well as general intelligence. A similar, more recently introduced test is the BRITISH ABILITY SCALES. Tests such as the AH4, AH5 and AH6 are designed to distinguish between university students, and most items are too difficult for the average person. Tests like the AH6 give separate measures of verbal, numerical and spatial intelligence, and discrepancies between the scores can be important.

The causes of differences in intelligence are controversial. Environmental theorists argue that IQ is mainly dependent upon differences in environment (diet, education, culture, etc.) whereas genetic theorists emphasize differences in genetic inheritance. Crudely, it is obvious that low IQ associated with cerebral palsy due to anoxia during delivery is environmental, whereas low IQ in untreated phenylketonuria is genetic. But the latter case shows the problems of attributing causality, for a phenylketonuric child in an environment with no dietary phenylalanine develops a normal IQ. There are no *absolute* answers to such questions, we can merely say genes or environment are *relatively* more important in a particular population at a particular time. Consider the less controversial topic of height. Half a millennium ago adult height in Britain was mainly a function of diet; now with no major nutritional deficits, differences in height are principally genetic. Ironically, it should be realized that the imposition of a uniform social and intellectual environment will result in all remaining differences being genetic; and in genetically identical clones, all differences must be environmental in origin.

A common method for assessing contributions of genes and environment involves monozygotic (MZ) twins. If a character is genetic, then since MZ twins have identical genes they should be more similar one to another than dizygotic (DZ) twins, who share only half their genes. However, MZ twins not only share genes, but also have more similar environments, being treated more similarly by their parents. In addition they sometimes develop PRIVATE LANGUAGES, which interfere with normal intellectual development. MZ twins have an average IQ of 95, compared with 100 for DZ twins and singletons. This discrepancy is not due to prenatal influences since if one member of the pair dies during childbirth, the IQ of the remaining twin averages 100. It is postnatal treatment that makes MZ twins have a lower IQ.

MZ twins separated at birth and reared in different families have identical genes but different environments, and hence any similarities ought to be genetic in origin. However, such twins are very rare (perhaps 300 cases in the world's literature), and their circumstances so special, often illegitimate or evacuated in war-time, or with retarded parents, that they cannot resolve the gene–environment controversy.

In the last two decades, a new method has resolved most of the problems by looking not at twins themselves, but at their children, who are mainly singletons. Think of two female MZ twins, each with children. The children of one twin are as closely related to their aunt as to their mother; and while in a normal family a child shares one eighth of a cousin's genes (half of the mother's genes, who has half the aunt's genes, who has half the cousin's genes), in MZ twin families a child shares a quarter of its cousin's genes. Cousins are raised in different families, and hence different environments, so it is possible, by using sophisticated statistical models to compare twin families with ordinary families and thereby find if intelligence has genetic or environmental components. Probably most researchers would now agree that about 40–50% of IQ variance has genetic origins, with the remaining 50–60% of environmental origin.

What then are the environmental influences upon IQ? Many factors contribute: for instance the FAMILY LEARNING ENVIRONMENT, parental provision of books, conversation and intellectual support, has an influence over and beyond the fact that parents of higher intelligence are more likely to provide a good environment. The differences in IQ between birth cohorts (see Chapter 17) also suggest an important role for environmental effects. Particularly interesting work has examined the influence of birth order and family size. Since genes cannot know the order in which they are born, or how many siblings they have, then effects of birth order and family size must be environmental. Later born children are of lower average IQ than firstborns, and children in smaller families have lower IQ, both effects being independent of social class (Fig. 7.1). Zajonc's CONFLUENCE MODEL accounts for findings of this sort. A first child initially has the undivided attention of its parents, and hence is exposed to undiluted adult intelligence. A second child necessarily receives less parental attention than its older sibling, since the parents' time is shared with the older sibling (although it does receive the partial compensation of being exposed to the rather lower intellect of its older sibling). The intellectual

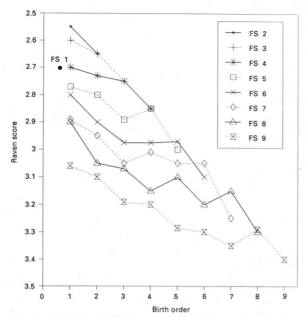

Fig. 7.1 Intelligence as measured by Raven's Progressive Matrices in 386 114 nineteen-year-old men who had been tested on entry into Dutch military conscription, in relation to the size of their family (FS) and their order in that sequence (birth order). Note that Family Size 1 is slightly laterally displaced to avoid confusion with the first born of family size 4. Because of the method of scoring used, low scores (e.g. 2.5) indicate *higher* intelligence than higher scores (e.g. 3.5). Adapted from Belmont L and Marolla F A (1973), Birth order, family size and intelligence, *Science*, **182**, 1096–1101.

environment of a second child is therefore less rich than the first child, and the first child's environment is also diluted; and so on for each additional child. The precise mathematical model predicts that first born children and children from smaller families should be more intelligent, as is seen in Figure 7.1. In the extended, non-nuclear families typical of developing countries, the last born in large families has a relatively increased IQ (see Fig. 7.2). The model copes well with this since although parental attention is further diluted, older siblings are now adult and continue to live in the parental home, where they can enrich the youngest children's intellectual environment.

The basic model needs one further refinement, since only children have a lower IQ than the first-born of families of two (see Fig. 7.1). This is ascribed to the beneficial effects to an older child of teaching their younger siblings: for teaching benefits teachers as much as pupils.

IQ is often criticized as a practical measure in that those with

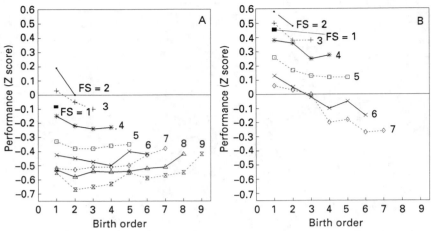

Fig. 7.2 Intelligence test scores (expressed as standard normal deviates, with mean of zero and standard deviation of one) of 191 993 Israeli school children, in relation to family size and birth order (singletons being indicated by a solid square). *a*) Students of predominantly Middle Eastern or North African origin (N = 109 304) and hence predominantly from extended families; *b*) Students of European, American and Australasian origin (N = 82 689) and predominantly from nuclear families. Adapted from Davis D J, Cahan S and Bashi J (1977), Birth order and intellectual development: the confluence model in the light of cross-cultural evidence, *Science*, **196**, 1470–2.

highest intelligence do not usually become leaders of society, politicians, captains of industry, etc. This is not due to intelligence being invalid as a measure, but rather reflects the complexity of the social psychology of leadership. Although high intelligence means greater reasoning power, and hence greater ability, this is of diminishing benefit as IQ increases; it matters little to be more intellectually able than 99% of the population rather than 98%. More importantly, if the arguments of those of high intelligence are not understood by those of lesser intelligence, then they will have no influence. Individuals typically only influence by argument those down to about ten or fifteen IQ points below themselves, and hence the highest intellects influence very few. Intelligence alone is not the only requirement of social success and influence, and hence the most successful are often of only moderately high intelligence (to the chagrin of the highly intelligent).

8

Personality

- TRAITS assess personality characteristics which are stable over long periods of time, whereas STATES assess short-term changes, as in the emotions.
- Behaviour is determined both by the personality of an individual and the situation in which they find themselves.
- METHODS OF ASSESSMENT tend to be less reliable and more difficult to interpret than PRODUCTIVE MEASURES, such as PERSONALITY QUESTION-NAIRES.
- The EYSENCK PERSONALITY QUESTIONNAIRE is an example of a DIMENSIONAL THEORY OF PERSONALITY, in which individuals are given scores on four separate personality dimensions, of EXTRAVERSION, NEUROTICISM, PSYCHOTICISM, and a LIE SCALE.
- Differences between extraverts and introverts can be explained in terms of extraverts having a lesser degree of cortical arousal, and hence being STIMULUS HUNGRY. This can explain the greater consumption of physical and social stimulation by extraverts.
- Personality measures can sometimes be more informative about an individual's personality than can the descriptions of a friend.

Personality is the behaviours that distinguish individuals and characterize them as specific people. Particularly distressing to relatives of a schizophrenic (see Chapter 30) is the DISINTEGRATION OF PERSONALITY, the sense of a different person inhabiting a familiar body.

TRAITS, the long-lasting behavioural characteristics of personality, must be distinguished from STATES, the more transitory behaviours of emotion. One might be anxious *today* because of an exam (state anxiety), or one might *generally* be an anxious person (trait anxiety).

Behaviours result partly from personality, and partly from situations. Thus two individuals might differ in their talkativeness in different situations.

| | Amount of talking in situation | | | |
	Discussion group	Lecture	Theatre	Funeral
Person A: talkative trait	+ + + +	+ +	±	−
Person B: non-talkative trait	+ +	+	−	−

The amount of talking depends both on the personality of A and B and also on the situation in which they find themselves. A knowledge of personality allows us to predict the behaviour of individuals in novel situations and to assess differences in that behaviour.

There are two broadly separate ways of asking questions about personality. One method asks questions such as 'What is X like as a person?' and 'How did X come to be the way they are?'; this is called an IDIOTHETIC approach, since it particularly concerns the single individual and their particular idiosyncrasies, and is primarily the province of the psychoanalyst, or psychodynamic theorist (see Chapter 11). A second type of question asks, 'How do X and Y differ?', or more generally, 'How does X differ from other people?'. This is the NORMOTHETIC approach that compares individuals with the rest of the population, and is the province of PSYCHOMETRICS.

Personality can be assessed in as many ways as there are situations and people. The METHODS OF ASSESSMENT involve observations of a subject in different situations. Thus in a CLINICAL INTERVIEW (or in its most extended form, psychoanalysis) a professional talks to a patient and forms a judgement; at its worst the method is lengthy, unreliable, idiosyncratic, unsystematic, and of dubious validity, and is often distorted by the theoretical preconceptions of the interviewer. Its great advantage is that it is unlimited in range, almost any questions can be asked and the answers evaluated. ASSESSMENT INTERVIEWS are more systematic, particularly if they ask for judgements on a series of rating scales, so that a range of behaviours may be systematically assessed; nevertheless reliability often leaves much to be desired. Finally, in NATURALISTIC OBSERVATION, a subject is watched or filmed while behaving in a natural setting, and the behaviours rated and assessed by a group of trained observers. In both these latter situations judgements are more reliable than in the clinical interview. The major theoretical problem of all three methods of assessment is that the personality of the subject is not assessed directly, but rather is filtered through the personality of the assessors, who themselves may have a distorted or biased view of the world. Nevertheless, with care, valuable results can be obtained.

PRODUCTIVE MEASURES of personality involve the subject producing responses to situations. The situation may be as straightforward as the humble but frequently used PERSONALITY QUESTIONNAIRE, which may contain between 10 and 200 questions, each requiring Yes/No answers or rating responses. The questions ask what the subject likes doing, feels about events, or would do in a particular situation, etc., so that the subject is asked to introspect on their own experiences in a systematic way. The advantages are the speed and ease of administration, reliability, quantitative results, and being standardizable; more problematic is that questionnaires are sometimes tedious to complete, are limited in range, obtaining answers only to questions that have been thought of in advance, and require cooperative and truthful subjects. PROJECTIVE TESTS, such as the famous RORSCHACH INK BLOTS, in which a subject is asked what they see in a random ink-blot, the TAT (THEMATIC APPERCEPTION TEST) in which subjects describe ambiguous cartoon stories, and WORD ASSOCIATION TESTS, in which subjects say the first word that comes into their heads in response to another word, are productive measures, which have the disadvantage that the answers require interpretation by a trained assessor. All tend to be biased towards a psychoanalytic perspective, and are little used in routine practice.

So-called OBJECTIVE TESTS involve subjects carrying out simple tasks such as blowing up a balloon, while automatic equipment records the rate of puffing, size of the puffs, size of the balloon, etc. Although undoubtedly people differ in the way they carry out the tasks, ultimately there is a mass of inchoate data, albeit 'scientifically' obtained, with so little theory to explain the differences that the results are of little practical use.

Since questionnaires are quite the commonest form of personality assessment, the rest of this chapter will be devoted to one of the most popular of them, the EYSENCK PERSONALITY QUESTIONNAIRE (EPQ), which demonstrates well the characteristics of a DIMENSIONAL THEORY OF PERSON-ALITY.

A dimensional theory says that individuals vary along a continuum, with a few individuals at either extreme, and the majority at intermediate positions. People are not divided into two or more separate TYPES, into which they are pigeon-holed, but instead the extremes act as convenient labels, although most individuals are not as extreme as these labels. (There is an old psychological joke about there being two types of people — those who divide people into two types and those who do not.)

The oldest dimensional theory goes back to Classical times and was codified by Galen (129–ca. 199) as part of his theory of the humours. Four separate humours, derived from the various physiological fluids, combined in differing amounts to produce two separate dimensions of personality (see Fig. 8.1); sanguine-splenetic (based on a relative excess of blood from the heart, or 'black bile' supposed to come from the spleen), and phlegmatic-choleric (based on the relative excess of phlegm from the head, or bile from the gall-bladder). Individuals had different mixes of these constituents, for various reasons, such as the season of the year or the place where they lived, and this resulted in a range of possible personality types, which are seen around the outside of Figure 8.1. Of course *l'homme moyen*, the typical person, was placed exactly at the centre. Eysenck's modern theory of person-ality builds upon the Greek example, but rotates the important axes through forty-five degrees, and relabels them EXTRAVERSION (E) *vs* INTROVERSION (I) and NEUROTICISM (N) *vs* STABILITY (S). An extreme extravert

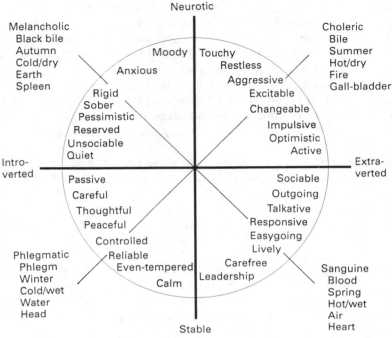

Fig. 8.1 The Galenic theory of the humours in relation to the modern dimensional theory of introversion – extraversion and neuroticism – stability. In Galenic theory, there were four principal personality types, indicated at the four corners of the diagram and by the lighter, diagonal axes; a range of intermediate types are also indicated on the inner circle. Each personality was felt to be due to an excess of a particular HUMOUR which came from a particular organ of the body. The humour was characterized by its predominant ELEMENT and by its associated QUALITIES, and these qualities relate directly to the personality type. Each humour was associated with a particular season of the year, and individuals born then were more likely to have the particular personality type. The modern theory of personality uses the same descriptions (although not the same theory of its origins) but rotates the axes by 45 degrees to the vertical position, to the positions shown by the solid lines. Adapted from Eysenck H J (1964), Principles and methods of personality description, classification and diagnosis, *Br J Psychol*, **55**, 284–94.

is a person who is sociable, cheerful, enjoys taking risks and is optimistic, in contrast to an extreme introvert who dislikes company, is overly careful, pessimistic and appears to lack enjoyment. The more typical AMBIVERT, in the middle of the range, has some of each of these characteristics. An individual with a high neuroticism score (which should not be taken as having the same meaning as a person with a neurosis, which is a psychiatric term – see Chapter 28) tends to be anxious, particularly about the minutiae of life, to worry unnecessarily, especially about health, and to be overly emotional, whereas a stable personality is calm, unflappable, steady and unemotional. Eysenck has also extended the original two dimensions of the Greek scheme with a third dimension, called PSYCHOTICISM (P), (again not to be taken as synonymous with psychotic, which is a psychiatric term, see Chapter 28, although there is some evidence that high P scorers are more likely to be psychotic). High P scorers tend to be solitary, uncaring, insensitive, aggressive and impulsive individuals, although of course only a very high scorer would be all of these things. Eysenck has also developed a fourth score, the LIE SCALE (L), which was originally designed to assess whether respondents were telling the truth or were trying to FAKE GOOD in order to impress. The L scale asks questions to which any ordinary person would normally have to answer a particular way, for instance asking if they have *ever* been late for an appointment, and assuming that an answer of 'no' is designed to impress or deceive, rather than tell the truth. More recently the L scale has been re-interpreted as a measure of SOCIAL ACQUIESCENCE and is being regarded as a measure of a separate personality dimension in its own right, reflecting a person's desire to please others and answer as they would find desirable. To give some idea of the range of scores, Figure 8.2 shows the personality scores of entrants to medical school compared with the norms for the population of that age; entrants are more extravert, less neurotic, less psychotic, and are lying slightly more than the average population. Since there are only minimal differences between those accepted and those rejected, the differences of entrants from the general population must be due to certain types of individual applying to medical school, rather than medical schools preferentially selecting certain types of student.

If a personality test is to be useful, it should also predict other aspects of behaviour, and this the EPQ does well. For instance in comparison with introverts, extraverts consume more tea, coffee, alcohol, and cigarettes, have earlier and more varied sexual behaviour, and are more likely to suffer from sexually transmitted diseases and to divorce. In contrast, high N scorers have increased rates of psychosomatic diseases and have more sexual problems, such as impotence and premature ejaculation, whereas high P scorers have increased rates of serious mental illness, criminality, alcoholism and drug abuse. The test therefore predicts a broader range of behaviours than the 90 Yes/No questions might lead us to expect.

If differences exist between individuals then there must be reasons for these differences. Eysenck has argued that extraversion is a result of differences in cortical arousal, neuroticism of differences in autonomic arousal, and psychoticism of differences in androgenic activity. These aspects of Eysenck's theory are not entirely uncontroversial, and therefore just the theory of extraversion will be described in more detail to give an idea of the way in which such a theory can be developed.

Sensory inputs have a dual input to the cortex: a direct route and

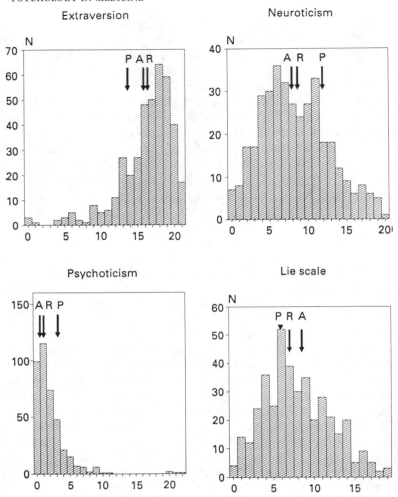

Fig. 8.2 The personality of 255 entrants to medical school. The mean scores of successful applicants to medical school (A) are compared with those of 99 rejects (R), and with the population norms for the same age-sex group (P). Unpublished data of I C McManus.

an indirect route whereby they activate the reticular activating system in the brain stem, which in turn activates the cortex (Fig. 8.3). In the presence of such activation there would be a danger of over-activation (and epileptic discharge) and therefore the cortex also inhibits its own activity by the process of REACTIVE INHIBITION. Eysenck proposes that extraverts have relatively low levels of cortical activation, via the reticular system, and have greater reactive inhibition than do introverts. The consequence is that in an extravert a sensory event produces less cortical activity than in an introvert. If sensory events are of less impact to an extravert, then greater levels of sensory

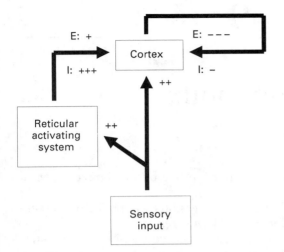

Fig. 8.3 Eysenck's theory of the relationship between extraversion and cortical arousal. The sensory input causes excitation (+ +) of the reticular activating system and the cortex. The cortex inhibits its own activity by reactive inhibition, either strongly in extraverts (E: − − −) or weakly in introverts (I: −). The reticular activating system excites the cortex either weakly in extraverts (E: +) or strongly in introverts (I: + + +).

stimulation would be needed to obtain the same level of cortical activation. Extraverts will therefore be STIMULUS HUNGRY and require greater stimulation (and hence also will ingest more stimulants such as tea, coffee, cigarettes, etc) and will obtain more social stimulation than do introverts. Introverts can be seen as chronically over-aroused, and extraverts under-aroused. The theory can also explain why extraverts have higher auditory detection thresholds, have higher pain thresholds, are slower at being conditioned, and are less able to carry out boring jobs or VIGILANCE TASKS, which involve the detection of rare events.

A final question concerning personality tests is whether they will tell us anything about a person that, say, their best friend could not have told us from their experience. An experiment looked at this by asking pairs of friends to complete an EPQ; each member of the pair was then asked to complete a second EPQ in the way that they thought their friend would have completed it. Comparison of the results showed that individuals were good at estimating the extraversion of their friends, but were poor at describing their friend's neuroticism or psychoticism. Personality tests therefore are useful at giving us information we would not necessarily have known in some other way.

9

Emotion

- EMOTIONS or AFFECTS are not purely cognitive but also have visceral components.
- Emotions as represented in facial expressions seem to be universal, being found in similar forms in all cultures.
- William James' theory, that emotions are caused by bodily states rather than bodily states being caused by emotions, is supported by the action of beta-blockers and by the diminished emotions of patients with a spinal transection.
- Schacter's TWO-FACTOR THEORY OF EMOTION has extended James' theory of emotion and said that visceral arousal is interpreted by the cognitive system as an appropriate emotion according to the context.
- The frontal and temporal lobes, and Papez's circuit in the limbic system, are probably important for emotion.
- The right hemisphere seems to be more important than the left in producing emotional responses.

A recent dictionary of psychology says:

> '*Emotion*: historically this term has proved utterly refractory to definitional efforts; probably no other term in psychology shares its indefinability with its frequency of use. Most textbook writers wisely employ it as the title of a chapter and let the material presented substitute for a concise definition.'

This book will be no different. This chapter will therefore consider a number of aspects of emotion, and Chapters 11 and 13 will also discuss emotional development in the context of Freud's theories, and in relation to Personal Construct Theory.

We all experience EMOTIONS (or AFFECTS or MOODS), such as anger, love, jealousy, hatred, joy, ecstasy, misery, and disgust, and we recognize them in others. They do not seem purely intellectual but have strong visceral components, arising not only in our minds but in our heart, bowels, limbs, etc. Sometimes they seem dissociated from cognition ('I knew in my mind it didn't matter, but still I felt angry'), suggesting a separate process from pure thought.

Classification is difficult and although 'primary emotions' have been differentiated from mixtures of those primaries, there is little consensus.

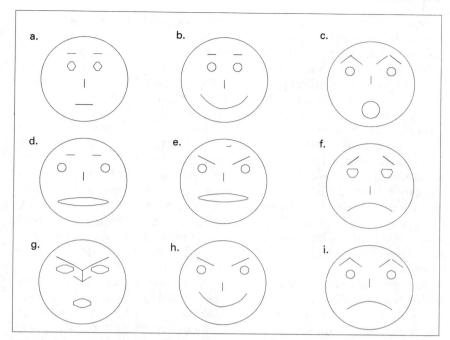

Fig. 9.1 Diagrammatic representations of six pure facial expressions of emotion (b–g), and two blended expressions (h–i). *a*) neutral, *b*) happy, *c*) surprise, *d*) afraid, *e*) angry, *f*) sad, *g*) disgusted, *h*) angry brow and eyes with happy mouth, *i*) surprised brow and eyes with sad mouth. Adapted from Lloyd P, Mayes A, Manstead A S R, Meudell P R and Wagner H L (1984), *Introduction to psychology: an integrated approach*, London, Fontana.

Ekman's work on facial expressions of emotion followed Charles Darwin's (1809–1882) *The expression of the emotions in man and animals* of 1872 in arguing for several basic emotions. Figure 9.1 shows facial expressions with six different emotions (happy, surprised, afraid, angry, sad and disgusted), and two of many possible combinations, ('happy anger' and 'sad surprise'). As well as showing how a cartoon can express complex states, similar figures and photographs have been used cross-culturally to assess Darwin's hypothesis of the UNIVERSALITY OF EMOTIONAL EXPRESSION. The emotions are recognized by people in all cultures tested, implying a biological coding of facial emotions rather than the simple cultural learning found with other non-verbal communications, such as head shaking, which has different meanings in different societies. Darwin also suggested that similar expressions were found in animals, particularly primates, presumably being the basis for attribution of emotions to pet cats or dogs (and perhaps why animals like fish are said to be unemotional because they cannot produce facial expressions; and hence the phrase 'They are a cold fish').

Figure 9.1 also shows another aspect of emotion. Look at Figure 9.1c, raise your eyebrows, and open your mouth in an 'o' shape; you *feel* something like surprise; and replicating Figure 9.1e produces a feeling like anger. Such observations on the role of FACIAL EFFERENCE raise an important question of causality: do we have emotions and our body then responds to them or are emotions the perceptions of bodily actions? The second theory was proposed by William James (1842–1910), when he said 'we are afraid because we run, we do not run because we are afraid'. The first, more commonsense hypothesis, ascribed to Walter Cannon (1871–1945), says emotions are states of mind resulting from cognitive analysis that firstly provides reasons for emotions such as fear (we might just have seen a tiger) and then activates the autonomic system (increased heart-rate, etc). Although counter-intuitive, the second theory has evidence to support it. It predicts that a lack of visceral sensations should reduce emotions, and that false visceral feedback should result in inappropriate emotions.

Anxiety, amounting almost to fear, occurs in young musicians taking examinations, the 'stage fright' ruining their performance, particularly due to hand tremor. Beta-blockers, which act by slowing the heart, diminish the fear and reduce the tremor; reducing the visceral sensation reduces the emotion, as James' theory predicts. Beta-blockers have become popular amongst junior doctors taking examinations, despite no evidence for improved performance and the possibility of impairment because some intermediate level of arousal is usually necessary for optimum performance.

Patients with a spinal cord transection lose a large proportion of their visceral afferents, higher lesions producing greater loss. The patients report reduced emotions of fear, anger and sexuality, as James' theory predicts. However the precise comments ('Seems like I get thinking mad, not shaking mad', 'It's a mental kind of anger', and 'I don't really feel afraid, not all tense and shaky, with that hollow feeling in my stomach like I used to') suggest central emotions are still present, but lack the visceral effects which make emotions so powerful.

BIOFEEDBACK can be used to make subjects aware of visceral processes, such as heart rate, by connecting ECG electrodes so that each heart beat produces an audible click. If such feedback is artificially speeded up or slowed down then the FALSE FEEDBACK modifies emotional interpretations of events. I remember once seeing the film *Earthquake* and during an exciting episode was impressed by my tachycardia of about 120 beats per minute; but a finger on the pulse showed my true heart rate was 70 beats per minute. The film's soundtrack contained false low frequency auditory feedback, which enhanced the excitement (a device exploited many times in film soundtrack music).

A different approach to emotion is Schacter's influential TWO FACTOR

THEORY OF EMOTION, bridging the gap between James and Cannon. Schacter says that visceral stimuli are like other sensory stimuli, requiring interpretation by the cognitive system, which tries to make sense of events. Schacter also says AROUSAL or ACTIVATION is the only activity that can be recognized in the visceral inputs. Consider the fear felt when running away from a tiger. Schacter says we see the tiger and start to run, which produces arousal, and the cognitive system then detects increased visceral arousal, which it explains by saying the emotion must be fear. The visceral activity is LABELLED as fear, the most reasonable explanation for all the phenomena. Identical visceral activity at some other time, as during vigorous exercise, would not be labelled as fear, but instead would be ascribed to the exercise and labelled as tiredness coupled with physical well-being. Emotion therefore requires *both* appropriate physiological arousal *and* an appropriate emotional context for the arousal.

Schacter has supported his theory with an ingenious experiment. Four groups of subjects in a laboratory supposedly received injections of 'suproxine', a hypothetical vitamin. One group (P) actually received a saline placebo, and the other groups (T, F & N) received adrenaline. Group T was told they might experience tachycardia, tremor, etc, the true side effects of adrenaline. Group F was told they might experience numbness of the feet, itching, etc, false side-effects of adrenaline. Group N and P were given no information about possible side-effects. After the injection subjects waited in a room, which they shared with another 'subject', actually a confederate of the experimenter. This stooge was conspicuously euphoric. Subjects later recorded their emotional state, and their pulse rate was measured to confirm the adrenaline had produced similar degrees of tachycardia in groups T, F and N. The amount of euphoria was greatest in group F, followed by N and P, and finally T. Schacter interpreted the result as follows: group T were aroused and had a cogent reason for the arousal, which they attributed to the injection and therefore felt no euphoria. Group F were similarly aroused but since they could not attribute it to the injection (it not being one of the possible side-effects), they attributed their arousal to euphoria induced by the confederate (and indeed acted appropriately). Group P felt little arousal, having received the placebo. Group N felt arousal but did not know if it might be the effect of the drug and hence were intermediate between groups F and T. Such experiments suggest emotions are not feelings independent of thought (like the coloured wash used to tint a monochrome engraving), but instead both influence and are influenced by thought itself (and hence are an integral part of the picture itself). The mind actively tries to understand the world in which it finds itself, and the body, with its physiology, is also a part of that world, a part in some ways as foreign as the world outside it.

Emotion, like all other behaviours, depends upon the brain, and attempts have been made to locate sites of importance in emotion. A popular image has the cortex as the seat of thought, and sub-cortical nuclei producing emotions, the 'higher' cortex inhibiting the 'lower', primitive, sub-cortical nuclei. (The model was most popular when Freudian theories were in the ascendant, and provided correlates of ego and id.) In the 1930s, Papez, an American anatomist, hypothesized that the LIMBIC SYSTEM (in particular the hippocampus, septum, hypothalamus, anterior thalamus, cingulate gyrus, and entorrhinal cortex) were a circuit (known now as PAPEZ'S CIRCUIT), responsible for emotional behaviour. The AMYGDALA is now also thought to be important, although there is still no coherent theory of the neuropsychology of emotion. Brain lesions in animals can nonetheless produce abnormal emotions, as in the KLUVER-BUCY SYNDROME, in which bilateral temporal lobectomy causes intense, labile emotions as also does bilateral frontal lobectomy. Patients with frontal or temporal tumours, or with TEMPORAL LOBE EPILEPSY, can present symptoms of emotional instability. Because of such observations, some neurosurgeons have attempted to control disturbed emotional behaviour in psychiatric patients by FRONTAL LOBOTOMY or FRONTAL LEUCOTOMY, or lesions to limbic system or subcortical nuclei. Because most such lesions have been made without adequate theoretical justification, and without controlled trials of efficacy, the pejorative epithet 'cerebral topiary' is not entirely without justification.

Recent work suggests emotions may depend more upon the right than the left hemisphere (see also Chapter 23). Patients with left hemisphere lesions (which 'release' the right hemisphere), often display CATASTROPHIC REACTIONS to illness, being fearful and depressed, whereas right-hemisphere lesions produce INDIFFERENCE REACTIONS or EUPHORIC REACTIONS, with denial of disease. Similar symptoms can be produced by unilateral intracarotid sodium amytal. Such effects are partly explained by aphasia after left-hemisphere lesions, and neglect after right-hemisphere lesions, although these are not entirely the explanation. Right-hemisphere lesions also impair judgements of emotion in others, and of humour in cartoons, whereas left-hemisphere lesions only produce defects secondary to language difficulties in describing emotions.

Emotion is the salt that gives savour to cognition; it is always present and should never be forgotten. But it is still far from well understood.

10

Child development

- Piaget's theory of intellectual development says that children pass through four separate STAGES OF DEVELOPMENT; in each of these thought is qualitatively different.
- In the SENSORIMOTOR PERIOD, the child develops the concept of an OBJECT, and learns to manipulate objects physically.
- In the PRE-OPERATIONAL STAGE, the child learns to attach verbal labels to objects and to manipulate names as if they were objects. The child is EGOCENTRIC, both intellectually and morally, and makes characteristic errors of thought, such as the failure of CONSERVATION.
- ATTACHMENT between parents and child starts with BONDING, and is particularly intense up to the age of five, when SEPARATION ANXIETY and FEAR OF STRANGERS are very strong. Differences in attachment can be measured in the STRANGE SITUATION test.
- Poor attachment can result in CHILD ABUSE, and a complete absence of attachment can result in the syndrome of MATERNAL DEPRIVATION.
- Attachment is the first stage in developing SOCIAL RELATIONSHIPS, which in childhood pass through Erikson's series of five CRISES, each of which be helped or hindered by different PARENTING STYLES.

The physical transformation of the single cell of a fertilized ovum into a newborn baby is complex and remarkable. No less complex and no less remarkable is the psychological transformation of that wriggling neonate into a sentient, intelligent adult that can write plays, paint pictures, drive cars, read newspapers, understand nuclear physics, or study medicine. In the same way as the fertilized ovum is not a *homunculus*, containing miniature versions of the various organ systems of the neonate, so neither is the mind of the neonate a miniature version of the adult brain, merely requiring a little more effort, a little more memory or a little more attention. As the fertilized ovum contains the essential plans for building a neonate, in the form of its DNA, so the mind of a neonate is not a TABULA RASA, a blank sheet, but contains the essential physiological and psychological equipment from which an adult mind can be *constructed*. The neonatal mind does not therefore contain any specific information about the nature of objects in the world or of three-dimensional space, about people, or about social relationships. The neonate looks out on a world which, in William James' words, is 'a blooming, buzzing confusion'; the neonate cannot *know* that the pattern of light and shade that sometimes appears in its visual field and the strange noises that accompany it are its mother talking to it, but it can learn about the association and then start to predict when the events will occur. And also it needs to learn such subtle, and apparently trivial and obvious facts, as that the pattern of light and sound come from an OBJECT that continues to exist even when not being observed by the child.

Adult human beings are not simply 'thinking machines', absorbing information which is then converted into other forms of information before being output; they are also, perhaps predominantly, individuals with feelings and emotions, which are attached to the objects around them, which have ideas about how those objects work, and which form social relationships with the particular objects which are other people. All of these different aspects develop in parallel during childhood, each assisting and interacting with the other aspects. In a book such as this, only a few basic ideas about child development can be presented, which are chosen to emphasize particularly important points: those concerning intellectual development, and Piaget's stage theories; the development of attachment; and the formation of social relationships. Other aspects of development are also considered elsewhere in the book, as for instance in Chapter 6 on language, Chapter 11 on Freud and emotional development, Chapter 17 on ageing, and in Chapters 28, 29 and 30 on psychopathology. In so far as adults have necessarily all once been children, so every part of psychology has its developmental aspect.

INTELLECTUAL DEVELOPMENT

The central figure in understanding intellectual development is JEAN PIAGET (1896–1980), a Swiss psychologist who regarded himself as a biologist studying the nature of mind and who developed the field he called GENETIC EPISTEMOLOGY (*genetic* in its original meaning of 'developmental' and *epistemology*, the study of knowledge and its origins). Piaget's theories have dominated education and developmental psychology throughout the twentieth century.

Piaget developed a complicated theory of development, a STAGE THEORY, which argued that the successive phases of development of a child are not just successively more complicated, as if the intellect were merely growing in size, but differed qualitatively one from another with the modes of thinking actually being different in type from each other; and in part this explains why children's thought is so difficult for adults to understand. Stage theories cannot be explained entirely by LEARNING THEORIES (see Chapter 3), which only allow for a gradual accretion of knowledge, without sudden changes in the STRUCTURE or FORM of thinking. As well as Piaget's, there are several other stage theories in psychology; Freud's theory of emotional development (Chapter 11), Erikson's theory of ego development (Chapter 17) and Kohlberg's theory of moral development.

Piaget argued that four major stages of development existed, for which approximate ages can be given. The order in which they are passed through is invariant and not all individuals reach the highest stages; not all adults reach stage 4, and some retarded children may only reach stage 1 or 2. Interestingly, gorilla infants pass through stage 1 more quickly than human infants, but then never reach stage 2. Although still central to developmental psychology, Piaget's theories are not now accepted in their entirety. A major distinction between Piaget and the NEO-PIAGETIANS is that Piaget considered *all* of a person's intellectual activities to be at the same stage, whereas neo-Piagetians accept that some activities can be at more advanced stages than others.

Stage 1: The sensorimotor period (0–2 years). Consider what it is like to be a newborn baby (that of course you must have been one at some time doesn't actually help much). You have sensations which are not organized, i.e. they are sensations without perceptions, so although aware of areas of light and dark you are not aware of 'objects' as such. Indeed you can have no concept of an object because you are encountering a new world; the very *idea* of an object is itself to be discovered. Similarly there are also noises that make little sense. You also have limbs, can move muscles and kinaesthesis tells you things are happening, but there is no sense of limbs moving *in space*, because the three-dimensional nature of space is not known to you. Finally, sensations arise from within your own body, from viscera, etc., although you cannot know these sensations particularly come from *you*, rather than a separate thing called the outside world, from which you receive no sensations and have no control over. Your only systematic behaviours are certain PRIMITIVE REFLEXES that turn your head towards sounds, or towards things touching your cheek or lips, and move your limbs in the undifferentiated STARTLE RESPONSE to sudden sounds or lights. Of course in saying 'you' or 'aware' I am not implying you have any such self-concept or self-consciousness or self-awareness; and indeed if such consciousness did exist then as adults we would probably be able to remember the earliest years of our life.

From such an unpromising start you, and only you, have to come to understand a strange and mystifying world. The world contains regularities, such as the presence of particular people (but again at that time you have no concept of a person, only of regular associations of sounds, smells and patterns of light); on these regularities you must build. Of course it cannot be emphasized enough that the one thing you do not have to help you is an adult, thinking, rational, self-conscious intelligence, with knowledge and experience.

Piaget argued that in the sensorimotor stage the child understands the internal logic of its sensory and motor systems, realizing such non-trivial conclusions as that certain patterns of light are related to certain movements that can be made, so that the thing seen is a hand, your hand, under your control. Additionally, you learn that other patterns of light, perhaps your mother, or the cot-sides, are regular, with certain sensations when touched although outside of your direct control, so that your body has certain distinct limits. Simple associative learning also teaches us much; objects are sucked and chewed, and some found to be associated with pleasant visceral sensations (food) whereas others are not and cease to be sucked. The first *intellectual* development, in which an explicit *idea* transcends mere reflex association of sense and movement, is the development of OBJECT CONSTANCY. Piaget suggested it had developed by eight months of age, and more recent work suggests about five months. Before that time objects exist only when they can be seen or touched, and their components of movement, position, colour, etc, are perceived independently; they are only *events* or *actions*. Once constancy has developed, they exist in the child's mind even when the sensations that produced them are no longer present. This is shown in a simple, elegant experiment typical of those carried out by Piaget on his own children. A small white doll moves along a track, goes behind a screen and emerges from the other side, stops and then returns to its starting point. Both young and old infants satisfactorily track the object with their eyes. The experiment is then changed so that a white doll disappears behind the screen but a red toy lion emerges on the other side. Younger infants continue tracking the moving object, apparently oblivious of its change of identity, whereas older infants show surprise and keep looking back to the screen, as if to await the reappearance of the doll. The older infant not only has a concept of the object which exists when the object is no longer visible, but also has an internal model of how the object should behave, and hence predicts or expects the doll to merge at a point and time. As an example of an implicit intellectual model of object constancy, imagine your surprise if you read the front page of a newspaper, then read an inside page, and on returning to the front page found a different story despite holding the newspaper the whole time. Our world model says that objects like newspapers simply do not behave in such a way (although such behaviours are allowed in television screens, which change images unpredictably). Such interpretations are not reflexes but are intellectual analyses in a pure sense. The sensorimotor period develops and elaborates such insights, with the development of SECONDARY BEHAVIOURS; a child may see a ball on a rug, want the ball and yet be unable to reach it; at 8 or 9 months of age the child pulls the rug to get the ball, and in so doing has put the actions together mentally before actually performing them.

Stage 2: The pre-operational stage (2–5 years). Towards the end of the sensorimotor stage, the young child has a sophisticated repertoire of motor acts and sensory analyses equivalent to those of most young mammals. In stage 2, the beginnings of linguistic development separate the intellectual development of the child from that of other animals.

Although object concepts have existed for the sensorimotor child, in the pre-operational stage those objects have *names* attached to them as labels. The names can then be manipulated in lieu of the objects themselves. Such SYMBOLIC THOUGHT, the manipulation of symbols which represent objects, dominates the next few years of development. Words and names are funny things, with strange properties. For instance, although 'Daddy' is a 'man', not every man is Daddy; OVER-INCLUSION, the failure of that realization, is a common problem for the early pre-operational child. Thus a child aged 2:1 (i.e. 2 years and 1 month) said 'That's not a bee, it's a bumble bee. Is it an animal?'. The causal relations between words also have to be learned and can be faulty, producing the error of TRANSDUCTION: 'I haven't had my nap, so it isn't afternoon' (4:10); and the mere existence of a name, or the juxtaposition of objects, is felt to be sufficient explanation for causation e.g.

Adult: 'What makes the [railway] engine go?'
Child: (4:0) 'The smoke'.
Adult: 'What smoke?'
Child: 'The smoke from the funnel'.

The pre-operational child also suffers from CENTRATION, a fixation upon one aspect of a stimulus, rather than upon relationships, so that in Figure 10.1a, the child will know there are equal numbers of eggs and egg-cups, but in Figure 10.1b will say there are more egg-cups than eggs, since the egg-cups take up more space. This problem, combined with a lack of understanding of reversibility, results in the failure of CONSERVATION (Fig. 10.2). A child is shown two identical glasses of water, A and B, filled with the same amounts of water. The water from B is then poured into C while the child watches, and the child is then asked which glass holds more water. The pre-operational child either says that C contains more water, because it is wider, or that A contains more water because it is deeper. The child uses the words 'more' and 'less' but they cannot be applied appropriately to a fluid, which can change its shape and yet still conserve its volume, and instead they are applied to the container itself. Therefore, although the pre-operatinal child has a large and rapidly expanding vocabulary

a).

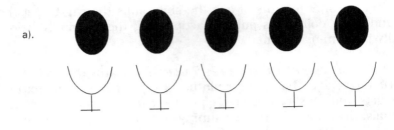

b).

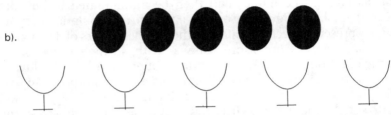

Fig. 10.1 Piaget's egg-cup experiment. Shown the situation in a) the pre-operational child will say that there are the same number of eggs and egg-cups, but after rearrangement as in b) will say that there are more cups than eggs.

to name its internal concepts (see Fig. 10.3), it is unable to use those labels accurately to make predictions about how objects will behave in the real world. The labels stand in isolation, and as such they can be extremely useful ('Give me a drink of water' or 'My head hurts'), but are limited in their effectiveness as tools for manipulation and prediction.

Stage 3: The concrete-operational stage (6–12 years). During this stage the child not only uses words correctly, but manipulates them as if they had the properties of objects, as it were, putting into words what it has already learned about actions during the sensorimotor period. Therefore, in the conservation task the concrete-operational child realizes that the volume of water is unchanged by being poured into another glass. The intellectual limitation in this stage is that such operations are only applied to real or CONCRETE objects; hypothetical or abstract objects cannot be considered. As a ten-year-old I well remember being told about algebra, and that the letter x in an equation could represent any number, and said 'Well it can't be *any* number, it must be some particular number'; a year later the concept posed no difficulty, and I had passed from concrete operations to *Stage 4: The abstract-operational stage (12 years onwards)*, in which symbols

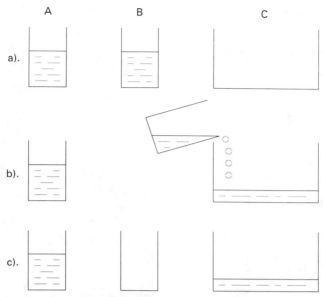

Fig. 10.2 Piaget's conservation test. *a*) A pre-operational child sees two identical beakers A and B which contain the same amount of water and the child says there is the same amount of water in each. *b*) In front of the child the experimenter pours the water from B into a wider, flatter beaker, C. *c*) When asked whether the beakers contain the same amount of water then the child says either that C contains more water (because it is wider) or less water (because it is shallower).

had properties, had arbitrary relations to one another and to the world, and could be manipulated via transformations to correspond as well as one wanted with the actual world.

This account of Piaget's thought has so far emphasized intellectual or cognitive skills. Piaget felt that such skills dominated our thinking, and themselves affected all other aspects of our psychological existence. As an example, Piaget described the pre-operational child as being EGOCENTRIC, seeing the world only from its own view-point; and intellectually this is shown in Piaget's MOUNTAIN TEST (Fig. 10.4), in which a child looks at a model of mountains and is asked whether a doll can see particular objects such as a house. A pre-operational, egocentric child cannot answer correctly, seeing the objects only from its own view-point. At this stage the child is also morally and emotionally egocentric, seeing problems entirely from the view-point of its own interests, and being unable to see the interests of other people; it is incapable of PERSPECTIVE-TAKING. The onset of lying and deception occurs also at the end of the pre-operational stage when the non-egocentric child realizes that others are not aware of its own

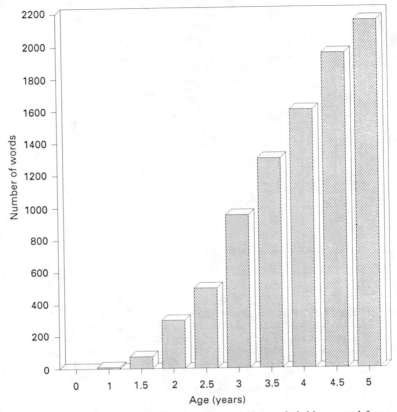

Fig. 10.3 The number of words in the vocabulary of children aged from one to five years. Adapted from Lispitt L P (1966), Learning processes of human new-borns, *Merrill-Palmer Quarterly*, **12**, 45–71.

thoughts. The dominance of intellectual processes over other activities is also seen in the games that children play. For the first two years, games are entirely related to sensual gratification, involving tickling, noises, and motor activity, such as knocking over bricks; in no sense does the *idea* of a game exist at this stage. Pre-operational games are egocentric, the child ignoring the rules, and using the game as a vehicle for its own amusement, independently of the other players. During the concrete-operational stage, the rules are strictly observed, being regarded as inviolate and immutable, with absolute authority, being almost concrete (as if graven on tablets of stone). Finally during the adult, abstract operational stage rules are seen as arbitrary, to be experimented with to produce better, more interesting games according to the needs of the participants.

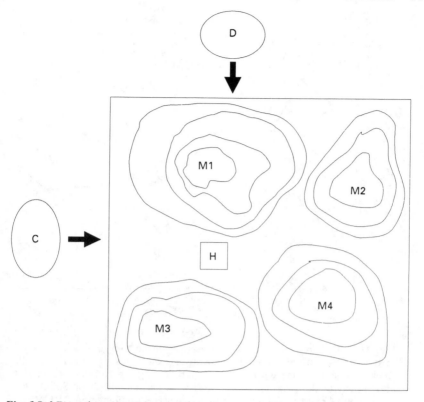

Fig. 10.4 Piaget's mountain test to show the egocentricity of the pre-operational child. Seen from above, the child, C, looks at a realistic model of mountains, M1, M2, M3 and M4, on which are placed various objects including a house, H. The child is asked if they can see the house and they say they can. They are then asked if the doll, D, can see the house, and if pre-operational then they will also say that it can, even though mountain M1 is actually blocking the doll's view of the house.

ATTACHMENT

From birth onwards, children begin to form the earliest of social relationships, that of attachment, in which they show BONDING to specific persons, typically the parents. Until about the age of six months the attachment is fairly undifferentiated, reacting to any smiling face. However, as object constancy develops, the child can differentiate adults, attachment strengthens to particular adults, and removal of the child from the parents is manifested as SEPARATION ANXIETY, a continuous screaming or sobbing, rejection of food or comfort offered by strangers, and clinging when the parent returns. The anxiety is particularly great when the child is left with *other* adults (see Fig. 10.5), FEAR OF STRANGERS. Separation anxiety and fear

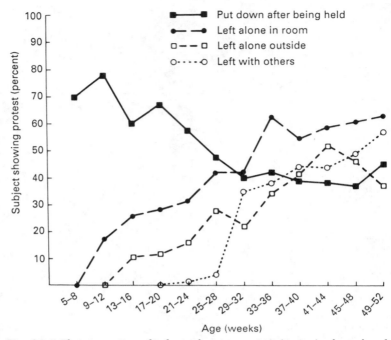

Fig. 10.5 The proportion of infants showing protest (crying) when placed in different situations. Note the sudden rise of protest in children at 29 weeks of age when left with *other* adults, reflecting separation anxiety, and attachment to the parents. Reproduced with permission of the Society for Research in Child Development, from Schaffer H R and Emerson P E (1964), The development of social attachments in infancy, *Monographs of the Society for Research in Child Development,* **29**, 3.

of strangers reach a peak at about one year of age, and then fall off, allowing relationships to be formed with siblings, grandparents, etc, and by the age of four or five the anxiety has almost disappeared. Admission to hospital for children under five can provoke severe separation anxiety, and it is now policy in most good paediatric units to allow parents of young children to stay in hospital with their children as long as they wish. Careful studies in both humans and monkeys suggest it is separation from a parent that is the principal source of distress, rather than being in a strange place, although distress is less if the infant remains in a familiar place while separation occurs ('mother goes to hospital' rather than 'child goes to hospital').

Not all children are attached in the same way, and empirically this has been particularly well studied by Mary Ainsworth, in the STRANGE SITUATION test. Children about eighteen months old play in a strange room with their mother present; the mother then leaves, returns, and departs again; a stranger enters and leaves; and the mother then returns. Most children show SECURE ATTACHMENT, exploring the room and playing when the mother is present and returning to her at intervals as a SECURE BASE, but are upset when she leaves or when the stranger enters, and cling to the mother on her return. Some children show ANXIOUS, AMBIVALENT ATTACHMENT, being distressed even when the mother is present and are ambivalent about using her as a secure base. A few children show AVOIDANT ATTACHMENT in which they avoid the mother, do not use her as a secure base, and show no distress on separation or when a stranger is present. These differences seem to arise from parents' treatment of their child, avoidant attachment being associated with cold, angry indifferent mothering, and ambivalent attachment being associated with warm mothering insensitively applied at inappropriate times. There is also evidence that these patterns continue into later childhood, and possibly adulthood, and produce abnormalities of emotional relationships.

Child abuse. Attachment is not a one-way process between child and parent, but is reciprocated, with obvious biological advantage to each side. Parental attachment to children is facilitated from birth by the appearance of the neonate, which like all young animals has a large head and large eyes which make it attractive to adults; by social interactions, in the form of imitation of parental actions; and after the age of one month or so, by smiling and laughing in response to parental actions. Occasionally, attachment by parents is severely impaired resulting in the syndrome of CHILD ABUSE, in which children are physically damaged, with broken bones and other NON-ACCIDENTAL INJURIES, or are severely NEGLECTED, resulting sometimes in death of the child. Abusers come from a wide range of backgrounds, but on average abusing parents tend to be from lower social classes, younger than average, with many children, and re-married, step-fathers being particularly likely to abuse. Interaction is abnormal in the strange situation test, showing avoidant attachment. Perhaps most important of all, abusers often have a history of abuse themselves in childhood, perpetuating a cycle of abuse from one generation to the next. Children are more likely to be abused if unwanted, physically or mentally handicapped, premature or treated in a special care baby unit, or if they are 'irritable' babies who seem to cry a lot.

Maternal deprivation. Infants and young children are often separated from their parents, but usually only for brief periods of minutes or hours. Occasionally, separation is prolonged and does not end, as when children are orphaned or abandoned and placed in institutions where they are cared for physically but cannot form emotional bonds with any particular carer. Separation from parents is followed by the behavioural sequence of PROTEST, acute distress and crying, DESPAIR, a period of misery and apathy, and finally DETACHMENT, in which the child is apparently contented and loses interest in its parents. However, the British psychiatrist, John Bowlby (1907–1990) has shown that children showing such parental deprivation are far more likely as adolescents and adults to become DELINQUENT, committing petty crimes, to be PSYCHOPATHIC, being unable to form affectionate relationships, and to be of diminished stature, so-called EMOTIONAL DWARFISM, or intellectually retarded. Although the syndrome was originally called *maternal* deprivation, it is far from clear at present whether mothers are especially important compared with fathers, or indeed whether the important factor is having *someone* who acts as a full-time carer. That early formation and maintenance of emotional bonds is important for subsequent development is not however disputed.

SOCIAL INTERACTIONS

Attachment is part of a broader process by which children learn to become part of the larger social world, and learn to interact with adults and other children. This process starts early in life. A study of nine newborn children awaiting adoption, who were cared for by one specific nurse for the first ten days of life, and then on day ten were cared for by a different nurse showed increased crying and distress after the change, suggesting that the infants had already adapted to the specific habits of their carer.

Social interaction occurs even in children two months old, often involving IMITATION, which acts as an important foundation for OBSERVATIONAL LEARNING (see Chapter 3), and also rewards the parents and helps bonding. Erikson has argued that psychosocial development passes through a series of stages, or DEVELOPMENTAL CRISES, in which the person encounters certain social problems, which must be coped with. Central to the developmental sequence is the concept of EGO IDENTITY, the person's sense of who they are and what they want to be (see also Chapter 17 and Figure 17.1). The first crisis, in the first year of life, is of BASIC TRUST VS. MISTRUST: the infant learns that there are other individuals in the world whom it can trust and who will care for it. The second crisis, between the ages of 1 and 3, is of AUTONOMY VS. SHAME AND DOUBT: the child attempts to become autonomous and if this independent behaviour is encouraged by parents then confidence in its own abilities is fostered. The third crisis, between the ages of 3 and 6, is of INITIATIVE VS. GUILT. The autonomous child starts to play on its own and with other children, and to help in the house: if initiative is encouraged by the parents then the child is rewarded, whereas if the initiative is not encouraged by parents then guilt is fostered. The fourth crisis, between the ages of 7 and 11 years, is of INDUSTRY VS. INFERIORITY: the child attends school, and within the much wider social world of its own peers and its teachers, finds both rewards and punishments for hard work and industry, often involving conflicts between the wishes of parents and teachers (to work hard and succeed), and peers (not to be 'a swot' or a 'creep'). The fifth crisis

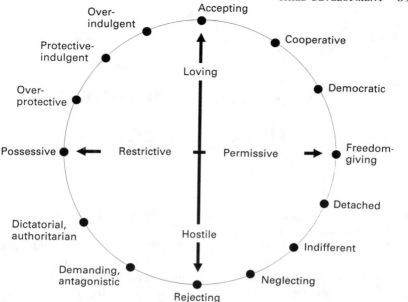

Fig. 10.6 A factorial model of the two major dimensions of parental style shown in rearing children, with some of the many combinations that can result. Adapted from Fischer K W and Lazerson A (1984), *Human Development: from conception through adolescence*, New York, W H Freeman, 409.

occurs in puberty and ADOLESCENCE, the final stage of childhood, and involves IDENTITY VS ROLE-CONFUSION: the child has to cross the social barrier and become a fully-fledged adult, with a sense of personal identity and direction in life, forming new, adult social relationships with parents and siblings, and taking responsibility in the outside world. Passage through all these crises is affected by the PARENTAL STYLE adopted by parents in dealing with their children (Fig. 10.6). Two major dimensions have been identified, of which all combinations are possible: on a LOVE-HOSTILITY SCALE, loving parents are warm, accepting their child's needs, and rewarding their achievements, whereas hostile parents are dissatisfied with their children, and either belittle or ignore them; on a PERMISSIVE-RESTRICTIVE SCALE, permissive parents rarely establish rules for good or bad behaviour, and do not enforce rules that do exist, whereas restrictive parents have strict rules, which are enforced intolerantly. There are many correlations between parenting style and subsequent child development: typical are findings that parents who are aggressive, particularly in their use of punishment, have children who are more aggressive; overly possessive or protective-indulgent parents have children who are dependent; restrictive, more authoritarian parents have children who are independent; and the children of permissive parents are often not achievement oriented.

11

Freud and emotional development

- Freud's ideas are difficult and best understood in the historical order in which they evolved.
- Studies of CONVERSION HYSTERIA, in which FUNCTIONAL SYMPTOMS could be related to psychological trauma in early life, and cured by CATHARSIS, suggested that unpleasant memories could be REPRESSED.
- The UNCONSCIOUS can be understood through the interpretation of dreams, in which the LATENT CONTENT of the unconscious mind is transformed by the DREAM WORK into the harmless but incomprehensible MANIFEST CONTENT.
- Many repressed memories arise from the stages of INFANTILE SEXUALITY, and in the case of patients with conversion hysteria, often take the form of fantasies about sexual seduction.
- The ORAL STAGE of infantile sexuality occurs first, and revolves around the passive pleasures of ingestion of food. FIXATION at this stage can result in an ORAL PERSONALITY.
- The ANAL STAGE, which emphasizes bowel control, is concerned principally with active control and of mastery. Fixation can result in the ANAL RETENTIVE or ANAL EXPULSIVE personalities with their emphases upon control, meanness and parsimony, or on florid generosity.
- Freud's final theoretical innovation was the tripartite division of the mind into the conscious EGO, and the unconscious ID and SUPER-EGO, the latter arising during the PHALLIC STAGE in response to the OEDIPAL CONFLICT.
- The EGO-DEFENCE MECHANISMS, such as DENIAL, REPRESSION and PROJECTION are common responses to threatening information, and are frequently found in patients who are ill.

Sigmund Freud (1856–1939) is still one of the most misunderstood figures in psychology, his ideas often being dismissed out of hand by psychologists and non-psychologists alike without any real knowledge of the theories. However, his influence upon psychology is immense, principally because he tackled the most profound problems of psychology, providing answers within a comprehensive theory, which has important implications for many problems of clinical practice. Freud therefore cannot be ignored in a book like this, although space prohibits any analysis of experimental studies investigating Freud's theories, of psychodynamics in general, or of the POST-FREUDIAN THEORISTS, such as Carl Jung (1875–1961), Alfred Adler (1870–1937), Anna Freud (1895–1982), and Donald Winnicot (1896–1971). If you are interested, there is a vast literature on these topics. The ideas of Melanie Klein (1882–1960) will be described in Chapters 29 and 30.

Freud's creation of PSYCHOANALYSIS is the present concern. My account is expository, encouraging understanding rather than scientific proof; the ideas are interesting enough to merit such an approach. Freud is best understood by following the evolution of his ideas as they developed in response to clinical and theoretical problems.

Freud trained as a doctor in Vienna, researched into the neurology of aphasia and infantile hemiplegia, and introduced cocaine as a local anaesthetic in ophthalmology and ENT surgery, and as a stimulant, to which he became addicted. During his neurology training Freud worked in Paris with the great French neurologist Charcot, who was hypnotizing patients suffering from CONVERSION HYSTERIA, in which psychological problems result in physical symptoms. Typical symptoms are an anaesthesia or paralysis unrelated to the region's actual innervation, as in GLOVE ANAESTHESIA, where the entire hand is anaesthetic up to the wrist, a defect not corresponding to the anatomy of dermatomes or cutaneous nerves. The deficit is FUNCTIONAL (i.e. due to disordered psychological processing) not STRUCTURAL (i.e. disordered anatomy). Charcot did not ask why his patients had these symptoms.

On returning to Vienna, Freud studied similar patients with Breuer, the physiologist (who had discovered the Hering-Breuer reflexes), and who had developed a 'talking cure'. He found that often a symptom could be traced back to a psychological trauma in early life, and that when revealed, strong emotional reactions were produced and the symptom disappeared. This, however, was not a cure because a new symptom subsequently emerged. Freud and Breuer concluded that conversion symptoms were caused by painful, unpleasant memories of traumatic events that had been REPRESSED into the unconscious, so patients no longer remembered them, and that symptoms were alleviated by making the memories conscious, thereby discharging the associated emotions (CATHARSIS).

Freud had the problem that if these memories were repressed, deep in the unconscious, then how could they be found? After trying several methods, such as hypnotism, he developed a technique in which the patient told him their free associations, dreams, slips of the tongue (PARAPRAXES), jokes, etc, and the analyst extracted the useful portions and systematically interpreted them until the repressed memory was found. The best method was the recall of dreams, and in *The interpretation of dreams*, of 1900, Freud called them 'the royal road to the unconscious'. Freud assumed that sleep had a biological (not psychological) function, and despite not knowing this function he argued for the importance of sleep not being disturbed. He also argued that repressed memories are not unique to the hysteric, but are found in everyone to some extent, that they particularly manifested during sleep, and would wake the sleeper if unpleasant or traumatic. Dreams acted as 'guardians of sleep', preventing repressed memories and wishes from breaking through and waking the sleeper. The DREAM WORK neutralized the true or LATENT CONTENT of the memory into the less harmful, non-threatening MANIFEST CONTENT by CENSORSHIP, using CONDENSATION (merging several events) and SYMBOLISM (transforming one event into another). Symbolism can be demonstrated experimentally by dripping water onto a sleeper's forehead and then waking them, when they report dreams of flooding, drowning, of ships at sea in a storm, etc. You yourself may have experienced an alarm clock, or an early morning phone call, being transformed into church bells, or whatever.

Dream censorship does not occur in young children, and wishes and memories may be observed directly, either waking the child from terrifying nightmares, or else being reported as direct fulfilments of wishes from waking life. To Freud an adult dream is the disguised fulfilment of a suppressed or repressed wish or fear.

Dream work, and dream interpretation, are well seen in the dream reported in his journal by the French literary critic, Edward de Goncourt on Bastille Day, July 14, 1883, several years before Freud published his theories:

'I dreamt last night that I was at a party, in white tie. At that party, I saw a woman come in, and recognised her as an actress in a boulevard theatre, but without being able to put a name to her face. She was draped in a scarf, and I noticed only that she was completely naked when she hopped onto the table, where two or three girls were having tea. Then she started to dance, and while she was dancing took steps that showed her private parts armed with the most terrible jaws one could imagine, opening and closing, exposing a set of teeth. The spectacle had no erotic effect on me, except to fill me with an atrocious jealousy, and to give me a ferocious desire to possess myself of her teeth just as I am beginning to lose all my good ones. Where the devil could such an outlandish dream come from? It's got nothing to do with the taking of the Bastille.'

Quoted with permission from Peter Gay (1985), *The Bourgeois Experience: vol 1: Education of the Senses*, New York, Oxford University Press, 198.

This dream has been interpreted in terms of the *vagina dentata*, the toothed vagina (a common anthropological symbol), representing fear both of castration and of declining sexual potency (falling away as Goncourt's own teeth fall out). The occurrence of the dream on Bastille Day is related to its revolutionary associations, of the young French republic rising up to kill the patriarchal power of its father, and invoking the threat of reprisal in the form of castration (a variant of the Oedipal complex — see below). If such an interpretation strikes one as bizarre it can only be emphasized that it is hardly more bizarre than the original dream itself; and clearly *some* explanation is required beyond mere laughter or sniggering.

The final principle from Freud's analysis of dreams was PSYCHOLOGICAL DETERMINISM. This says that all mental events, however strange, have causes that can be discovered. There are no random, trivial, or meaningless psychological events, just failures of understanding.

If we all have repressed memories and wishes, then what are these wishes? Early in his career, Freud had found that most female hysterics reported sexual assaults or seductions as children, often by relatives, the SEDUCTION THEORY of hysteria. Freud later withdrew the theory (in circumstances which are now controversial) when he realized that most such seductions had not actually occurred, but were FANTASIES, or WISH FULFILMENTS. Because of the sexual nature of these fantasies, as well as of the latent content of many dreams, Freud developed his most misunderstood idea, the THEORY OF INFANTILE SEXUALITY, which analyses the development of emotions connected with SENSUAL GRATIFI-CATION, the pleasures and pains derived from sense organs. During a series of stages, different EROTOGENIC ZONES act as the focus for emotional gratification which dominate emotional development, and which, if not properly worked through, result in FIXATION, with effects occurring long into adult life.

To understand infantile sexuality, we must put ourselves into the mind of the infant, forgetting all we know as adults, and see the child's world through its own eyes, and with its knowledge and experience. An infant in the first few months of life has little control of its limbs and only a rudimentary analysis of sensations. The world is a strange, confusing place in which some events cause pleasure or gratification, of which the most consistent is feeding. This ORAL STAGE continues into the second year of life. Pleasure comes from food, and all that goes with it, causing secondary associations, particularly with the mother and the mother's breast, the provider of bounty. This pleasure is entirely *passive*, appearing and disappearing out of control of the infant. The infant feels itself the victim of apparently arbitrary fate, sometimes rewarding, sometimes punishing by its absence, and always beyond real understanding.

By the second and third years of life the child has adequate muscle control and good perception. To the parents the child's development is dominated by an important social behaviour, toilet training, which also dominates emotional development, for the bowels are a source of pleasure in the ANAL STAGE. The bowels are the first internal organ requiring mastery (without which they act reflexly and spontaneously), and such control gives both reward, in the parent's pleasure, and punishment, in the parent's displeasure at lack of control. More importantly the pleasure is *active*, the child realizing *it* controls whether reward is received, and realizing it can punish the parents by defecating inappropriately. The parents' responses to defecation show that faeces are in some sense a valued SYMBOLIC GIFT.

At this stage you may well be repelled by this apparently bizarre turning in Freud's theorizing. Freud realized this and countered it well in his *Introductory lectures on psychoanalysis*, of 1915:

'I know you have been wanting for a long time to interrupt me and exclaim: 'Enough of these atrocities! You tell us that defecating is a source of sexual satisfaction and already exploited in infancy! that faeces is a valuable substance and that the anus is a kind of genital! We don't believe all that but we do understand why paediatricians and educationists have given a wide berth to psychoanalysis and its findings.' No, Gentlemen. ... Why should you not be aware that for a large number of adults, homosexual and heterosexual alike, the anus does really take over the role of the vagina in sexual intercourse? And that there are many people who retain a voluptuous feeling in defecating all through their lives and describe it as being far from small? As regards interest in the act of defecation and enjoyment in watching someone else defaecating, you can get children themselves to confirm the fact when they are a few years older and able to tell you about it. Of course, you must not have systematically intimidated them beforehand, or they will quite understand that they must be silent on the subject.' Freud S. *Introductory Lectures on Psychoanalysis*, Standard edition, vol 16, 315–16.

The fourth and fifth years of life are the PHALLIC STAGE, when the child finds that the penis or clitoris is a source of pleasurable sensations, that the two sexes not the same, and the child is attracted to the parent of the opposite sex. Masturbation occurs, is suppressed by the parents, and responding to social rewards and punishments, is suppressed by the child. The child then enters the long LATENT STAGE, from five to puberty, when there are no apparent erogenous zones. At puberty the child enters the adult GENITAL STAGE, with sexual pleasure manifesting primarily from the genitals, and secondarily through all the senses, intercourse being only part of the broader pleasures of sexuality.

If the stages are not worked through properly then fixations occur, to some extent occurring in all of us. ORAL FIXATION results in undue pleasure from passive consumption, particularly of food, but from any object in the mouth (and many of us chew pencils while writing ...).

ANAL FIXATION produces two separate symptom complexes; the ANAL RETENTIVE personality, emphasizing control, and often meanness and parsimony, and the ANAL EXPULSIVE personality, with its florid emphasis upon giving.

Analysis of the sexual stages of development led Freud to his final contribution, a comprehensive theory of the mind, particularly of the unconscious. The sexual stages are the result of unconscious processes, reflecting the PLEASURE PRINCIPLE of immediate gratification. These pleasures conflict with others which are conscious and controlled largely by social factors acting on the REALITY PRINCIPLE, of deferred gratification for subsequently greater rewards. CONFLICTS between conscious and unconscious processes are a major cause of symptoms.

Freud's theory of the mind has three parts. The ID, the lowest, unconscious, instinctual part of the mind, containing sexual motivations and drives such as hunger, thirst, and sleep, is driven entirely by the pleasure principle of immediate gratification. It is the only mind of the newborn infant. The EGO is the conscious mind, which splits off from the id in the first months of life, is rational and accepts the reality principle that pleasures must sometimes be deferred. The SUPER-EGO, also unconscious, and formed during the phallic stage, acts as morality or conscience. It arises from what Freud called the OEDIPAL CONFLICT, named after the character in Sophocles' tragedy *Oedipus Rex*, who inadvertently killed his father and married his mother. Freud said the phallic stage pushes the child towards the parent of opposite sex, resulting in family conflict and sexual jealousy. The conflict is resolved by the developing super-ego, which responds to social and moral pressures to restrain the wishes and desires of ego and id. Unsuccessful Oedipal resolution results in undue IDENTIFICATION with one parent.

Freud's theory of the mind has the ego as the only conscious part (the 'I', the internal voice which seems to be 'us', ourselves). It is bombarded from below by the animal drives of the id, and from above by the moral restraints of the super-ego. The ego is protected from these unconscious demands, which often conflict with one another and with the ego, by the several-fold EGO DEFENCE MECHANISMS, whose importance transcends specifically Freudian theory, and apply to any situation in which ego is threatened. Table 11.1 lists the mechanisms and shows how they might appear in a patient with a possible diagnosis of cancer. All doctors should look out for these mechanisms (both in themselves and other doctors as well as in patients) and then should ask about the *real* underlying problems.

In this necessarily abbreviated account of a major western thinker, you may have found it difficult to accept many of the ideas. At a personal level, the processes cannot possibly seem to apply to you or to the people around you. Freud responded to such criticism by pointing out in psychoanalytical therapy the revelation of unconscious

Table 11.1

The ego defence mechanisms, with examples of their applications in a patient with malignant disease.

– – – – – – – DEFENCE MECHANISM – – – – – – –   – – – – – – EXAMPLE – – – – –

Altering the facts

DENIAL	Pretend the facts are wrong	"No, I can't feel a lump"
REPRESSION	Forget the facts	"No, no complaints"
ISOLATION	Accept the facts, but deny the feelings	"Oh, only a small lump of no importance"

Altering the feelings

PROJECTION	Attribute own feelings to others	"My husband is so worried about it"
REACTION-FORMATION	Excessive feelings of the opposite sort	"I've never felt calmer and more relaxed"
SUBLIMATION	Liberating unacceptable feelings through socially acceptable actions	e.g. sudden, excessive and atypical work for charity
DISPLACEMENT	Transfer emotions from one person to another	"The nurse [i.e. you, the doctor] is so unsympathetic"

Altering the interpretation

REGRESSION	Retreat to a previous stage of development	"I'm in your hands completely, doctor"
INTELLECTUALIZATION	Analyse problem in general, rather than in relation to you specifically	"What is the quality of the scientific evidence that this treatment is necessary?"
RATIONALIZATION	Explain the serious in terms of the trivial or mundane	"I always tend to lose some weight during the summer"

processes always produced RESISTANCE and emotion, and that meant one was nearing an essential truth. On intellectual grounds the theories are also threatening, and we can now see Freud's theory as the third great revolution in western man's thought about human nature; the Copernican revolution said man was not the centre of the universe; the Darwinian revolution said man was not different from other animals; and the Freudian revolution said the mind of man was not his own, being influenced by uncontrollable unconscious processes. Such ideas are threatening and denial is tempting. Nevertheless, Freud's theories provide insight into a range of psychological phenomena needing explanation, and which form problems for many patients; how it does that we will see in Chapters 28, 29 and 30.

12

Attitudes

- ATTITUDES have EVALUATIVE, AFFECTIVE and CONATIVE components, and must be distinguished from OPINIONS, VALUES, BELIEFS, INTENTIONS and BEHAVIOURS.
- STEREOTYPES are erroneous beliefs about the world, which sometimes contain a kernel of distorted truth.
- Attitudes can be measured by questionnaire, using LIKERT SCALES, with a number of alternative answers which cover the range of feelings.
- In the THEORY OF REASONED ACTION behaviours depend upon intentions, which are themselves determined by attitudes and by NORMATIVE BELIEFS.
- Attitudes can be formed by classical conditioning, or by MERE EXPOSURE, but more often are influenced, in the INFORMATION-PROCESSING MODEL OF ATTITUDE CHANGE, by PERSUASIVE MESSAGES.
- COGNITIVE DISSONANCE, which occurs when attitudes and behaviour are inconsistent, is unpleasant and results in a change in either attitude or behaviour.

People differ not only in their personality, which is relatively fixed over long periods of time, and in their emotions, which are transitory, but also in their attitudes, which do change but over a fairly slow time period, from days to weeks to years. Attitudes and beliefs underlie many major life decisions, as in a patient's decision to visit (or not visit) a doctor, to take treatments, to change to a healthier life-style, etc., and they also underlie many decisions by *doctors* to use treatments or to abandon old ones, to use particular treatments for particular patients, etc. Important decisions are often necessarily based on incomplete information, and attitudes help to rationalize and justify our decisions.

ATTITUDES must be distinguished from OPINIONS, BELIEFS, VALUES and INTENTIONS, although sometimes attitude is also used to describe the whole complex of terms (as in the title of this chapter). One definition of attitude is as follows:

'A relatively enduring cluster of feelings, emotions and behaviours relating to persons, objects and issues, which constitute a mental 'state of readiness', and which are derived and organized from experience.'

An attitude is therefore related *to* a particular behaviour, and involves an EVALUATION of the behaviour as good or bad in terms of some ultimate criterion. Thus one might have an attitude that 'People should be discouraged from smoking cigarettes'. This attitude might exist because one has BELIEFS (i.e. knowledge or facts about the world), which say that 'Cigarettes lead to a premature death', and a set of VALUES (i.e. ultimate goals of life), which say that people should live healthy lives because lives should be lived to the full. Having an attitude that people should be discouraged from smoking does not, of course, perfectly predict behaviour; I may hold such an attitude and be willing to tell people not to smoke in my office, or to ask them to stop smoking in No Smoking compartments of trains, but still not be willing to destroy cigarette advertisements or commit arson on tobacconist shops. For each actual BEHAVIOUR I also have an INTENTION as to whether or not to perform it. Intentions are related to attitudes, but are also influenced by NORMATIVE BELIEFS, which are a set of social beliefs concerning how other people think about the behaviour; or rather, what we *think* other people think about the behaviour. Thus if a stranger lights a cigarette in a railway No Smoking compartment I am more likely to protest if my travelling companions are four fellow doctors than if they are strangers. My attitude remains the same, but its relation to actual behaviour has been altered by how I perceive the normative beliefs of my companions. There is therefore a long chain between values and the behaviours derived from them. The chain is fragile and easily broken, particularly by social pressure. Figure 12.1 summarizes this model which is based on Fishbein's THEORY OF REASONED ACTION, although other models also exist.

Attitudes do not only have an EVALUATIVE dimension, and a CONATIVE or behavioural dimension, they also have an AFFECTIVE or emotional component, so that we may feel angry, happy or sad according to whether or not our attitudes are consistent with the events of the world, and it is this which accounts for much of the importance of attitudes. I might therefore not only *think* that people should be discouraged from smoking, but also *feel* angry that they are not. In this way mere OPINIONS are distinguished from attitudes by the absence of conative or affective components; so that, if asked 'Do you think that more money should be spent on research into particle physics?', you may have an opinion about it (Yes or No), but will probably not have any strong, passionate feelings.

Why do we have attitudes? The world is a complex place, in which decisions continually need to be made and frequently sufficient information is not available, or we do not have time to allow us to obtain such information in order to make a fully informed, rational judgement. In such cases, which can be about everyday events, as well as about more complex MORAL or ETHICAL judgements, attitudes act as a pre-packaged, off-the-peg set of behaviours which we have

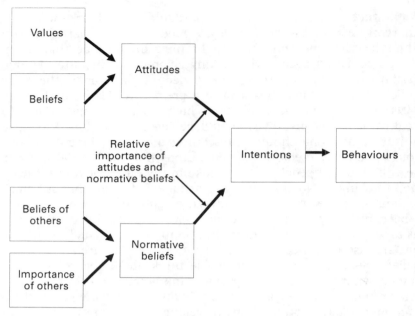

Fig. 12.1 A summary of the Theory of Reasoned Action. Adapted from Ajzen I and Fishbein M (1980), *Understanding attitudes and predicting social behaviour*, New Jersey, Prentice-Hall.

used in previous situations and on which we can rely to some extent. They are therefore convenient and efficient, although no one would claim that they are perfectly reliable.

A variant on the attitude is the STEREOTYPE, which is an erroneous pseudo-factual belief about the world, which when combined with particular values necessitates particular attitudes. Stereotypes can distort the average position — 'Psychiatrists are very left-wing'; and they may reduce the variance — '*All* psychiatrists are very left-wing'. As a matter of empirical fact, psychiatrists are indeed more likely to vote Labour than are surgeons, but this neither justifies describing them as *very* left-wing, nor as assuming that they are *all* left-wing; indeed many psychiatrists vote Conservative. But this example also reveals another feature of stereotypes, that at their heart they often contain a kernel of statistical truth, which has been distorted and exaggerated. Like attitudes, stereotypes are useful in creating a simplified world, which allows action in the absence of better information.

The measurement of attitudes is easily and straightforwardly carried out by questionnaires, although the apparent simplicity of their construction often belies problems encountered in measuring precisely what is intended. Typically, attitude questionnaires like LIKERT SCALES in which are indicated the strength of an attitude using a 5- or 7-point scale, ranging from 'Strongly in favour...' to 'Strongly opposed...'. Table 12.1 shows the attitudes to abortion in applicants to medical school, assessed on a four-point scale.

Normative beliefs can be assessed by a similar method but asking individuals to complete questions that start 'Most people who are important to me think that...', rather than 'I think that...'. And beliefs can be assessed by questions starting 'It is true that...'.

Attitudes do not just exist, but must have come from somewhere, and since, as social phenomena, it is inconceivable that they are genetic, they must be acquired by learning. And once formed they can also be changed. If health education is to be successful, that process of change must be understood.

Attitudes can be learned by classical conditioning, simple association inducing an attitude. The object (say, a packet of cigarettes or the brand name) is the conditioned stimulus (CS), which is repeatedly paired with an unconditioned stimulus (US), such as a picture of a racing car, which induces an unconditioned response (UR) of excitement, interest or a generally positive feeling, perhaps by secondary conditioning. Eventually the CS, the cigarettes, produce a similar response, the conditioned response (CR). As legislation restricts cigarette advertising so such sophisticated advertising is more common; indeed some adverts are now so cryptic that the pleasure of solving the problem is itself the UR to the CS.

Attitudes can also be changed by MERE EXPOSURE. Repeated presentations of a stimulus make it preferred when a choice is allowed — a psychological process also exploited by cigarette manufacturers who emblazon logos or motifs on the clothes and equipment of sports stars.

Nevertheless, most attitudes are not formed by simple learning, but result from more complex cognitive analysis. People are continually receiving MESSAGES on aspects of the world about which we have attitudes. Whether or not these messages change our attitudes depends on several things; the CONTENT of the message — does it seem reasonable, well-argued, consistent with the known facts? the SENDER of the message — is it a source which we usually trust (such as a particular friend or our regular newspaper) or one which we distrust (a particularly suspect politician or an advertiser), so that we reject the content entirely as unreliable? and is it CONSISTENT with our current attitudes — and if not, but is a well-reasoned message from a source we trust, what do we do? This is the INFORMATION-PROCESSING MODEL of attitude change; like an idealistic mental Parliament we listen to debate, assess the worth of arguments, and change our attitudes accordingly. Sometimes however change does not occur when it should; individuals with particularly strong, polarized political attitudes may deny the validity of all messages thereby avoiding the need for change. Alternatively, if particularly enamoured with the sender of a message, huge changes can occur so that attitudes are consistent with those of the sender.

Table 12.1

The attitudes to abortion of 325 applicants to St Mary's Hospital Medical School in 1981, who indicated their feelings using a four-point response scale. In 1986, another 1937 applicants were asked three of the questions, and the percentage replies are indicated in brackets, to show the remarkable consistency over a five-year period. The items were originally asked in random order, but here have been rearranged in order from those for which most are in favour to those for which most are opposed.

"In which of the following situations in which an abortion has been requested would you think that it should be performed?"

	Definitely yes	Probably yes	Probably no	Definitely no
A woman with congenital heart disease who is unlikely to survive the rigours of childbirth.	76%	20%	2%	2%
A 13-year old girl who has been raped.	75% (74%)	19% (19%)	3% (4%)	3% (4%)
A 25-year old woman who has been raped.	59%	28%	9%	4%
A woman known to be definitely bearing a fetus with spina bifida.	49% (44%)	38% (38%)	7% (11%)	5% (8%)
A woman who might have had German measles earlier in pregnancy.	20%	47%	24%	9%
A 38-year old mother of six.	19%	39%	28%	14%
An unmarried woman who is pregnant as a result of failed contraception.	16%	33%	33%	18%
A woman who has failed to use any form of contraception.	5% (6%)	23% (24%)	38% (39%)	34% (31%)

Inconsistencies between attitudes and behaviours have provoked much research, especially into the problem of COGNITIVE DISSONANCE, in which two separate attitudes or beliefs are held, each mutually inconsistent with the other. Dissonance is unpleasant and induces change in order to reduce the tension. A time-worn but nonetheless pertinent example from Leon Festinger, the founder of COGNITIVE DISSONANCE THEORY, considers a person who smokes cigarettes but knows that cigarettes cause cancer. The statement 'I smoke cigarettes' is inconsistent with the statement 'Smoking is dangerous to health'. There are many ways to reduce the dissonance: to deny the evidence ('there is no proper *experimental* evidence in man, only correlations' or 'My grandfather smoked until he was 95 and was then run over by a bus'); to deny that one's own form of smoking is dangerous ('I only smoke 10 a day' or 'I smoke filter cigarettes'); to invoke social support ('All my friends smoke so it can't be very dangerous'); or to deny the fundamental values involved ('I'd rather have a short pleasurable life than a long miserable one'); finally, smoking may be used as a positive virtue, flaunting the machismo, devil-may-care aspects ('The dangers don't worry me, I'm man enough to cope with them'). In all such cases, defence mechanisms (see Chapter 11) have been used to reduce dissonance. From such a perspective man appears not to be a ration*al* animal but a ration*alizing* animal.

Cognitive dissonance theory has stimulated a series of ingenious experiments to test its predictions. Some experiments study FORCED COMPLIANCE, in which a person behaves inconsistently with their attitudes (as when a teenager smokes to impress friends, even though feeling it to be wrong). In the laboratory, subjects have acted as subjects in a long, tedious and very boring psychological experiment. Dissonance is then induced by asking the subjects to tell the next group of subjects that the experiment was very interesting. Subjects were paid $1 or $20 for taking part. As part of the debriefing, subjects were asked how interesting they found the experiment. Surprisingly, those paid $1 rated the experiment as far more interesting than those paid $20. The group paid $20 had no cognitive dissonance; they had done a boring experiment, had lied about it, and had been paid well, which justified their attitude and they could therefore truthfully say the experiment was not enjoyable. However, the $1 subjects were in a different situation; they had wasted a lot of time on a tedious experiment, had lied, and had been paid a paltry one dollar, which hardly justified their effort. Their only way of reducing the dissonance between effort and reward was to claim the experiment *was* actually interesting, thereby justifying their exertions. Many a doctor looking back on the long hours of learning the endless facts of anatomy or biochemistry, or contemplating the long sleepless hours of the pre-registration year, also justifies it retrospectively by arguing for its actual interest or real utility; and once more cognitive dissonance has altered attitudes.

13

Personal construct theory

- Personal construct theory is a comprehensive theory of human action and perceptions, which takes as its central metaphor that man is a scientist, collecting data about the world, and forming and re-forming hypotheses about the nature of the world.
- The repertory grid is both an autonomous measurement instrument and an integral part of personal construct theory. It allows subjects to evaluate systematically a set of ELEMENTS in relation to a set of BIPOLAR CONSTRUCTS.
- Analysis of a repertory grid, by techniques such as cluster analysis, allows the construction of a pyschological map which shows the relationship between the various elements and constructs used by the subject.
- Repeated use of repertory grid allows assessment of change, as might occur in therapy.
- Personal construct theory is not only a cognitive theory, describing ways in which the world is perceived, but is also a theory of emotions, which arise when change occurs or is imposed upon the construct system.

Most psychological tests of personality inevitably impose upon the subject the preferences and prejudices of the creator of the test. As a result not only the person taking the test, but also the person administering it, feel the test has missed out the things 'really' defining the person. Could we, for instance, distinguish our friends and relations solely from their standardized extraversion and neuroticism scores? The essence of personality, why Bill is Bill and not Ben, is bypassed by conventional tests. That is not surprising, for the problem of assessing that essence is that it differs in all of us, all having had different experiences, and hence viewing the world in different ways; not a situation that encourages uniformity of testing. Not all psychologists suffer from this problem. Psychoanalysts view each person as a separate individual, assessing their personality by detailed interviews over months or years. But that is hardly a viable alternative to questionnaires for a busy practitioner wanting an assessment of a patient, and it is almost impossible to do statistical analysis of the material from several hundred hours of psychoanalytic sessions.

One method of steering between the Scylla of the standardized questionnaire and the Charybdis of the long, unstructured psychoanalytic interview, which will allow sophisticated and structured testing of an individual, tailored to their special needs and problems, along with formal statistical testing when required is REPERTORY GRID TECHNIQUE.

The repertory grid was invented by the American psychologist George Kelly (1906–1966) as a part of his THEORY OF PERSONAL CONSTRUCTS. Although an integral part of Kelly's theoretical framework, the grid may also be used as an independent, generalized method of assessment. But it is best described along with Kelly's theory.

Kelly saw people as scientists trying to *understand* their world, to *predict* that world, and *control* it. Some people though are bad scientists, produce bad theories, and make wrong predictions. Science, good or bad, is based upon data, which are either valid or invalid. The data of the 'human scientist' are the events occurring around us, particularly people and their social interactions. Kelly accepted, as do philosophers of science such as Popper (see Chapter 5), that no observation is theory-free. We see the world through the spectacles of our prior theories as to how it is organized, and such theories can distort our image of the world. Like the botanist or any other natural historian we also simplify observations by dividing things, and people, into two groups: 'good' or 'bad', 'lucky' or 'unlucky'. Although the world is not of course really just black and white, but a thousand shades of grey, Kelly argued it is convenient, and perhaps psychologically *necessary*, to use CONSTRUCTS which are BIPOLAR.

Not only do individuals have different bipolar constructs, they also differ in *what* and to *whom* they apply those constructs, the combination defining our personalities. In grid technique the things to which constructs are applied are called ELEMENTS. Individuals may differ not only in their constructs but in the elements to which they apply them. Constructs also differ in their inter-relationships; 'good' and 'friendly' may be synonymous to one person, whilst almost independent or orthogonal to another.

Kelly's theory has strictly organized postulates, assumptions and corollaries, so that its theoretical basis is made clear. Here we consider just the FUNDAMENTAL POSTULATE, from which the remaining theory is derived: 'A person's processes are psychologically channelled by the ways in which they anticipate events'. That is, its purpose is *anticipation*, predicting events in the world, and the predictions are special to each particular *person*, the predictions affecting everything else the person does; individuals therefore do not have an infinite repertoire of possible behaviours, but run within certain channels, dependent upon their past, and affecting their future. The channels within which an individual runs are the CONSTRUCT SYSTEM, which differs between individuals, and which is ORGANIZED hierarchically; some constructs, ·the SUPER-ORDINATE CONSTRUCTS, being at the top, and implying the truth or falsity of others below them. The constructs not only *are* the individual's personality in some strict sense, but also are chosen by the individual themself, as being those dichotomies which are most useful *for that person* to predict events in *their world*. Note at this point that the theory is REFLEXIC in that it entails its own origins (in a way that no other psychological theories do: Skinnerian learning theory was not formed in Skinner's mind due to stimulus-response contingencies, and Freudian theory did not develop in Freud's mind due to his own infantile sexual experiences, but Kelly's theory did develop out of his own attempts to construct a model of the world which predicted behaviour). Likewise individuals also build their own future construct systems from their present systems. Construct systems are not fixed, but change continually in response to experience, according to whether particular predictions are useful or wrong, in which case the constructs from which they derive are INVALIDATED.

A construct system is of limited size with a finite number of dichotomous constructs (for it could hardly be infinite). The nature of these constructs depends upon the needs and interests of the particular person. To a cook the construct 'hot-cold' may be more useful in construing saucepans than the construct 'brightly coloured-dull', whereas to an internal designer the converse might be the case. Constructs can only be applied to a limited range of events, their RANGE OF CONVENIENCE. Some constructs, such as 'good-bad' are highly PERMEABLE, applying to many objects, whereas others, such as 'fluorescent-incandescent' are IMPERMEABLE, being really only useful when applied to different types of light-bulb. The range of convenience of the CORE CONSTRUCTS includes the person as they see themself; thus I might see myself as good rather than bad, but neither fluorescent nor incandescent.

Constructs can be related to one another. I might think that 'fluorescent' means 'economical' and hence 'good' (and of course then 'incandescent' must mean 'not economical' and therefore 'bad'). Such inter-relationships need not be strictly logical, instead displaying only 'psycho-logic'; so that I might also believe that 'gives to charity-does not give to charity' implies 'generous-mean' and hence 'not economical-economical', which I construe as 'good-bad'. But note that now 'economical' implies 'bad' whereas earlier, with respect to light-bulbs it implied 'good', a logical but not a psychological inconsistency.

THE CONSTRUCTION OF A REPERTORY GRID

A repertory grid systematically assesses the relationships between a set of CONSTRUCTS and a set of ELEMENTS (things, objects, ideas, or people). The technique has many variations, and the particular form depends upon the problem and on the ingenuity of the investigator. Figure 13.1 shows a small, easily comprehensible grid elicited from an adolescent who was describing the books they had read recently, and what they thought about them. In clinical practice the repertory grid is most frequently used for understanding human relationships; Figure 13.2 shows a grid discussed by Kelly, which assessed the perception of people.

The first step is the choice of elements. In Figure 13.2, Kelly has strictly delineated certain choices (self, mother, father, etc.), but allowed some freedom in choosing others (e.g. number 7, pal, 'your closest present friend of the same sex as yourself', or 14, 'the teacher who influenced you most when you were in your teens'), and others are hypothetical or idealized (e.g. 19 'the person known to you personally who appears to meet the highest ethical standards'). The choice of elements could also be broadened, by asking the subject to add other important or relevant people. The important thing is that all the elements should *matter* to the subject.

In the second stage the constructs are elicited. Kelly recommends selecting triplets of elements, and asking in what way any two of the elements differ from the third. The choice of three elements may be random, or it may be systematic, as in Kelly's grid, so that relationships of interest are not omitted. In Figure 13.2, the elements included in triplets are shown in circles. Thus construct 1 compared a successful person, a happy person, and an ethical person. The subject thought that the successful and happy person were alike because they didn't believe in God (the EMERGENT POLE of the construct, indicated by a cross inside the circle) and are contrasted with the ethical person who does believe in God (the IMPLICIT POLE, indicated by the open circle). The choice and labelling of emergent and implicit poles can give valuable information about the subject's feelings. Although some of the constructs in Figure 13.2 have identical names, they are derived from different triplets, and are used in somewhat different ways, and illustrate the poverty of words to describe subtle distinctions which the subject makes with little difficulty.

The repertory *grid* derives its name from the third stage in which each element is systematically construed on each construct, a tick indicating elements to which the emergent pole of the construct applies (and by implication blank cells refer to the construct's implicit pole, although an additional symbol can indicate elements outside a construct's range of convenience).

A repertory grid can be interpreted at several levels. The simplest is 'eye-balling', just looking for relationships. Thus in Figure 13.2 it is apparent that the subject is religious (construct 1), but that rejecting, threatening but also successful and happy people (including his ex-flame) do *not* believe in God, implying a source of conflict and ambivalence between the ethical virtues of religion and worldly

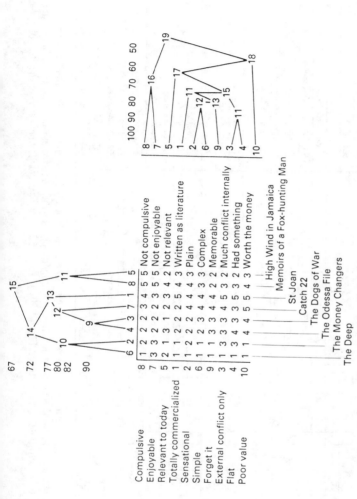

Fig. 13.1 A simple repertory grid in which an adolescent gave constructs of a number of books that they had read. The elements (the books) are arranged along the bottom, and the constructs are arranged down the sides of the table. A score of 1 indicates that the left-hand pole of the construct applied, and a score of 5 that the right-hand pole applied, with scores of 2, 3 and 4 indicating intermediate positions. At the top is shown a cluster analysis of the structure underlying the elements, the tree indicating the degree of similarity of the elements (so that 'The Dogs of War' and 'The Odessa File' are seen as very similar, whereas 'The Deep' and 'Memoirs of a Fox-hunting man' are seen as very different). The figure on the right hand side shows a similar analysis of construct inter-relationships, with constructs such as 'External vs internal conflict' and 'Flat vs had something' being highly related, and constructs such as 'compulsive vs not compulsive' and 'poor value vs worth the money' being almost unrelated. Reproduced with permission of authors and publishers from Pope M L and Keen T R (1984), *Personal Construct Psychology in Education*. London, Academic Press, 59.

CONSTRUCTS

SORT NO.	EMERGENT POLE	IMPLICIT POLE
1	Don't believe in God	Very religious
2	Same sort of education	Complete different education
3	Not athletic	Athletic
4	Both girls	A boy
5	Parents	Ideas different
6	Understand me better	Don't understand at all
7	Teach the right thing	Teach the wrong thing
8	Achieved a lot	Hasn't achieved a lot
9	Higher education	No education
10	Don't like other people	Like other people
11	More religious	Not religious
12	Believe in higher education	Not believing in too much education
13	More sociable	Not sociable
14	Both girls	Not girls
15	Both girls	Not girls
16	Both have high morals	Low morals
17	Think alike	Think differently
18	Same age	Different ages
19	Believe the same about me	Believe differently about me
20	Both friends	Not friends
21	More understanding	Less understanding
22	Both appreciate music	Don't understand music

Elements:

1 Self · 2 Mother · 3 Father · 4 Brother · 5 Sister · 6 Spouse · 7 Ex-flame · 8 Pal · 9 Ex-pal · 10 Rejecting person · 11 Pitied person · 12 Threatening person · 13 Attractive person · 14 Accepted teacher · 15 Rejected teacher · 16 Boss · 17 Successful person · 18 Happy person · 19 Ethical person

Fig. 13.2 An illustrative repertory grid of interpersonal relationships. Crosses in circles indicate the two elements forming the emergent pole of each construct and open circles indicate the element forming the implicit pole of the construct. Ticks indicate other elements which are also assessed as being at the emergent pole of a construct. From Kelly G A (1955), *The psychology of personal constructs*, vol 1, New York, WW Norton, 270.

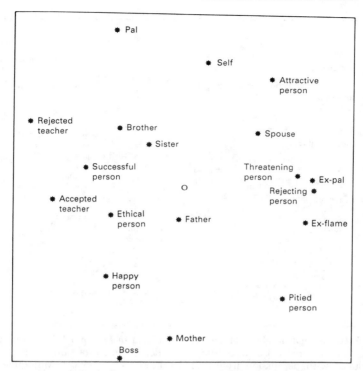

Fig. 13.3 Statistical analysis of the repertory grid of Figure 13.2 to illustrate the positions of the elements on the two principal dimensions underlying the grid. Reproduced with permission from van der Kloot W A (1981), Multidimensional scaling of repertory grid responses, in Bonarius H, Holland R and Rosenberg S, *Personal Construct Psychology: Recent advances in theory and practice*, London, MacMillan, 177–86.

success. Looking down the columns one can systematically compare individuals. The subject sees himself as more like his father than his mother (5 differences in constructs versus 9), and more similar to his spouse (6 differences) than to his ex-flame (11 differences). The spouse is perceived as more similar to the subject's mother (9 differences) than was the ex-flame (12 differences), and so on. And a similar analysis can be carried out across the rows. Thus having high morals (row 16) is generally associated with being more religious (row 11), although the subject's brother and the spouse are exceptions to that, perhaps deserving further exploration.

More systematic, statistical analysis compares the relationships between all pairs of elements, or all pairs of constructs. Figure 13.3 and Figure 13.4 show the two principal dimensions resulting from cluster analyses. Figure 13.3 shows the positions of the individual elements on these two dimensions, and Figure 13.4 shows the

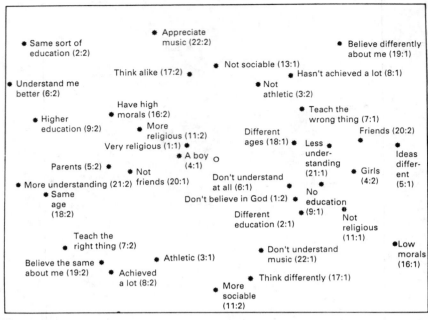

Fig. 13.4 Statistical analysis of the repertory grid of Figure 13.2 to illustrate the positions of the construct poles on the two principal dimensions underlying the grid. Reproduced with permission from van der Kloot W A (1981), Multidimensional scaling of repertory grid responses, in Bonarius H, Holland R and Rosenberg S, *Personal Construct Psychology: Recent advances in theory and practice*, London, MacMillan, 177–86.

positions of the construct poles on the two dimensions. The horizontal dimension is an evaluative dimension, the left hand end being evaluated positively and the right hand negatively. Teachers are thought of highly, and the ex-flame is disliked intensely. Figure 13.4 shows that highly evaluated means being educated and understanding, whereas poorly evaluated means having different ideas to the patient, being female, and being uneducated. The vertical dimension assesses personal or social proximity, those at the top being close and those at the bottom being distant. Figure 13.3 confirms that the patient feels closer to his mother than to his father, who is very distant; the ex-flame is more distant than the spouse. Being close to the patient means liking music, being religious, not being athletic and not being very sociable (Figure 13.4). This mathematical analysis therefore produces a detailed psychological map of the patient's perceptions of those around him.

An important statistical property of factor analysis, which will be used in Chapters 28, 29 and 30, is an assessment of the number of statistically independent dimensions which are needed to explain the relationships between constructs. Figure 13.2 can be well summarized by just two construct dimensions, as is seen in Figures 13.3 and 13.4. More complex data may require three, four or more dimensions.

Repertory grid analysis can give a sophisticated description of how a person sees the world, and of what they think is important in that world. It can be applied to almost any topic (social relationships, subjects in a school curriculum, national stereotypes, medical specialities, wines, etc.), and can be applied in different ways. Elements can be RANKED in importance on each construct, or RATED on each construct (say, on a 7-point scale). The same grid can be repeated on different occasions to assess change, as in therapy. Figure 13.5 shows the elements of an obese patient before and after treatment. Component 1 is a measure of social adjustment. Before weight loss the patient sees herself as poorly adjusted, and after treatment as well adjusted. The position of 'self when overweight' varies in relation to weight (Fig. 13.6), and improves only after weight has begun to be lost, and then deteriorates before weight is put on again, suggesting that self-perception is more resistant to change than is weight itself. In IMPGRIDS, the hierarchical relationships between contrasts are assessed by a grid indicating whether constructs imply the truth or falsity of other constructs (e.g. does 'religious-irreligious' imply 'good-bad' or vice-versa, for implications need not be symmetric). Finally 'duo grids' are used in marital therapy, couples completing grids individually and then together, so that the relative dominance of each partner's views can be assessed. For research purposes many individuals may complete grids with identical elements and constructs.

EMOTION AND CONSTRUCT CHANGE

Personal constructs are dynamic structures, changing continually as constructs are validated (and hence strengthened), or invalidated (and hence rejected). Change also occurs in the relationships between constructs, so that perhaps after a bad experience 'blonde' is no longer construed as parallel to 'fun'. Kelly argues that emotion occurs when constructs change, different emotions resulting from the nature of the change, its origin, and the constructs affected.

ANXIETY is the consequence of recognizing that events are occurring which are outside the range of convenience of the construct system. Events are therefore unknown in their consequences, and their results are beyond prediction.

HOSTILITY occurs when a person perceives that the predictions of their construct system have failed, but they still try to validate the system by forcing other people or events to behave in a manner more consistent with the system.

THREAT and FEAR occur in response to externally imposed changes of the *core* construct system, THREAT occurring when a person becomes

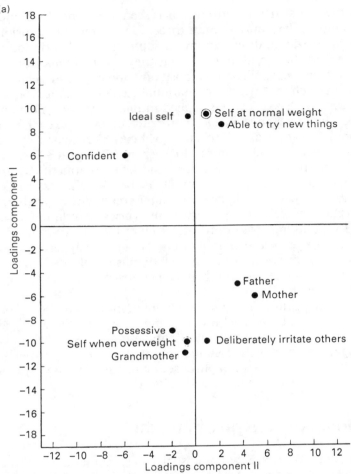

Fig. 13.5 An example of the change in relationship between the elements and constructs of a repertory grid in an obese woman *a*) at the start of treatment and *b*) after five months of treatment. The first principal component (the vertical axis) is a measure of the patient's social adjustment. Reproduced from Bannister D and Fransella F (1971), *Inquiring Man: the psychology of personal constructs*, Penguin.

aware that some external agency is forcing a change in their construct system, and FEAR occurring when incidental changes, usually without obvious cause and hence inherently unpredictable, force a change in core constructs.

GUILT, SHAME and EMBARRASSMENT relate to the perception of self in the core constructs, GUILT occurring when we become aware that our behaviours are not consistent with our own construction of ourself, SHAME when we realize that our behaviour is inconsistent with someone

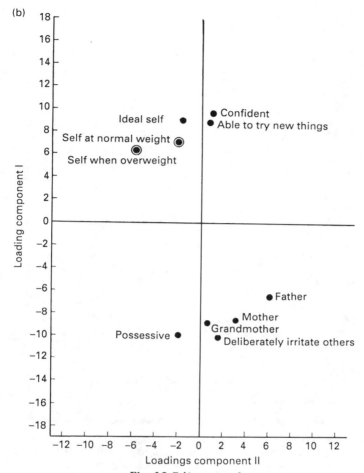

Fig. 13.5 *b) continued*

else's construction of us, and EMBARRASSMENT being the anticipation of another's perception of us in ways inconsistent with our own core constructs.

Positive emotions, which should not be forgotten, occur when the construct system is changed to make it more effective, to reflect further understanding, wider knowledge, or additional validation. SELF-CONFIDENCE and PRIDE reflect an awareness of the validation of our core constructs, and HUMOUR occurs when we realize that our construct system has several interpretations of the same event, some more plausible than others. LOVE is perhaps an awareness of a concordance between our own construct system and that of another person, with similar ideals, intentions and evaluations.

Personal construct theory and the repertory grid technique therefore provide powerful, general methods of understanding a broad range

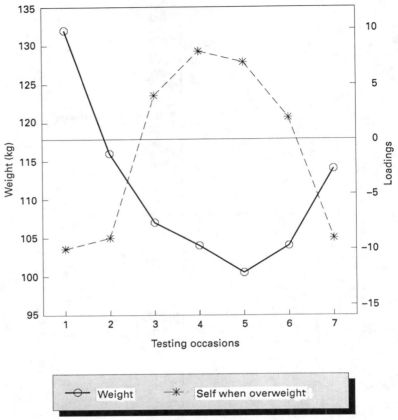

Fig. 13.6 For the same patient as Fig. 13.5, showing the position of the element 'self when overweight' (right-hand axis) in relation to changes in actual weight (left-hand axis) during the course of treatment. Adapted from Bannister D and Fransella F (1971) *Inquiring Man: the psychology of personal constructs*, Penguin.

of psychological processes, and are also readily implemented within the context of ordinary clinical practice, both for assessment of individual patients and as a research tool. In Chapters 28, 29 and 30 we will see how personal construct theory can be applied to understanding neurosis, depression and schizophrenia.

14

Group processes

- Man is a SOCIAL ANIMAL; people who are not members of SOCIAL NETWORKS show an increased mortality.
- ALTRUISTIC or HELPING BEHAVIOUR depends upon the ATTRIBUTIONS that are made for the person needing help; help being given if the causes are felt to be EXTERNAL rather than INTERNAL.
- The FUNDAMENTAL ERROR OF ATTRIBUTION is that individuals attribute their own behaviour to external causes whereas observers attribute it to internal causes.
- SELF-ATTRIBUTION is used to understand our own behaviour when it contradicts that of others around us, as in the ASCH EXPERIMENT.
- Groups differ in their purpose according to whether their goals are OPEN-ENDED or SPECIFIC, and INTRINSIC or EXTRINSIC, but nonetheless usually go through a similar evolutionary sequence of FORMING, STORMING, NORMING and PERFORMING.
- Groups sometimes have a single LEADER, but will often have both a TASK SPECIALIST and a SOCIO-EMOTIONAL SPECIALIST, who perform different ROLES.

Man, like most primates, is a SOCIAL ANIMAL, continually interacting with other individuals. An extensive social group provides SOCIAL SUPPORT, from a SOCIAL NETWORK. Epidemiological studies find that individuals with least social support have a higher mortality than those who are well connected within a network (Fig. 14.1), partly because social isolation is stressful, and partly because supportive, caring relationships provide informal psychotherapy for minor psychopathology and encourage healthier behaviours such as less drinking or smoking.

As groups get larger so the complexity of their interactions increases until finally they are the province not of psychology but of SOCIOLOGY. Small groups do however have particular psychological features of their own, and since they are very common in the social world, such as teams, committees, juries, hospital wards, general practices, etc. we must consider them.

Groups differ in their effects according to their size. Groups of two, or DYADS, are the smallest possible, and immediately show an important problem: should the individuals cooperate, and if so, how to decide if

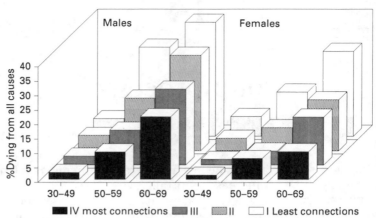

Fig. 14.1 Mortality during a nine-year period in relation to the age, sex and size of an individual's social network, those with most connections having large, complex networks, and those with least connections having few individuals within their social network. Adapted from Berkman L S and Syme S L (1979), Social networks, host resistance and mortality: a nine-year follow-up study of Alameda County residents, *Am J Epidemiol*, **109**, 186–204.

it is worthwhile? A much studied situation is the PRISONER'S DILEMMA game.

You and your accomplice in a serious crime have been arrested and are in separate cells. Each is told that if neither confesses then each will receive a three year sentence on minor charges. However, if you confess and turn Queen's evidence then you will only receive a 1 year sentence while your accomplice will get 20 years. The twist is that the same option is also given to your accomplice, and if you both confess then neither party will need to be Queen's evidence, although in mitigation for confessing you will only receive eight year sentences. What do you do, given that you cannot communicate with your accomplice? The dilemma is that your best outcome, to confess, is only best if your accomplice does *not* confess. Should your accomplice think of confessing then the *joint* best strategy is for neither to confess, when each receives a three year sentence. However, since you cannot rely on your partner cooperating (because if certain that you will *not* confess then his best strategy is to confess) then the best individual strategy overall is to confess, meaning that each receives an eight year sentence.

The game illustrates the central problem for group processes. If individuals optimize their own benefit then they might not attain the maximum benefit achievable with optimal cooperation. Many social situations are similar NON-ZERO-SUM GAMES, in which losses to one player are not gains to another; in a theatre fire, it is to each individual's benefit to run for the exit, but if everyone does so, the resultant panic benefits no one; similarly, individual investors may decide to sell shares to avoid a Stock Market crash but *en masse* they precipitate the crash; and likewise when motorists park on yellow lines, thereby blocking the traffic system which they will later wish to use. Many social rules evolve precisely to avoid the catastrophes that result from individual maximization of benefits. In experiments, the likelihood of cooperation depends upon the individual personalities of the players (are they both trusting or suspicious?), on the previous response of the other player (one successful strategy is TIT-FOR-TAT: cooperate this time only if the other player cooperated last time), on the details of the rewards and losses and their consequences, and on the ability of players to communicate with each other.

A variant on the prisoner's dilemma concerns ALTRUISTIC or HELPING BEHAVIOUR. A person collapses in the street. You are in a hurry, and in some sense it would cost you to stop whereas you would gain by hurrying past, perhaps by reaching an appointment on time. In the future though it might be *you* who needs help, and therefore it may be to your long-term benefit to help now. Social psychologists started investigating such situations, often using stooges who would 'collapse' while hidden observers watched the behaviour of passers-by, after a notorious incident in March 1964. A New York woman, Kitty Genovese, was attacked and killed in the street, the half-hour long incident being witnessed from windows by 38 people, none of whom went to help, or even telephoned for the police. One explanation, of the DIFFUSION OF RESPONSIBILITY ('Somebody else will have phoned by now'), is rejected by experiments in which passers-by were *certain* that only they had witnessed the incident, but still did not help. A better explanation invokes a cognitive analysis of justice and fairness. All other things being equal, an unconscious person in a street is assumed to be 'responsible', or to 'deserve' being in that condition ('Just another alcoholic'), unless there is evidence otherwise, such as a white stick, or smart city clothes, when it is then felt unjust for a person to be in that condition, and help is given. Of course such an analysis does not explain the implicit moral calculus used by the passers-by. The origins of morality and conscience are complex but from empirical studies it seems that a well developed conscience develops when parents use withdrawal of attention and love rather than physical punishments, when parents reason with children about moral issues, are consistent in their attitudes and behaviour, and when there is warmth, mutual trust and esteem within the family.

Situations like the prisoner's dilemma and helping behaviour emphasize that responses in social contexts are not simple reflexes. Instead people interpret the origins of the situation and the actions of other people: they try to make CAUSAL ATTRIBUTIONS about the situation, to explain the *reasons* for the situation occurring and for the behaviour of the persons present.

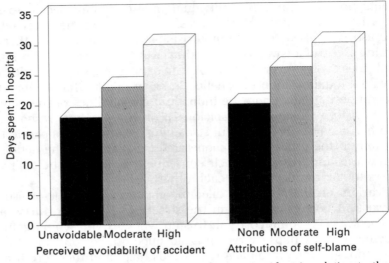

Fig. 14.2 Days in hospital recovering from an accident in relation to the patients' attributions of responsibility for the accident. All mean values are adjusted statistically to take account of differences in severity of accidents. Adapted from Frey D and Rogner O (1987), The relevance of psychological factors in the convalescence of accident patients, in Semin G R and Krahe B, Eds, *Issues in contemporary German social psychology*, London, Sage.

The nature of patients' explanations of illness or injury, of their attributions of blame and causality, can affect recovery, as is seen in a study of hospital patients recovering from accidents at work, on the road or at home. Those who felt their accidents were highly avoidable and blamed themselves took longer to recover in hospital than those who felt the accident was unavoidable or not their fault (Fig. 14.2). Individuals with less perceived control over their world (who did not avoid 'avoidable' accidents or who were to blame for accidents) also have less control over their own recovery processes, and hence recovered more slowly.

To understand attributions more clearly, consider the case of a student interrupting a lecture and asking a question. How can the situation be interpreted? Consider the information available. There are EFFECT DATA, describing the event itself. *What happened?* 'A question was asked about a topic mentioned by the lecturer.' What was the *outcome?* 'The lecturer replied and the student asked a subsidiary question'. How was it *experienced* by the questioner? 'They felt embarrassed and anxious, but angry that the lecturer hadn't answered their question properly'. There are also CAUSE DATA: What in the *environment* stimulated the behaviour? 'The lecturer was unclear and the student who had disliked the way the lecturer answered a previous question, had also misheard what was said'. What were the questioner's *intentions?* 'To show the class that the lecturer was wrong, to clarify the situation and to display their own superior intellect'.

In attributing causes for events, different types of information are available to an ACTOR, the person carrying out the action, and to an OBSERVER, a person watching the action. *All* five types of information are available to an actor, whereas only two types of information, about the *event* and the *outcome*, are available to an observer, the other types being private to the mind of the actor.

The FUNDAMENTAL ERROR OF ATTRIBUTION results from this distinction between the knowledge available to actors and to observers: actors, being privy to all information, particularly about their own perception of the environment, make attributions that are EXTERNAL, in which they ascribe causes to the specific environment — 'I asked the question because the point was unclear and because I thought the lecturer had paused for a question'. In contrast an observer's limited information means attributions are typically INTERNAL, in which causes are ascribed to factors intrinsic to the actor involved — 'that sort of person is always asking questions, likes the sound of their own voice, and craves attention'. In other words, *I* perceive myself as carrying out an act in response to events in the world around me, but I perceive *you* as doing the same act because you are that sort of person.

Attributions (and mis-attributions) underlie many social behaviours. After failing to take their tablets a patient (the actor) will attribute failure to specific side-effects, such as nausea, whereas a doctor (the observer) will blame the personality of the patient — they don't care, lack will-power, etc. Likewise smokers (actors) attribute smoking to SITUATIONAL FACTORS such as being under stress, whereas non-smokers (the observers) attribute smoking to DISPOSITIONAL FACTORS, smokers being weak-willed, self-indulgent, inconsiderate, etc. Altruistic behaviour occurs when attributions are external rather than internal (so that help is deserved since the person is not responsible for their condition): is the person *drunk* (internal cause, the sort of person they are) or have they had a *heart attack* (external, situation-specific cause)?

The human desire to attribute causes is so strong that patients and relatives will often search for causes when no rational basis can exist for one. Parents of children with leukaemia often cannot accept medical assurances that the disease is the result of a random mutation, without real cause, and instead will blame the illness upon themselves, for not treating the child properly, or upon local factors such as a nuclear power station or a chemical plant, and will apparently gain reassurance from such attribution. Attribution is important in maintaining a sense of CONTROL, in maintaining SELF-ESTEEM, and in SELF-PRESENTATION or IMPRESSION-MANAGEMENT. As doctors we may regard such attributions as irrational or stupid; nevertheless we should follow the advice of George Bernard Shaw in *The Doctor's Dilemma*: 'When the patient has a prejudice, the doctor must either keep it in countenance or lose his patient ... If he gets ahead of the superstitions of his patient he is a ruined man'.

Attributes derive not only from observing an event, but also from observing other people's responses to that event. Since these other observers are also making attributions, we try to make our own attribution consistent with others. If everyone else ignores a person who is slumped on the ground then as a lay person we assume this is not a heart attack or *the others* would have helped, and hence their absence of involvement supports our own attribution of drunkenness. However as doctors we will feel entitled to ignore these other lay attributions as ignorant or ill-informed, and will use the ashen face, blue lips, shallow breathing and expression of pain to diagnose a myocardial infarction. Our specialist knowledge permits us to ignore the erroneous attributions of others.

Attributions are not only made about other people, but also about ourselves, by observing both our own and other people's behaviour. This process has already been seen in cognitive theories of emotion (see Chapter 9), and is also seen in laboratory studies of the ASCH EFFECT. An experimental subject in a group of 'subjects', who are actually stooges, has to make a simple perceptual discrimination, saying which of three clearly different lines is the same length as a standard. The other subjects report their decisions before the experimental subject, and unanimously report what is clearly and blatantly the wrong answer. The experimental subject will then, in about a third to half of cases, also report the wrong answer. The degree of YIELDING depends on the group size and on the extent of unanimity between the stooges, one dissenter 'immunizing' the experimental subject against yielding. Yielding occurs even in groups of two if the other person has high status or authority. In a famous variant of the experiment, Stanley Milgram asked subjects to assist a scientist in a 'learning experiment' by giving increasing electric shocks to a supposed 'learner' in another room (actually an actor simulating the effect of shocks). Most subjects complied, giving shocks far above the voltage marked 'Danger', for as long as the experimenter insisted, and despite the cries and pleas of the learner, and indeed of the protests of the subject themself.

The Asch and Milgram experiments can be understood in terms of SELF-ATTRIBUTION. In the Asch experiment the subject tries continually to account for their own behaviour, and make attributions for the continual disagreements. The subject might think all the other subjects are wrong, but in so doing they have to attribute each one's behaviour to blindness, stupidity, or malevolence, an unlikely situation in each of these apparently random chosen subjects. The only rational conclusion must be that the other subjects are right and they themself are wrong; and then appropriate self-attributions have to be made to explain the discrepancy: 'I am sitting at an awkward angle', 'Perhaps

I misunderstood the task', etc.

Self-attribution is also seen in an experiment involving placebos (see also Chapters 20 and 21). Base-line pain threshold is measured and a subject then given a placebo injection which they are told is an analgesic. When retested the pain threshold is then higher. The subject is then told that the injection was actually a placebo, and that there was no active drug to account for the higher pain threshold. Finally the subject is tested a third time, without a further injection, in a condition which should be equivalent to the base-line, but the threshold is found to stay at the raised level. From the subject's point of view the raised pain threshold after the injection cannot be attributed to a drug (an external cause), since only a placebo was given, and hence the only possible attribution is the subject's own actions which have raised the threshold (an internal cause); and if those actions could cause the threshold to rise once then they could raise it again, producing the high threshold on the third testing.

Individuals differ in the way they typically choose to explain events in the world, and this applies also to symptoms and disease states. Individuals with an INTERNAL LOCUS OF CONTROL believe they are responsible for and control their own bodies, and that diseases arise due to a failure of control, which can be reinstated as a part of therapy. In contrast, those with an EXTERNAL LOCUS OF CONTROL believe they cannot influence their own bodies, and that disease is due to events from outside that are beyond their control, seeing themselves as hopeless victims of circumstance, beset by fortune.

The prisoner's dilemma and helping behaviour are unusual in that small numbers of people are involved, who do not know each other and can only communicate little with each other. However, most groups do know each other, if only for a few hours, and can communicate to some purpose. Groups have many reasons for existing, and have different objectives. Groups differ in their SPECIFICITY (are they there to solve a specific problem or to produce an open-ended form of result?), and in their FOCUS (an extrinsic goal or the group's own interpersonal relations?). Thus a works committee to increase output is *specific* with an *extrinsic* goal; a therapy group for drug addicts is *specific*, to treat the addiction, but *intrinsic*, trying to change the members' own behaviour; a scientific committee of a professional society has an *open-ended* but *extrinsic* aim (solving a broadly-based problem with many possible answers, such as decreasing the incidence of heart disease); and an ENCOUNTER GROUP is *open-ended* and *intrinsic*, trying to increase awareness of interpersonal relations within the group perhaps in order to help the members in their normal social roles, be it as managers or therapists. In each case, the GROUP DYNAMICS, the inter-relations of individuals, will be different, reflecting different means and ends. Certain processes do seem to be common in most groups, irrespective of their *raison d'être*. Groups evolve in a fairly standard series of stages, particularly if all members are new at the same time; FORMING, in which the members orient themselves to their task, and to each other; STORMING or REBELLION in which hostility develops between members as they resist the formation of particular structures; NORMING, where resistant disappears and members accept the norms of the group, and become a cohesive unit; and PERFORMING or COOPERATION in which interpersonal problems have been resolved, and the group can get on with its main task.

Groups carry out most activities by talking, and the structure and relations between individuals can be assessed by taking detailed measurements, preferably from video-tapes, of the amount of time that each individual spends talking, to whom they are talking, and what sort of thing they are saying, in a general sense, looking not at the specific CONTENT but rather at its FORM; the *way* things are said rather than *what* is said. A popular scheme for analysis is Bales' INTERACTION PROCESS ANALYSIS (IPA, Table 14.1), in which statements are categorized either in terms of the group's TASK AREA (producing questions or answers) or its SOCIO-EMOTIONAL AREA (is it positive, helping the group work better, or negative, attacking other members of the group?). When group members are asked who guided the discussion most, who had the best ideas and who stood out as leader, there is general agreement that the three tasks are all carried out by one individual called the TASK SPECIALIST, who makes most task area statements. Alternatively when asked which individual was liked best then the task specialist is often not liked, but a second person, the SOCIO-EMOTIONAL SPECIALIST, emerges, who makes most positive socio-emotional comments. Task specialists often produce hostility, monopolizing discussion and concentrating single-mindedly upon the task objectives, and this hostility, which might endanger the group's existence, is neutralized by the socio-emotional specialist. Not all groups develop two leaders, and one person often fills both roles, particularly in FORMAL or LEGITIMATE groups (such as a committee with an appointed chairman rather than an AD HOC group), or if there is one individual with both greater status and knowledge than the other members. Failure to achieve a socio-emotional leader, or for a formal chairman to adopt such a role, can lead to a group failing to achieve its objectives.

In any group of any size a DOMINANCE HIERARCHY tends to form, which is analogous to the PECKING ORDER that is formed in most social animals, and at the top of which there is a LEADER. There is some evidence that leaders have particular sorts of personality. Compared with other group members they tend to be more intelligent, more extraverted, more dominant, more masculine, show better personal adjustment and sensibility to the needs of other people, and to be more liberal in their outlook; although of course there are many exceptions. There are also tendencies for them to be taller, better educated, more verbal

Table 14.1

The observation categories of the Bales Category System. Reproduced with permission from Gahagan J (1975), *Interpersonal and group behaviour*, London, Methuen, 103.

<u>Socio-emotional orientation</u>

A. Emotionally positive responses.

a.   <u>shows solidarity,</u> raises other's status, gives help rewards.

b.   <u>shows tension release,</u> jokes, laughs, shows satisfaction.

c.   <u>Agrees,</u> shows passive acceptance, understands, conceives, complies.

B. Emotionally negative responses.

a   <u>Disagrees,</u> shows passive rejection, formality, withholds help.

b.   <u>Shows tension,</u> asks for help, withdraws.

c.   <u>Shows antagonism,</u> deflates other's status, defends or asserts self.

<u>Task orientation</u>

C. Problem-solving responses: Answers.

a.   <u>Gives suggestion,</u> direction, implies autonomy for other.

b.   <u>Gives opinion,</u> evaluation analysis.

c.   <u>Asks for suggestion,</u> direction.

D. Problem-solving responses: Questions.

a.   <u>Asks for orientation,</u> information, repetition, confirmation.

b.   <u>Asks for opinion,</u> evaluation analysis.

c.   <u>Asks for suggestion,</u> direction, possible ways of action.

and of higher social class. Leaders can also show different styles of leadership. In one experiment, carried out with teenage boys, a leader allocated to each group adopted one of three styles; AUTHORITARIAN, allocating specific tasks to each group member, allowing little choice, and permitting little extraneous activity, and not providing information on the purposes of the group; DEMOCRATIC, in which members chose their own project, allocated tasks amongst themselves, and were allowed to communicate freely with one another; and LAISSEZ-FAIRE in which the leader provided materials and general instructions but otherwise was passive and did not intervene. The authoritarian and democratic groups were similar in terms of actual production of end results, and superior to the laissez-faire group. In social terms, the democratic group performed better, there being less aggression or oppression between members, and the democratic group also performed better in the temporary absence of its leader. The laissez-faire group performed poorly in every respect. The role of the leader is therefore best exercised when the abilities of the individual members are maximally utilized, rather than all control and decision-making coming from the top. Groups are also more successful when the particular styles of the individuals are consonant. In one study experimental groups of four individuals were made up either of an authoritarian or non-authoritarian leader, and three members, all of whom were authoritarian or non-authoritarian, and the groups functioned best when the leader and the group members all had the same style.

Very often the role of a group is to make a decision of some sort. Because each individual in a group will arrive at the group with their own particular opinions, it is tempting to assume that the group's overall decision will simply be the average of the individual decisions. A series of experimental studies seemed to falsify that assumption, as committees seemed to make decisions that were chancier, or less cautious, than those made by the individuals, the so-called RISKY SHIFT PHENOMENON. Thus a group would be more likely to recommend that an individual should leave a steady but boring job and take up an exciting but uncertain post in a smaller company, where failure was a real possibility. Further research showed that the risky shift only occurred if most members of the group were the sort of people who would tend to take chances anyway; if instead most group members are staid, solid, non-risktaking individuals then the group would be *less* likely to recommend taking a chance. This phenomenon, of POLARIZATION, the tendency to move to a position away from the population norm, and beyond the average position of the group members, can readily be seen at the annual meetings of political parties, where conferences vote for more extreme policies than the members present would support individually (and certainly more extreme than their voters would support).

Groups can encourage loyalty amongst their members, and this produces COHESION, and a sense of group identity. Cohesive groups tend to meet frequently, to interact a lot, to contain members of similar interests and attitudes, and to have a purpose or task that requires cooperation for its successful completion. An external threat to the existence of the group can also increase the cohesion as the members rally around one another.

Cohesive groups are regarded as in EQUILIBRIUM, able to resist external forces and changes, such as the loss and replacement of members by others who slot into the vacant place. If groups are very large, or alternatively if members have well-defined activities within groups, as for instance do doctors, nurses, etc. in the hospital ward then individuals have ROLES to play, the allusion to acting and the theatre being intentional. If played strongly then roles can restrict the behaviour of other individuals; for instance it is difficult *not* to play the role of 'patient' if all other group members act their roles.

In a psychiatric setting one of the most important, and relatively recent, uses of groups is in GROUP PSYCHOTHERAPY, in which a number of patients, perhaps four to ten in number, often with a range of different problems, will meet regularly under a group leader or FACILITATOR, whose purpose is to maintain order, motivate members, guide discussion as appropriate, interpret when necessary, and observe. Conventional psychotherapy involves a single patient talking to a therapist about their problems. Group therapy aims not only to be more cost-effective, by treating several people at once, but also has theoretical advantages over conventional therapy, since the increased number of individuals will produce a greater flow of ideas, and of free associations, and will also allow SOCIAL SKILLS to be developed, so that a patient can observe responses of other people to their statements and actions, as well as observing the problems and needs of other people.

General applications
to medicine

15

Doctor-patient communication

- A majority of doctors think they are good communicators, whereas a majority of patients are dissatisfied with the outcome of consultations.
- Communication skills can be improved by effective teaching, particularly with video-taped feedback. The most important component of such teaching is probably SENSITIZATION to one's own behaviour and its effects.
- Patient satisfaction can be broken down into a COGNITIVE COMPONENT dependent upon the doctor's verbal communication, and an AFFECTIVE COMPONENT dependent upon non-verbal communication.
- Interviews should be STRUCTURED, both so that the patient knows what to expect, and so the doctor can obtain the information they need from the consultation.
- Patients remember more information from interviews if the material is EXPLICITLY CATEGORIZED, is specific, uses short words and phrases, is repeated, uses POSITIVE ATTRIBUTION, and if the important items are presented first.

Learning communication from a book is as forlorn an enterprise as learning to ride a bicycle by reading about it; success requires practice rather than theory, and is best learnt from a skilled teacher who can see the problems, and help with difficulties. Bicycle books instead try to persuade that cycles are useful objects, that people differ in their skills on two wheels, that accidents can result from poor riding, that the machine is more enjoyable and effective when ridden with understanding, and that life is easier for all if a few social rules are observed; in other words, to help you realize it is more difficult and sophisticated than you first thought, but that the difficulties are surmountable.

Most doctors believe they communicate well (just as 80% of motorists think their driving is above average). Regrettably, surveys of patients suggest the opposite; a majority of patients are dissatisfied after consultations. Most doctors qualifying before 1970 had no training in communication, and those qualified since have received only a few hours. Surveys of interviewing suggest that students at the end of their clinical course are no more EMPATHIC (able to share emotion) than those beginning their course, and are often worse at eliciting information.

Studies of communication skill courses show that they improve students' abilities to organize a consultation, to elicit important information, to establish rapport and form an empathic relationship, and to improve patient satisfaction. More importantly, those skills are still improved five years later when compared with controls. Probably the most effective teaching uses video-taping, followed by playback and discussion of problems, the feedback provided by the tape and the teacher being absent from conventional interviews. Nevertheless, all training seems to be helpful, suggesting that an important aspect of training is SENSITIZATION, becoming aware of one's own actions, of having control over the interview, of finding ways to change, and of assessing the impact of changes. To look at one's own behaviour as would an external observer, realizing where it succeeds and where it fails.

The Royal College of General Practitioners has defined good communication in general practice as follows:

'The doctor creates a receptive and calm atmosphere in the consulting room, and the patient is encouraged to communicate freely. He communicates his interest in the patient and his story. He actively explores the patient's view of the problem, and seeks to achieve a high degree of agreement between it and his own view of the problem. He gives evidence of his own commitment to the patient now and in the future. There is clear and adequate information on the services provided by the practice. The doctor's communication with the patient helps him to define the reasons for the patient's attendance at the surgery, to manage the patient's problems, to educate the patient on relevant health care problems, to offer support to the patient and to promote health in its broadest sense.'

For research purposes each part of such a definition can be assessed separately, trained observers rating interviewers for 'self-assurance', 'warmth', 'empathy', and 'competence'.

Patients can also be asked about how satisfactory was an interview. Broadly speaking, satisfaction has two components; *cognitive*, the doctor's verbal ability at conveying information and answering questions clearly; and *emotional* or *affective*, depending on non-verbal communication, to do with manner, attitude, warmth, friendliness and concern.

Success in communication can also be assessed in terms of effectiveness at achieving an outcome. Does the patient take the pills, lose weight, or stop smoking? If not, then there is a lack of COMPLIANCE, and at some level the consultation has failed. Poor compliance is common (Table 15.1), 44% of patients not adequately complying with a doctor's advice.

Table 15.1

Failure of compliance with medical advice in a range of studies. From Ley P (1977), in Rachman S, Ed, *Contributions to Medical Psychology, vol 1,* Oxford, Pergamon.

Type of advice		No of studies	Median percent of patients who did not follow advice
A.	Medicine taking		
i.	TB drugs	20	35
ii.	Antibiotics	8	50
iii.	Psychiatric drugs	9	44
iv.	Other medicines	12	58
B.	Diet	11	45
C.	Other advice e.g. child care, antenatal exercises	8	15
D.	All advice	68	44

A consultation is a complex social occasion. Lasting from five to fifteen minutes, each party brings their own expectations and hopes to achieve a specific result. The doctor hopes to understand the patient's problems, make a coherent diagnosis if possible, provide treatment as appropriate, and produce a satisfied patient. Medically, the most important component is the diagnosis, since from it all other decisions follow. Experimental studies suggest that a good history will provide 85% of the information for making a diagnosis, and examination and tests only about 10% and 5% of the information; the key to a good history is good communication. The patient has a different perspective. They have a problem, although it may not be the one they are telling the doctor (perhaps because they are too embarrassed or shy to mention their sexual or psychiatric problems). They want it diagnosed efficiently, thus inspiring confidence, to receive reassurance and honest, comprehensible information, and to obtain treatment as necessary.

Doctor and patient both make assumptions about the rules to be observed during a consultation. A recent study asked individuals what rules should be observed in particular social situations, including those for doctor and patient (Table 15.2). Although these are generally observed, it must be emphasized that if the patient's rules are broken, the doctor's social role is still to help the patient as far as possible; by contrast the doctor has a professional duty not to break the rules. If the doctor-patient relationship is compared statistically with other social interactions, then the doctor's role is seen as like both teacher and repairman, whereas the patient's role is similar to that of pupil and of householder (as it were, the owner of property needing repair).

Table 15.2
The social rules that a majority of the public feel should be observed by doctors when seeing a patient, and by patients when visiting a doctor. Reprinted with permission of the copyright holders from Argyle M and Henderson M (1985), *The anatomy of relationships*, Harmondsworth, Penguin.

By the doctor

1. Listen carefully to the patient.
2. Always explain very clearly.
3. Counsel on preventive medicine.
4. Be frank and honest.
5. Hold information obtained from the patient in strictest confidence.
6. Keep confidences.
7. Respect patient's wishes.
8. Don't criticize the patient publicly.
9. Look the patient in the eye during conversation.
10. Respect the patient's privacy.
11. Show emotional support.
12. Don't engage in sexual activity with the patient.
13. Come to a clear diagnosis.
14. Appear neatly or smartly dressed when with the patient.
16. Don't become personally involved with the patient.
18. Strive to present yourself to the patient in the best light possible.
19. Don't ask the patient for material help.

By the patient

1. Question doctor if unclear or uncertain.
2. Give doctor all relevant information.
3. Follow the doctor's instructions carefully.
4. Be completely honest.
5. Ensure cleanliness for the medical examination.
6. Don't waste the doctor's time.
7. Don't make unreasonable demands on the doctor's time.
8. Have confidence in the doctor.
9. Respect the doctor's privacy.
10. Present problems at one time.
11. Look the doctor in the eye during conversations.

Verbal behaviour. Systematic studies of students communicating with patients find several common problems. INSUFFICIENT INFORMATION is elicited, important symptoms are missed, or whole areas are simply omitted, particularly about social background, psychological response to illness, or occupation. Sexual or marital problems are mentioned by patients but then not followed up by an embarrassed doctor, despite being the patient's main concern. Many problems of elicitation arise because the doctor FAILS TO CONTROL THE INTERVIEW, letting the patient ramble on about irrelevancies, or because of LACK OF CLARIFICATION, hints not being followed up when they are made. Alternatively, the interview may be UNSYSTEMATIC, with no set topics to be covered in any interview. Information may also not be elicited because the wrong questions are asked: they may be LEADING QUESTIONS ('And I suppose there is nothing wrong with the bowels?') in which a particular answer is anticipated; they can be too complex because of TECHNICAL LANGUAGE or JARGON ('Any recurrence of the melaena?'); they may use EUPHEMISMS which are not understood ('How are the waterworks?', 'Oh, you mean my urinary tract!'); or they may use verbal constructions, involving passives, double negatives, or unusual words which are beyond the patient's intellect. Finally, many questions in natural speech are unintentionally several questions, without a simple, obvious answer: 'Any problems with the chest...or heart...or the circulation?'

Problems also arise when patients do not know what to expect. Particularly in hospital, patients do not know *who* is talking to them, *why* they are talking, *how long* they will be talking, and *what* the interview is for. Patients may have something they wish to say, or questions they want answered, but find the opportunity never arises, as the interview suddenly finishes without warning.

Non-verbal behaviour. Non-verbal behaviour (see Chapter 6) reveals many subtle nuances of meaning, as in the tone of voice, a look in the eyes, head position, the holding of arms, etc. Freud suggested, 'he that has eyes to see and ears to hear may convince himself that no mortal may keep a secret. If the lips are silent, he chatters with his finger tips...'. Such non-verbal communication occurs in both directions, with the patient also receiving messages about the doctor's attitudes: warmth is perceived from leaning forward toward the patient rather than sitting back in the chair; firmly folded arms indicate coldness, rejection and inaccessibility; gazing around the room, or writing while the patient talks, indicate indifference and lack of concern; and an occasional sympathetic smile or nod of the head, along with a muttered 'Hmmm...' are FACILITATIVE and indicate willingness to listen further. The most difficult non-verbal signal is silence. After asking a difficult direct question, particularly about emotionally disturbing problems, then CONFRONTATION, a sustained silence, accompanied by direct, prolonged eye-contact, will help a patient to talk, but only if the doctor resists the overwhelming desire to break the almost unbearable silence, which can almost be cut with a knife. Psychiatrists and psychotherapists are masters of the art of the FACILITATIVE SILENCE, and an expert should be carefully observed at work.

The placing of doctor and patient also sends non-verbal messages; the patient in a hospital bed or on a trolley, especially lying flat, feels inferior, subservient and unimportant, making communication difficult, and the patient likely to use the ego-defence of REGRESSION. Sit the patient up in bed, support them with pillows, and sit yourself on the edge of the bed, or in a chair, so your heads are at the same level; literal talking down easily becomes metaphorical talking down. Some medical students spend time as surrogate patients, experiencing the disorienting effects of confinement to bed, of being wheeled on trolleys, of being talked over and about by professionals apparently unaware of the patient's existence. Such experiences are recommended to all students. Alternatively, talk to colleagues or relatives who have been in-patients.

Much that is important, both verbal and non-verbally, concerns what is *not* said. Parents of newborn children with Down's syndrome describe how they first knew the problem, long before formal communication:

> 'I knew something was wrong as soon as he was...born. They all looked at each other and then went very quiet. Some other people then came in...but when I asked was he all right, they said he was fine and not to worry...but I knew they knew all the time, so why didn't they say something instead of keeping me wondering and worrying all that time?'

> 'I guessed she wasn't all right. She was always the last baby brought up from the nursery for feeding and people, doctors, students and nurses and all that, kept popping in to see us but never seemed to want anything...'

The medical consultation is unique in allowing close physical proximity between strangers, the examination involving intimate looking and touching. Physical intimacy without psychological intimacy is legitimized by the formality of the relationship, and the professional demeanour of the doctor. Needless to say it should be respectful, unhurried and careful. A patient will be more relaxed if the doctor starts by examining the least sensitive parts, such as eyes, face, and hands and gradually moving to chest, abdomen, groins and perineum. Patients should not be naked, for thus lies humiliation and severing of confidence, and should be covered with a sheet as far as possible. Many patients are fearful and nervous because they do not know why certain things are being done; a few words will calm.

Patients also know that some things *should* be done; the application of stethoscope and sphygmomanometer inspires confidence even when the complaint is of an ingrowing toe-nail, and avoids the accusation of 'Well, I wasn't examined properly!', and a thorough examination occasionally reveals the real concern to be for a lump in breast or scrotum.

Patients have their own ideas about how doctors should act, how bodies work, about what is important for health and about treatments. Such HEALTH BELIEFS may be wrong, or even absurd, but must not be ignored or laughed at; instead they should be exploited to help the patient. As an example of erroneous beliefs, Figure 15.1 shows the ideas of four patients about the location of organs within their bodies. Needless to say, ideas about physiology and pathology can be far more confused.

The therapeutic benefit of a consultation often derives from the implicit psychotherapy carried out by the doctor, and its power should not be neglected. In recent decades such skills have been neglected at the expense of increasing prescriptions for psychoactive drugs. It is now accepted that a doctor's sympathy and concern, coupled with genuine, understanding reassurance are often suffient to treat minor psychosomatic and neurotic complaints without drugs; as Michael Balint put it, the doctor is a powerful active drug whose specific effects should be used whenever possible.

Successful doctor-patient communications have STRUCTURE and are not just a rambling chat. The structure helps the *patient* orient themselves, know why the interview is taking place, and helps them remember the important parts. The structure helps the *doctor* obtain necessary information systematically, and emphasizes the doctor's professional competence. Maguire's model of a clinical interview distinguishes CONTENT (the information obtained) and TECHNIQUE (the means of getting the information). The doctor should obtain *information* about:

i. *The main problem*: there may be several and the first mentioned may not be the real one.

ii. *The impact of the condition on patient and family*: social and psychological consequences, which may be of more *practical* consequence than the physical problems.

iii. *The patient's ideas about the problems*: serious or trivial? Why do *they* think they have it? What might make it better or worse? What treatments should be used?

iv. *Predisposition to developing similar problems*: is there anything in the patient's background that the *patient* thinks is relevant, either physically (family history, occupation) or psychologically (early experience, etc.)?

v. *Screening questions*: a systematic (but perhaps brief) history

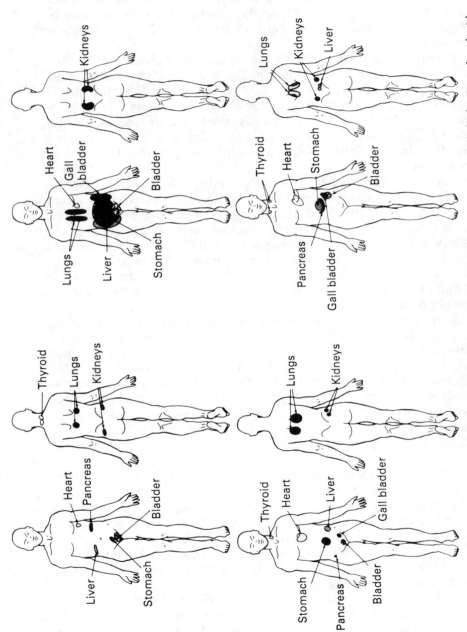

Fig. 15.1 Patients' diagrammatic descriptions of their ideas on the location of various organs of the body. Reproduced with permission from Burnett A C and Thompson D G (1986). Aiding the development of communication skills in medical students. *Medical Education,* **20,** 424–31.

covering the bodily systems, and social and psychological factors, to avoid omission or suppression of relevant information.

The technique for obtaining the information is:

i. *The beginning.* The interviewer greets the patient, shaking hands if appropriate, and introduces themselves both by name and status (but do not expect them to understand the convoluted medical hierarchy of consultants, registrars, SHOs, etc.). Particularly in hospitals, doctors often appear in scrub gear, or plastering apron, and the patient will not know that they are a doctor, as so many persons in a modern hospital wear a white coat. Patients should be greeted by name, both as a common courtesy, and to avoid confusion between patients. The first name should not be used, unless the patient is genuinely well-known to the doctor, and the patient would also call the doctor by the first name; false, 'chummy' use of the first name is off-putting, and is offensive to older patients, for whom the spouse may be the only person who calls them by their first name, and to any one who ordinarily uses their second name.

ii. *Explanation of the structure of the interview.* The doctor should indicate why they are there (the patient may have seen several other doctors or students), what sort of information will be elicited, and the reasons for it. This stage not only puts the patient at ease, but allows them to compose their thoughts, and organize themself for the interview.

iii. *The interview proper.* Although primarily designed to elicit information (at least from the doctor's point of view), also listen carefully for hints of hidden or unacknowledged problems. Many doctors are too ACTIVE or DOMINANT, asking questions when they would better be listening. Much psychotherapy and NON-DIRECTIVE COUNSELLING requires almost *only* that the doctor be a good listener, the patient resolving their own problems, by bouncing them off the doctor.

iv. *Ending the interview.* This can be surprisingly difficult. Make the patient aware that the interview is finishing, summarize what the patient has said, check salient facts for accuracy, and give the patient a clear opportunity to ask further questions, or volunteer further information. Finally, thank the patient for their time, and indicate when doctor and patient are likely to meet again.

Consultations frequently end with a diagnosis, advice and, perhaps, a prescription. Such information is designed to be remembered (if not remembered, it is pointless). Much is actually forgotten, and Ley's recommendations, based on experimental studies in general practice, increase recall.

i. *Explicit categorization.* Put material into clear categories, a proven method for helping memory in many situations (including exam preparation).

'I am going to tell you:
— What is wrong with you;
— What tests will be needed;
— What will happen to you;
— What treatment will be needed;
— What you must do to help yourself.

Firstly, what is wrong with you . . .
Secondly, what tests we are going to carry out . . .
Finally, what you must do to help yourself . . .'

This simple technique increased patient's recall of advice from 28% to 65%, of miscellaneous information from 46% to 70%, and of the diagnosis from 60% to 66%.

ii. *Specific rather than general statements.* 'You must lose two stone in weight', or 'You must take two weeks' holiday', rather than 'You must lose some weight' or 'You must relax more'. Recall increased from 20% to 50%.

iii. *State important pieces of advice first.* The primacy effect (see Chapter 4) means that early items are remembered better than later items. Most consultation summaries start with the diagnosis, which is very salient and remembered well anyway, and advice on life-style comes later. If life-style advice is important then placing it first aids recall. 'You must lose more weight . . . because the arteries to the heart are being affected' rather than 'The arteries to the heart are being affected . . . and so you must lose more weight'.

iv. *Use short words and short sentences.* Studies of patient information leaflets, included with drugs, or given before X-ray examinations, show that those containing easier reading material, and hence readable by more of the population, are understood and remembered better. The same applies to verbal material: keep sentences short and use common words. Such advice seems so self-evident as to be unnecessary, except that much literature for patients actually requires a reading ability possessed by only 5% of the population (Fig. 15.2).

v. *Repetition.* Repeated items are remembered better. If an item is important, repeat it. Important items should be repeated. Repetition emphasizes the point.

vi. *Positive attribution.* Persuasion or advice often contains implicit criticism, which is threatening ('You must lose weight [and I have to keep telling you because of your lack of self-perception, will-power, and intelligence]'). Positive attributions convert advice into a compliment, which is more likely to be remembered and to be acted upon: 'I'm sure that a sensible person like you realizes the health hazards of overweight, and will be keen to lose some weight'.

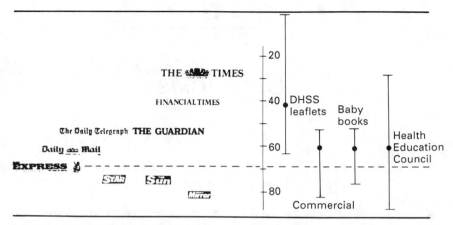

Fig. 15.2 The 'readability' as indicated by the Flesch score of a range of daily newspapers, as compared with patient information leaflets issued by various bodies. The dashed line is the average reading ability for the population. Reproduced with permission from Polnay L and Hull D (1985) *Community Paediatrics*, Edinburgh, Churchill Livingstone, 48.

There are no simple formulae: the attribution must be made to measure.

This chapter has introduced the problems of communication, particularly of oral doctor-patient communication. It has not talked much about written communications, and has not considered communication with other health personnel, such as other doctors, nurses, paramedical staff, etc. Nevertheless, I hope it has convinced you that communication matters, that it can be improved, particularly with skilled help, and that the most important step towards improvement is *realizing* that it matters; doctors who are bad communicators on leaving medical school probably remain bad communicators throughout their careers.

16

Diagnosis

- Diagnosis rarely uses deductive logic, but instead uses inductive logic to make diagnoses from imprecise, uncertain, probabilistic data.
- BAYES' THEOREM can be used by computer programs to calculate the probability of particular diseases given that particular symptoms are present.
- Computers can be more accurate at diagnosis than skilled physicians, not because doctors do not use Bayes' theorem appropriately but because doctors have an inaccurate data base of symptom and disease probabilities.
- When making diagnoses doctors start out with a very rapid EARLY HYPOTHESIS GENERATION, which is followed by CUE INTERPRETATION, and finally HYPOTHESIS EVALUATION.
- Experienced diagnosticians do not manipulate information differently from beginners, and neither do they consider a broader range of disease alternatives; instead they are like chess grandmasters in having a broader range of experiences against which to match the particular symptoms that they find in a patient.
- Inexperienced clinicians are often misled by FORCEFUL FEATURES; precise, easily analysed symptoms which are not strictly relevant to the actual, rather vague, symptoms with which patients have presented.

Hippocrates (ca. 460 BC–ca. 377 BC) recognized that diagnosis is the core of the entire medical enterprise. If an accurate diagnosis is made then, and only then, can an accurate prognosis be given, and appropriate treatment instituted. Surprisingly, diagnosis as a skill has hardly been studied until the past two decades. As one researcher put it:

'There is no more important field in medicine than diagnosis. Without it, we are charlatans or witch doctors treating in the dark with potions and prayers. Yet there is no field more difficult to teach. Strange that this art and science has not attracted innumerable theorists to make it more teachable! Thousands are studying membrane transfer, yet few strive to make a science of diagnosis.' (Cutler (1979) *Problem solving in clinical medicine. From data to diagnosis*, Baltimore, Williams and Wilkins)

The recent renaissance of interest in diagnosis has two origins: a growing interest by cognitive psychologists in the high level skilled activities involved in decisions and judgements by experts (and which are more 'natural', 'realistic' and 'ecological' than the sometimes artificial laboratory studies); and a demand fuelled by cheap, powerful microcomputers for programs to help with complex (and hence error prone) skills such as diagnosis. This demand for EXPERT SYSTEMS, imbued with ARTIFICIAL INTELLIGENCE, has focused attention upon the mechanisms used by real experts with 'natural intelligence'. The problems of understanding diagnosis as a skill can be seen by considering one popular form of expert system, which has been used for diagnosis, and comparing it with the same process as carried out by real doctors.

The earlier quotation by Cutler mentioned 'this art and science'. These terms are used in many ways, but one is that the *science* uses logical deduction, in which certain premises imply particular consequences (see Chapter 5). 'If, and only if, this patient has fresh blood in the cerebrospinal fluid, then subarachnoid haemorrhage can be diagnosed'. Such situations are fairly rare in clinical practice, and diagnosis in general uses not deductive logic but a form of inductive logic, in which a specific diagnosis is inferred from data which are only probabilistic. This manipulation of probabilities, likelihoods, relative risks, and the making of judgements under uncertainty, is the *art* of medicine. Consider the case of a patient with appendicitis. The appendix may simply be inflamed or it may have become gangrenous, a more serious condition needing immediate surgery, and having a greater morbidity and mortality. In one series of patients with appendicitis, the appendix was gangrenous in 29%. Patients with a gangrenous appendix are less likely to have audible bowel sounds, and hence it is routine examination in cases of acute abdomen to use a stethoscope to listen for bowel sounds. If a patient had appendicitis then, knowing nothing else about them, they have a probability of 0.29 of having a gangrenous appendix. Auscultation reveals no bowel sounds. Must the patient have a gangrenous appendix? No: many patients without bowel sounds have a normal appendix. However, the new information does make it *more likely* that our patient has a gangrenous appendix. If we have some background information then how much more likely can be calculated from BAYES' THEOREM (first formulated by the Rev. Thomas Bayes (1702–1762). Amongst all patients with appendicitis, 10% do not have bowel sounds, and in those with gangrene, 21% do not have bowel sounds. Bayes' theorem can be stated formally as:

$$p(disease \mid symptom) = \frac{p(disease) \cdot p(symptom \mid disease)}{p(symptom)}$$

The vertical line or 'solidus' means 'given that', and p(disease | symptom) is the conditional probability that a patient has a particular disease given that they have a particular symptom. Such abstract quantities are not easy to comprehend, and a more concrete form is:

$$p(gangrene \mid no\ bowel\ sounds) = \frac{p(gangrene) \cdot p(no\ bowel\ sounds \mid gangrene)}{p(no\ bowel\ sounds)}$$

We can now substitute the specific numbers mentioned above and calculate the probability that our particular patient has gangrene:

$$p(gangrene \mid no\ bowel\ sounds) = \frac{.29 \times .21}{.10} = .61$$

Knowing that our patient lacks bowel sounds therefore substantially increases the probability of a gangrenous appendix, making it twice as likely, although still not a certainty. The addition of further symptoms and signs, such as generalized abdominal tenderness, fever, and leucocytosis could all be included in the equation in a similar way, until eventually a sufficiently high probability is reached that we would decide to operate on the patient.

Computers have been programmed to use Bayes' theorem to diagnose many conditions, using basic information collected by non-medically qualified staff. One study looked at all patients in accident and emergency with an 'acute abdomen' (abdominal pain of recent onset). Although many diagnoses were made by the computer, here we need only differentiate two classes, those requiring immediate surgery and those not. In 45% of cases a correct diagnosis was made by the casualty officer, in 55% of cases by the surgical house-officer, in 70% of cases by the surgical registrar, and in 81% of cases by the consultant surgeon (in each case using identical information to that available to the computer). These differences between doctors can be explained in terms of different experience. Most interestingly, the computer was correct in 91% of cases, more accurate even than a consultant surgeon.

It may be felt that the computer had an unfair advantage in being presented with all the available information, much of which would be redundant and not normally collected by an astute doctor. However, computers using Bayes' theorem can also examine information sequentially, at each step choosing the item which is most informative (and if their cost differs, selecting the item with the best cost-benefit ratio). Figure 16.1 shows such an analysis, in a patient with jaundice, eleven categories of liver disease being considered. At each step the computer chose a piece of information from a list of 45 symptoms, signs and laboratory tests which gave the maximal amount of information. In Figure 16.2, in a study of non-toxic goitre, only three classes of diagnosis need be considered, and hence the relative probabilities of the three conditions can be plotted within a triangle. The computer (dashed line) moves in a smooth path from its initial position to the final diagnosis. Clinician 5 behaves similarly, whereas clinicians 3 and 6 take no note of much information they have asked

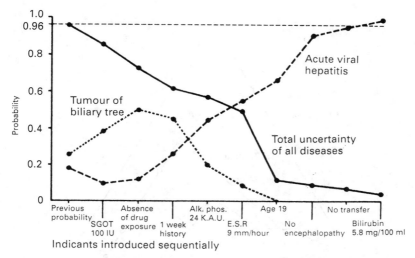

Fig. 16.1 An example of a computer sequentially selecting items of information in order to differentiate maximally between eleven different causes of jaundice using Bayes' theorem at each step, and calculating the conditional probability of each condition. Only two diseases are plotted here (for clarity). The 'total uncertainty' is an estimate of the amount of ignorance remaining at each step. 'No transfer' on the abscissa indicates that the patient had not been transferred from another hospital to this particular specialist unit. Reproduced with permission from Knill-Jones R P, Stern R B, Grimes D H, Maxwell J D, Thompson R P H and Williams R (1973), Use of sequential Bayesian model in diagnosis of jaundice by computer, *Br Med J*, **1**, 530–3.

for, and clinician 6 in particular asks for six tests from which no information at all is apparently derived. Given such results we cannot say that the difference between computer and clinicians in the acute abdomen study was due to clinicians making sequential use of information.

Since the computer and clinician receive identical information before making a diagnosis, two possibilities arise. Either clinicians do not have an adequate set of base-line probabilities (i.e. $p(D)$, $p(S)$ and $p(D|S)$ in Bayes' theorem), or else they have such information but fail to integrate it optimally with Bayes' theorem. That the former is the case is shown by two studies. Firstly, clinicians are frequently in error when asked to estimate probabilities. In one study, de Dombal asked six clinicians to estimate the proportion of patients with acute appendicitis in which pain is aggravated by movement; they estimated 26, 29, 30, 35, 43 and 54%, whereas in a series of 221 patients 62% had actually shown the symptom. A second study modified the earlier study of acute abdomen. Computer implementations of Bayes' theorem use a data base of probabilities calculated from all previous patients with that disease. Such a data base could also be estimated by a clinician drawing on their knowledge and experience. The study found

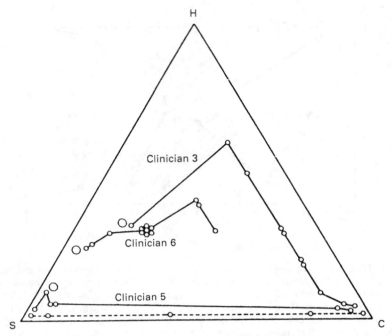

Fig. 16.2 Three clinicians and a computer (dashed line) diagnosing a patient with a non-toxic goitre, for which there are three main principal diagnoses possible: simple goitre (S), carcinoma of the thyroid (C), and Hashimoto's autoimmune thyroiditis (H). At each step, the clinician or computer asked for the results of a specific investigation and then stated what they thought were the relative probabilities of each diagnosis, and that judgement was entered as a single point in the triangle, the closer a point being to one corner then the more likely being that diagnosis. The patient in question actually had a carcinoma of the thyroid. Reproduced with permission from Taylor T R, Aitchison J and McGirr E M (1971), Doctors as decision makers: a computer-assisted study of diagnosis as a cognitive skill, *Br Med J*, **3**, 35–40.

that using its own data base the computer was correct in 91% of cases, the clinicians were correct in 80% of cases, and the computer using the clinicians' data base was correct in 82% of cases. We can conclude that clinicians are failing, relative to the computer, because they have an inaccurate data base, although Bayes' theorem was being applied adequately to those erroneous data.

An accurate data base of conditional probabilities does not just happen, but instead must be acquired, a process taking time and requiring experience of many patients, which probably explains the improved accuracy of the more senior, more experienced doctors. Of course mere exposure to patients does not necessarily produce an *accurate* data base, and as we have seen in Chapter 5, estimates of probability often err due to using faulty heuristics such as availability and representativeness.   If lack of experience is the problem shown by students and junior doctors we may ask how experience can be improved. Seeing more actual patients is one possible solution, although in practice it might be difficult to implement, work load already being great. Reading stereotyped or exaggeratedly typical case histories would not help, as the errors of availability and representativeness would then be exaggerated further, as most patients are not 'typical', and it is the *variability* that produces diagnostic problems. Case conferences and grand rounds may also exaggerate problems, since patients are often presented *because* they are atypical, having particularly bizarre or unusual features, which make them very available for recall but would distort the overall data base. One effective solution is to simulate patients on a micro-computer, so that they have characteristics randomly drawn from the true population. Fifty or a hundred different 'patients' could be seen in a morning, with a diagnosis required for each one, and feedback being provided on errors and misconceptions. In the same way as much flying experience of pilots is now obtained in flight simulators, particularly for dealing with emergencies, so patient simulators will probably play a similar role in the future. The final way of acquiring the crucial probabilities is to examine the data base of the computer itself, as it has been put:

> 'Next to the fusty volumes in the...library, with their loving descriptions of common, not uncommon, not so rare and rare disorders, will be the crisp new books that list the prior and the conditional probabilities of different states of health or illness. We need those books.' (Emerson P A (1979) *J Roy Coll Phys*, **13**, 185)

This chapter started by considering the problem of diagnosis as carried out *by doctors*, but has rapidly become side-tracked into a consideration of one very special way in which computers *can* make diagnoses. However, this does not provide any guarantee that such methods are the way in which doctors *actually* make diagnoses; indeed the abstruse nature of the equations, coupled with the very non-mathematical nature of many doctors, would seem to make Bayes' theorem a most unsatisfactory method of describing the behaviour of experienced doctors. The latter argument is in fact invalid (in the same way that when I catch a ball I must at some logical level be solving the appropriate equations of physical motion, although I may be profoundly ignorant of mathematical physics); nonetheless the criticism serves to highlight questions about the ways in which actual experts approach complex problems, albeit that their own introspections may not actually be an accurate guide to their true methods of solving the problems.

A range of studies have observed doctors making diagnoses in situations of differing degrees of realism. Some have video-taped real consultations and subsequently asked doctors to give a running commentary on their thought processes. Other studies have used actors who simulate patients, the doctors being asked to 'think out loud' as they talk to the 'patients'. A further variant adapts the game of 'Twenty Questions' and allows physicians to ask questions of a pseudo-patient, one item at a time, until a diagnosis is reached. The latter technique shows that clinicians who are more experienced ask less questions and get more information from each question than do inexperienced clinicians. A characteristic of all methods of study is that clinicians, be they experienced consultants or junior clinical students, show EARLY HYPOTHESIS GENERATION, with a list of four or five possible diagnoses being formed within the first few minutes of the consultation. This list frequently includes the final (but perhaps erroneous) diagnosis made by the clinician. The *number* of such hypotheses is unrelated to experience, and seems primarily to be limited by the capacity of working memory. The *nature* of the hypotheses, however, depends heavily upon experience and knowledge, experienced clinicians generating more hypotheses which usefully explain the patient's symptoms. The early hypotheses follow an initial process of CUE ACQUISITION, key items being extracted from the opening words of the patient. I only have to say 'A 58 year old man with a history of indigestion and weight loss' for experienced clinicians to be thinking 'carcinoma of the stomach/oesophagus; peptic ulceration; carcinoma of the pancreas' and they then ask specific questions to expand upon these and other related possibilities. Very many possible diagnoses will already have been implicitly excluded (e.g. prostatic hypertrophy, Alzheimer's disease, cystic fibrosis, Fallot's tetralogy, and diabetes inspidus), although those diagnoses might conceivably be returned to if necessary. The third stage, after cue acquisition and early hypothesis generation, is CUE INTERPRETATION; further information is collected by questioning and examination, to expand upon the early hypotheses and support or refute them, before the final stage of HYPOTHESIS EVALUATION. The hypotheses are systematically assessed and a final diagnosis reached, perhaps after creating further intermediate hypotheses. Experienced clinicians differ at each stage, although not in the way that they think or manipulate information, in the logic that they use, or in the range or depth of alternatives that they consider, but in the memory resources founded in experience that they apply to the task.

A similar process is clearly seen in a favourite subject for analysis of expert thought: the game of chess, with its most infinite numbers of variations and tactical subtleties. Grand masters do not think ahead more moves than amateurs, and neither do they try more combinations of moves, but rather for any specific situation they bring to bear a broader and deeper range of experience of similar situations, so that experience and practice can literally make perfect. This memory of previous games must not only be formed but also organized in a coherent manner reflecting the true possibilities of the game. As an example, chess masters are far superior to amateurs at remembering the positions of pieces placed in the middle play of a game of chess, but are no better at memorizing the positions of the same pieces placed *at random* on a chess board. The masters' experience of previous strategic play helps them understand, recall and organize the positions of the pieces only if those pieces are arranged in a manner truly compatible with an actual game of chess. A similar process occurs with experienced clinicians: patterns of symptoms fit together and evoke the recall of similar patterns from a well organized memory, derived from a lifetime of experience.

Diagnosis can sometimes be subverted, particularly in junior clinicians, by a FORCEFUL FEATURE, a piece of information that seems to suggest a particular range of hypotheses which are too constrained and do not include the actual diagnosis. This particularly occurs when a patient presents with diffuse symptoms (such as weakness or tiredness, for which there is a vast range of possible diagnoses). During history taking, another more forceful symptom is elicited (perhaps the suggestion of lower abdominal pain, for which specific hypotheses are readily generated), and much of the remaining consultation concentrates upon this all too forceful symptom. It was not a symptom that the patient presented with, but it is one with which the clinician feels comfortable (particularly if it includes an area of special expertise).

The problem with diagnosis as a skill is that it is highly ILL-DEFINED; it is not like solving Rubik's cube or doing The Times crossword, where the problem is well-defined, the relevant information and materials are specifically set out, and the solution is visible from afar. The diagnostician has to select the information that seems most useful from a vast range of possible items, must decide where to put most of the diagnostic effort, and must accept that much of the information which can be used is only probabilistic rather than absolute. Computers are only really good at solving well defined problems, as in the case in the programs described earlier for analysing the acute abdomen, jaundice or non-toxic goitre. Within such delineated areas, Bayes' theorem works well, and the processes of cue interpretation and hypothesis evaluation can be reasonably regarded as taking place in a similar way. The earlier stages though, of cue acquisition and early hypothesis generation, are not carried out well by computers, and they are the major stumbling blocks for junior, inexperienced clinicians who are lacking a conceptual data base in memory with which to derive adequate hypotheses for a subsequent more detailed analysis.

17

Ageing

- Erikson has identified three separate PSYCHOSOCIAL STAGES during adulthood, each with its associated CRISIS.
- CROSS-SECTIONAL studies of change during adulthood confound age differences with cohort difference, and are better replaced by CROSS-SEQUENTIAL studies.
- Intelligence and brain size are constant during adult life until about the age of 60, when a decline begins.
- The elderly suffer from a range of physical and sensory deficits which can exacerbate intellectual problems, and result in specific problems.
- SENILE DEMENTIA is a common problem in those over 75, and shows a characteristic sequence of decline in interests and abilities.
- Psychological treatment for senile dementia aims to be ameliorative, utilizing those abilities which are best preserved, minimizing inadvertent sensory deprivation, and using the environment as a COGNITIVE PROSTHESIS for failing memory and thought process.

Many things change with age, and the changes occur from early adulthood onwards. Some are physical and some psychological; some are continuous and others occur in stages, akin to child development. Life is continual change and adaptation, reflected in LIFE-SPAN DEVELOPMENTAL PSYCHOLOGY.

The American psychologist Erik Erikson (1902–) has identified eight PSYCHOSOCIAL STAGES OF DEVELOPMENT from birth to old age (Table 17.1), the first four being Freud's psychosexual stages (see also Chapters 10 and 11). Each stage has a critical problem or CRISIS to be overcome, successfully or unsuccessfully. Thus adolescence shows the well-known IDENTITY CRISIS, when individuals experiment to attain a firm and distinctive adult personality, copying from role models (friends, pop or sports stars, or ideals from philosophy or literature). Successful resolution of a crisis results in a BASIC STRENGTH, of long-lasting benefit for future stages. Table 17.1 also shows other characteristics assigned by Erikson to each stage.

Adulthood consists of three stages: EARLY ADULTHOOD, in which the major crisis is intimacy with others, in the form of love; MIDDLE ADULTHOOD, where caring is the basic virtue, and the crisis is the need to be GENERATIVE, producing objects of worth or quality for posterity

Stages	A Psychosexual stages and modes	B Psychosocial crises	C Radius of significant relations	D Basic strengths	E Core-pathology basic antipathies	F Related principles of social order	G Binding ritualizations	H Ritualism
I Infancy	Oral-respiratory, sensory-kinaesthetic (incorporative modes)	Basic trust vs. basic mistrust	Maternal person	Hope	Withdrawal	Cosmic order	Numinous	Idolism
II Early childhood	Anal-urethral, muscular (retentive-eliminative)	Autonomy vs. shame, doubt	Parental persons	Will	Compulsion	'Law and order'	Judicious	Legalism
III Play age	Infantile-genital, locomotor (intrusive, inclusive)	Initiative vs. guilt	Basic family	Purpose	Inhibition	Ideal prototypes	Dramatic	Moralism
IV School age	'Latency'	Industry vs. inferiority	'Neighbourhood' school	Competence	Inertia	Technological order	Formal (technical)	Formalism
V Adolescence	Puberty	Identity vs. identity confusion	Peer groups and outgroups; models of leadership	Fidelity	Repudiation	Ideological worldview	Ideological	Totalism
VI Young adulthood	Genitality	Intimacy vs. isolation	Partners in friendship, sex, competition, cooperation	Love	Exclusivity	Patterns of cooperation and competition	Affiliative	Elitism
VII Adulthood	(Procreativity)	Generativity vs. stagnation	Divided labour and shared household	Care	Rejectivity	Currents of education and tradition	Generational	Authoritism
VIII Old age	(Generalization of sensual modes)	Integrity vs. despair	'Mankind' 'My kind'	Wisdom	Disdain	Wisdom	Philosophical	Dogmatism

Table 17.1
The eight stages of development, from infancy to old age, in Erikson's account of psychosocial development, showing the psychosexual stages (A), the psychosocial crisis characterizing each stage (B), the significant persons who will help with that crisis (C), the basic strength (D) that will be achieved if the crisis is successfully surmounted, and the basic antipathies or pathologies (E) that can result from inadequate resolution of the crisis. In addition the table also shows Erikson's ideas on the social principles that predominate at each stage (G), and the ritualizations (H) associated with each stage. Reproduced with permission from Erikson E (1982), *The life cycle completed: a review*, New York, W W Norton, by permission of W W Norton & Co, Inc, Copyright 1982 by Rikan Enterprises Ltd.

(children, social structures, intellectual or aesthetic products); and LATE ADULTHOOD in which the crisis is developing an EGO IDENTITY, of a life well lived, with biological and social fulfilment. Failure at these crises results in SOCIAL ISOLATION in early adulthood, in STAGNATION, of failure to achieve in middle life, and of DESPAIR, of a life ill-spent, and inability to accept the inevitability of death during later life.

Erikson emphasizes the importance of *social* pressures in adolescence and adult life. However ageing is also a *biological* process, with inevitable changes. Strictly, ageing starts at about three to four months of age, when neurones cease dividing and after which only neuronal loss occurs. Nevertheless, the brain continues developing into adult life with an increased neuronal connectivity.

The decrease in neurones in the adult brain has led to a series of myths, unsupported by adequate evidence, of declining intellectual ability in adulthood. The myths result from two errors. The first reflects the venerable but erroneous assumption that intelligence relates to brain size, brain size and IQ being empirically uncorrelated. The second error is more subtle. Early studies measured overall brain size as well as histological measures, such as total neurone counts and neurone density. CROSS-SECTIONAL STUDIES, examining brains from individuals of different ages (e.g. 10, 20, 30...80, 90) found that brain size and neuronal number decreased with age. Other cross-sectional studies had also found a continuous decline in intelligence from age twenty onwards. Putting the studies together, intelligence was assumed to decline with age because of decreasing brain size. That conclusion is not justified though because cross-sectional studies confound age with date of birth. If in 1990 I compare the brains of a 30 year-old and a 70 year-old, I am also comparing brains born in 1960 and 1920. The social, educational and nutritional changes occurring between 1920 and 1960 might have affected the brains as much as has ageing. The methodological solution is to carry out a LONGITUDINAL STUDY, although there are practical problems; for intelligence we would have to wait half a century until we got any results, and studies of brain morphology are problematic in that post-mortems can only be carried out once. A compromise in studying intelligence is a CROSS-SEQUENTIAL study, which starts as a cross-sectional study, but then the *same* individuals are reassessed a few years later. Figure 17.1 shows a cross-sequential study in which intelligence was tested 7 and 14 years after initial testing in 1956. The cross-sectional data for 1956 suggest that intelligence declines steadily from age 32 to age 60, whereas the longitudinal data show that only after age 60 is there a genuine decline in IQ. In studying brain size the methodological problem is solved by comparing brain size with total cranial capacity (for a larger brain at an earlier age must still have fitted inside the skull, and the skull does not shrink); a genuine decline in brain size only seems to occur after age 60.

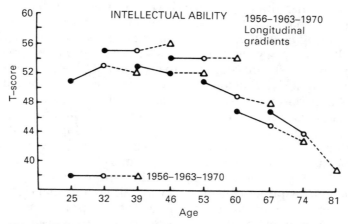

Fig. 17.1 Shows cross-sequential changes in intellectual ability of a group of adults assessed in 1956, 1963 and 1970. Solid circles represent measurements made in each cohort in 1956, open circles measurements made in 1963 and open triangles measurements made in 1970. The abscissa shows the age of each group of subjects at the time the measurement was made. Reproduced with permission from Schaie K W and Labouvie-Vief G (1974), Generational versus ontogenetic components of change in adult cognitive behaviour: a fourteen-year cross-sequential study, *Developmental Psychology*, **10**, 305–20.

Though the elderly undoubtedly show a declining IQ, the reasons for it are not obvious, not necessarily reflecting a simple decrease in information processing ability. In part the elderly perform less well on IQ tests because they fatigue more easily, are overly cautious in responding, and because of a NEGATIVE SELF-EVALUATION, believing themselves incapable of doing such tests; together these factors mean performance does not reflect competence. The decrease in IQ is also affected by many factors which are 'pathological' in some sense, but are so frequent in the elderly as to be seen as part of normal ageing. Those elderly with poor health have lower IQ scores, as do those with raised blood pressure or hearing defects. IQ also falls in the year or two before death, the TERMINAL DROP. Much of the intellectual deficit observed in the elderly therefore disappears if only the healthy, fit, normotensive, hearing elderly are assessed. The non-homogeneity of the elderly as a population is emphasized by greater range of IQ scores obtained in the elderly as compared with the young; many elderly persons are the intellectual equals of individuals 60 years younger. Indeed overall the effects of age are small compared with the large interindividual differences that occur at any age.

Intellectual deficits in the elderly particularly affect NON-VERBAL (or PERFORMANCE tasks) rather than VERBAL abilities. The distinction is also characterized in terms of FLUID rather than CRYSTALLIZED INTELLIGENCE, or

CONTROLLED rather than AUTOMATIC PROCESSING; well-consolidated, over-learnt and automatic skills such as language being less impaired than tasks requiring flexibility, novel thought or action, or the learning of new skills. Many non-verbal skills also stress response speed, and although the elderly are suggested to do less well because they cannot respond as quickly, that does not explain the results because the elderly still perform less well with unlimited time.

The elderly also show other physical deficits relevant to psychological functioning, particularly in vision and hearing. Visual acuity worse than 6/18 (i.e. objects are only visible at 6 feet which should be visible at a distance of 18 feet) occurs in 10% of 60–69 year olds, 30% of 70–79 year olds, and 35% of those over 80, due principally to glaucoma, cataract, macular degeneration and diabetes. About 30% of those over 65 have hearing deficits. Sensory deficits do not only restrict physical activity but also produce social isolation, with restriction to the home, and reduction in the circle of friends, and decreased intellectual stimulation. Social isolation is stressful and can precipitate psychiatric illness, particularly if a predisposition is present. The syndrome of PARAPHRENIA, a form of paranoid schizophrenia marked mainly by delusions (see Chapter 30), and which occurs in the elderly, is especially common in those with visual or auditory deficits, presumably due to impaired communication with others. Such problems of sensory deficits are not confined to the elderly, but occur at any age; in one experiment, students wore ear-plugs to produce a 30–40 dB hearing loss and showed symptoms of irritability and feelings of alienation and inferiority.

Changes also occur with age in non-intellectual functioning. Retrieval from long-term memory is less good, although a signal detection analysis (see Chapter 2) shows this to be due to greater caution rather than worse memory, RECOGNITION being less impaired than RECALL. On learning tasks the elderly perform less well because they do not use deep information processing if superficial processing is possible, although when encouraged to use deep processing they do perform better. The adoption of different strategies by the elderly reflects a broader personality change of old age, DISENGAGEMENT, which is a greater degree of introversion, coupled with a withdrawal from other people and activities. Although imposed by society to some extent, with enforced retirement in many cases, restricted opportunities for developing new activities, and diminished income and resources, it is also an active choice by the elderly to meet their own needs, and allow a reflective acceptance of life and its meaning.

In medical and psychological terms, the major challenge of old age is SENILE DEMENTIA, a progressive loss of intellectual ability, usually accompanied by cerebral pathology in the form of ALZHEIMER'S DISEASE or MULTI-INFARCT DEMENTIA, although there are other causes. There is a decrease in brain size and widening of the sulci, narrowing of cortical convolutions, decreased white matter and enlarged ventricles. The psychological deficits of dementia are not merely an exaggeration of normal ageing, although performance tasks are more impaired than verbal tasks, but there are also deficits in iconic, primary, and secondary memory (which are relatively unimpaired in normal ageing), and problems in learning, conditioning, and the use of language, particularly for object naming, and there is POVERTY OF SPEECH (restricted vocabulary, expression and spontaneous speech). Together these suggest a separate defect from that of normal ageing. Deficits progress fairly rapidly and in a predictable order, so that a scale of disability may be created. The condition starts with loss of hobbies and participation in social events, and then an inability to wash and to dress, followed by a disorientation in space and an inability to recognize other persons and to communicate; finally there is loss of control of bladder and then of bowels, an inability to move and finally an inability to eat. Dementia is common, *severe* dementia occurring in 0.6% of 65–74 year olds, 5.5% of 75–84 years olds, and 17.8% of over 85 year olds, while *mild* dementia occurs in 7.3%, 27.8% and 42.9% of the same age groups.

Psychological *treatment* of dementia cannot be curative because lost cortex cannot be replaced. However, careful consideration of psychological factors can reduce the burden on carers, reduce institutional care, and make life more acceptable to the patient; the intention is to *ameliorate* problems where possible. The benefits of reducing incontinence from six times per day to once per day are vast, both for patient and carer. Since intellectual deficits are least for automatic processing, it is such remaining skills that should be exploited to the full. Therefore, if possible, the mildly demented patient is kept in their own home or an environment they know well, so they know their way around, can find things, carry out basic tasks, etc. Much support involves providing aids for a failing memory (so that, as one worker put it, the whole environment becomes a cognitive prosthesis for the missing intellectual skills). Such simple devices as ensuring that a purse is always kept in the same place, or using large print for lists, can make the difference between success and failure at simple tasks, which is the difference between dependence and independence. Within institutions, it is being realized that INSTITUTIONALIZATION can exacerbate dementia. Many patients suffer sensory deprivation, in part due to hearing or vision loss, but also due to a lack of social interaction and a reduced need for physical action, since all needs are met, and this can exacerbate problems. Staff can also reinforce inappropriate behaviour, feigning interest or understanding when a patient's speech is confused, and thereby increasing such behaviour. Treatment programmes have used two techniques: STIMULATION AND ACTIVITY PROGRAMMES, which aim, through occupational therapy and social and domestic activities, to stimulate the deprived patient, and thereby restore purposive behaviours, and REALITY ORIENTATION in which the intention is to make patients aware that their actions have results which are of consequence to them, thereby reinforcing such actions. Both forms of treatment have been shown to be of benefit in improving behaviour.

18

Death, dying and bereavement

- ATTACHMENT, a normal social process, is eventually broken either temporarily in SEPARATION or permanently in LOSS, as occurs at death.
- A dying patient typically passes through five successive stages, DENIAL AND ISOLATION, ANGER, BARGAINING, DEPRESSION and ACCEPTANCE.
- GRIEF, the psychological response to BEREAVEMENT, is a process with its own successive stages of DENIAL, PINING, DEPRESSION and finally ACCEPTANCE.
- Bereavement is highly stressful and is associated with impaired immune functioning and a raised mortality, particularly from cardiovascular disease.
- Grief occurs after all forms of loss, not only those involving death, and takes similar if less extreme forms in all cases.

Death is a normal part of life and its inevitable outcome. Ultimately we must all accept the inexorable demise of ourselves and those around us. Necessarily, it will be upsetting and unpleasant, and neither intellectual detachment nor analysis can make it less so. ATTACHMENT is the mortar that binds together our social system (see Chapter 10). Although attachment is principally to other individuals, parents, siblings, family, spouse, children, and friends, attachment can also be to pets, objects such as car, house or garden, or even to abstract ideas. Our attachment binds us to them, and with other people that attachment is reciprocated, strengthening the relationship. Attachments eventually are broken, either temporarily in SEPARATION, or permanently in LOSS. The most traumatic loss is DEATH, although similar processes occur, to greater or lesser degree, after job loss, exam failure, divorce, limb amputation, bankruptcy, rape or other abuse. A loved object disappears from the person's life. For the dying person that loved object is life itself, and the psychological process of dying is similar to bereavement.

BEREAVEMENT, loss of a loved object, and GRIEF, the psychological condition associated with that loss, are not states, or emotions, but are PROCESSES, with a natural evolutionary sequence to be worked through. As C S Lewis (1893–1963) put it in *A grief observed*, a moving account of his own responses after the loss of his wife:

'[the book] turns out to have been based on a misunderstanding. I thought I could describe a *state*; make a map of sorrow. Sorrow, however, turns out to be not a state but a process. It needs not a map but a history ...'.

Bereavement and grief require the cognitive and emotional re-working of memories, and the comprehension of a future without the lost object and its many concomitants (perhaps loss of income, interests, and friends in the case of a spouse). To quote C S Lewis once more,

'... grief feels like suspense ... because of the frustration of so many impulses that had become habitual. Thought after thought, feeling after feeling, had H [his wife] for their object. Now their target is gone. I keep on through habit fitting an arrow to the string; then I remember and have to lay down the bow. So many roads lead thought to H. I set out on one of them. But now there's an impassable frontier-post across it. So many roads once; now so many *culs de sac*'.

Bereavement is also a *social* process, with death registration, funeral service, and burial or cremation representing the formal, outward acts of MOURNING, which help the bereaved to adjust to loss, and to accept movement into a new stage of life, with a different social role, as from wife to widow. Mourning acts as an anthropological RITE OF PASSAGE, helping the bereaved individual in the transition, and proclaiming it publicly.

DEATH AND DYING. Death comes in many ways. For some it is sudden, clean, immediate and unexpected; for others it is slow, drawn out, and long anticipated by patient, relatives, doctors and nurses, and it needs to be coped with. Elizabeth Kubler-Ross describes five stages in accepting one's own death:

i. DENIAL AND ISOLATION. Ego defence mechanisms reject the diagnosis and its implications. The patient may become isolated from friends, relatives and carers.

ii. ANGER. The patient is angry with staff and relatives, envies others who will live, resents their own suffering, and looks for explanations, trying to attribute blame for the disease's cause. The anger often results in accusations of incompetence by doctors, who should realize the psychological basis for such charges, and that they are not genuine criticisms of the standard of care. An overly officious defence of medical practice only makes things worse for all concerned; instead sympathy and compassion are required.

iii. BARGAINING. Patients bargain with carers, perhaps offering money in the hope of improved care and a greater likelihood of survival.

iv. DEPRESSION. As death becomes foreseeable, patients become depressed and tearful, weeping not only for their own loss, but for the future suffering of those around them. The temptation to provide false encouragement and assurances of recovery should be avoided, and instead the patient helped to work through the process, with the assistance of those around them.

v. ACCEPTANCE. The final stage when the patient accepts the inevitable, becomes resigned and passive, and often becomes detached emotionally from those around them.

Dying patients present many problems, some purely medical, as in the prescription of adequate quantities of analgesics to alleviate suffering. Other problems are personal for the doctor as dying patients often threaten one's own sense of well-being: death can wrongly be seen as a professional failure; it can upset directly if a close relationship has been formed; and it can be a chilling reminder of one's own mortality, for as John Donne said, 'No man is an island...any man's death diminishes me, because I am involved in mankind'. Ego defence mechanisms may make the doctor cultivate a professional detachment, or a cynical indifference to the problems of the dying, redoubling efforts for the treatable, and even denying the possibility of death in a patient. Such behaviours diminish the humanity of both doctor and patient, for death is both natural and inevitable, and should be seen as a normal part of caring. Although difficult at first for doctors, appropriate care of the dying can be very satisfying, and almost paradoxically, can itself be life-enhancing, increasing one's awareness of the good things that life has to offer.

The five stages of Kubler-Ross assume the patient knows their illness is terminal. Doctors often prefer not to break bad news, choosing to deceive rather than carry out the disagreeable and stressful task of telling the prognosis, and also fearing that the patient 'doesn't really want to know', and that induced feelings of hopelessness will produce a worse prognosis. Doctors can also be under pressure from relatives not to tell the patient, so that relatives themselves can avoid similar pressures. When well, 90% of the population say they want to be told if they are terminally ill (as do almost 100% of medical students and doctors); by contrast, during the 1960s, 90% of doctors thought patients *shouldn't* be told when terminally ill. Since then practice has changed, and many more patients are now told their diagnosis. Even if not told, most patients have a shrewd idea of their prognosis, and doctors and patients may engage in elaborate play-acting, each side pretending the other 'doesn't know that they know...'. Patients are very sensitive to social cues, particularly non-verbal, such as lack of eye-contact, shorter visits on ward rounds, evasive answers, false bonhomie, etc., and rapidly make an appropriate diagnosis for themselves. Perhaps the safest rule is to tell the truth, particularly if asked a straight, direct question ('Am I going to die?'), and only if certain that the patient is repressing, denying, or is asking for false reassurance, should one withhold the truth. Whatever the patient is told, do record it in the notes, so other carers know the situation, avoiding embarrassing and unnecessary contradictions.

Most people are inexperienced or uncertain when discussing death and illness, and avoid it if possible. One survey found that only a third of married couples in which a member's imminent death was known to both partners had actually discussed that death together. Those couples had found warmth and reassurance from sharing, and found it had assisted both of them, whereas those who did not talk subsequently had regrets. The doctor's role is to facilitate such sharing. It is not easy in a general hospital ward, but far easier in a HOSPICE, a hospital specializing in terminal or CONTINUING CARE, where experience helps not only with physical caring, but with open psychological caring, both of patient and relatives.

Ultimately the doctor must realize that little positive can be done to avert psychological suffering, for in part it is inevitable; however, many actions of omission and commission can exacerbate the suffering of patients and relatives. If in doubt, a useful rule of thumb, as in all psychological care, is to place yourself in the position of the patient or relative and ask what *you* would want; for beyond doubt you will be in a similar position one day.

BEREAVEMENT AND GRIEF. Bereavement is a process with a succession of stages which have to be worked through. As Gorer has pointed out, '[it is not] a weakness, a self-indulgence, a reprehensible bad habit, [but is] instead a psychological necessity'. An important part of one's life has been removed, and this requires a substantial cognitive reordering. The future has changed irrevocably, and many of the presumptions of the present have become the past. Memories, often of a life-time spent together, can no longer be shared, and must now be relabelled as referring only to the past and not to the future. Life itself will indeed change, because bereavement not only entails loss, but also deprivation of companionship, security, shared responsibilities, a sexual partner, a confidante, income, a specific role in life, and a particular future. This rethinking and readjustment is the process that Freud called the 'grief-work'. An empty space has appeared in our view of the world which must be filled, and the emotions which would have been discharged onto that object have to be discharged onto other objects. Nevertheless, as Freud said, 'no matter what may fill the gap...it remains something else. And actually this is how it should be. It is the only way of perpetuating that love which we do not want to relinquish'.

As with dying, bereavement passes through a series of successive stages, commencing with DENIAL, often accompanied by PSYCHIC NUMB-NESS in which there is a sense of unreality and lack of acceptance of the death. This stage can often be helped through if relatives can view the dead body, particularly if it appears calm and at rest. Death without a body, as in loss at sea, or in war, is particularly difficult to mourn appropriately, and leads to subsequent problems. That is also true with death or stillbirth of infants, where if mothers can hold their baby, and grieve for it openly, then adjustment occurs more easily. By contrast, viewing of a mutilated body, as after death by accident, can produce a recurrent vision which is discrepant with memories of the living person, and can make grief more prolonged. The formal processes of a funeral, and burial or cremation, can also help prevent denial.

The stage of denial can also be accompanied by ANGER; as with dying, this can be directed at hospital staff, in the form of accusations of incompetence or negligence, which should be treated not with overly defensive responses, but with a sympathetic understanding of the origins of these accusations. Parkes has called the second stage, which occurs after a few days or weeks of bereavement, PINING; there is a continuing process of SEARCHING for the loved one, frequently in acute episodes, the PANGS OF GRIEF being accompanied by severe anxiety, psychological pain, crying, and a sense of acute loss of the person. 'No one ever told me that grief felt so like fear ... the same fluttering in the stomach, the same restlessness, the yawning. I keep on swallowing ...', to quote C S Lewis once again. Initially frequent, these pangs decline in frequency, but are often triggered by tiny events in life, a casual comment, the memory of a shared event, a photograph. This searching is in many ways the equivalent of a young child or animal restlessly looking for a lost parent, and in evolutionary terms may be seen to be generally adaptive, although without hope of success in the case of death. Parkes has characterized the components of searching as:

1. Alarm, tension and a state of arousal.
2. Restless movement.
3. Preoccupation with thoughts of the lost person.
4. Development of a perceptual set for that person.
5. Loss of interest in personal appearance and other matters which normally occupy attention.
6. Direction of attention towards those parts of the environment in which the lost person is likely to be.
7. Calling for the lost person.

Notice that this is not the retarded picture associated with a depression (see Chapter 29), but is closer to the clinical picture of anxiety.

There is then often, but not always, a DEPRESSIVE PHASE, accompanied by a period of apathetic withdrawal, with a sense of hopelessness, of giving up, a preoccupation with thoughts of loss, a painful, repetitious recollection of the circumstances of the loss, and a sense of incomprehension of a world in which such events can be allowed to occur.

Bereavement can be a lengthy process, and ultimately is never truly complete, there always, as Freud suggested, being a part of our heart

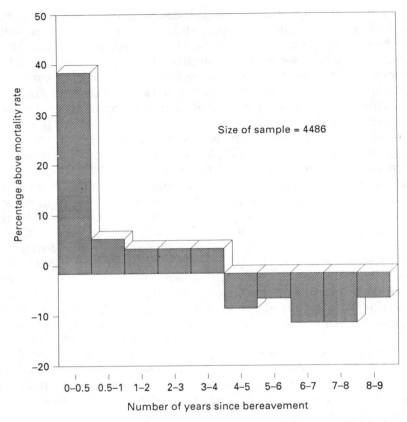

Fig. 18.1 The mortality of widowers aged over 54 compared with their expected mortality rate for men of the same age, for the first nine years after being widowed. Adapted from Parkes C M (1975), *Bereavement*, Harmondsworth, Penguin, 227.

which is forever elsewhere. Nevertheless normal life does resume again, although grief pangs can occur even years later. The 'normal' life will necessarily be different from that before loss, a reconstruction from the remnants of a previous stage of life. Several factors can prolong the grief reaction: AMBIVALENT RELATIONSHIPS (in which there is a mixture of love and hate towards the lost person) take longer to grieve adequately; sudden and unexpected deaths prolong grief, suggesting that in chronic illness much of the grief-work may be carried out in anticipation; and grief lasts longer in the absence of *social support* from friends or relations, or of other interests in life such as a job, or of opportunities for developing a new life-style (because of age, poverty, etc.).

Bereavement involves a failure to cope with the events of the world, and as such is extremely stressful, and results in a morbidity in its own right. Figure 18.1 shows data from a study by Parkes in which he compared the mortality of widowers with that expected on an actuarial basis. Mortality was higher than expected for the first four years after loss, primarily as a result of cardiovascular disease (almost literally 'a broken heart'). Bereavement is also associated with depressed immunological functioning for six or more months after loss. Patients often cope with stress by resorting to drugs, not only of those prescribed for them, minor tranquillizer use being common, but also the 'social' drugs, of tobacco and alcohol, which can result in medical problems in their own right.

As in the case of the dying patient, we may ask how the doctor can help with bereavement. Perhaps the most important way is in realizing the existence of the problem. The bereaved consult their doctors at an increased rate during the first year of loss, and an awareness of their needs, and of the real reason for their visits, is often of great comfort. Just talking is beneficial; 'Give sorrow words. The grief that does not speak, knits up the o'erwrought heart and bids it break', says Malcolm to the bereaved MacDuff in *Macbeth*. This is particularly important a month or two after loss, when grief is at its height, but the social support networks of family and friends have diminished as mourning ceases. Help is often available from voluntary self-help organizations, such as *Cruse*, which is particularly concerned with the problems of young widows with children, or the *Society of Compassionate Friends*, for parents who have lost children. The grieving are searching for something that cannot be found, and are not finding that which is available around them; support networks of any sort will help them find what is to be found in life, and to start living again.

Most of this section has been devoted to the most severe form of bereavement, of a spouse. However much loss involves grief, albeit on a lesser scale, and Parkes has summarized the seven major characteristics of bereavement reactions of any form, which are common to many situations of loss, not only in medicine, but in life in general; a failed love-affair, failure at an exam, moving house, illness or accident, or even the simple process of ageing, all involve loss of something, and can be the subject of grief.

'1. A process of realisation i.e. the way in which the bereaved moves from denial or avoidance of recognition of the loss towards acceptance.

2. An alarm reaction—anxiety, restlessness, and the physiological accompaniments of fear.

3. An urge to search for and to find the lost person in some form.

4. Anger and guilt, including outbursts directed against those who press the bereaved person towards premature acceptance of his loss.

5. Feelings of internal loss of self or mutilation.

6. Identification phenomena—the adoption of traits, mannerisms, or symptoms of the lost person, with or without a sense of his presence within the self.

7. Pathological variants of grief, i.e. the reaction may be excessive and prolonged or inhibited and inclined to emerge in distorted form.'

19

Sleep

- Sleep shows several stages; QUIET SLEEP (stages 1, 2, 3 & 4), shows large waves in the EEG, whereas ACTIVE SLEEP, associated with dreaming, shows an EEG pattern similar to that of waking.
- SLEEP DEPRIVATION, whether overall, or specifically of active or deep sleep, shows REBOUND, implying a specific function for each type of sleep.
- Comparative studies suggest that quiet sleep is associated with metabolic recuperation, whereas active sleep relates to the ecological niche occupied by the animal.
- Active sleep is associated with learning and memory.
- INSOMNIA is a common sleep problem and can be treated either with drugs or by psychological techniques such as RELAXATION THERAPY, STIMULUS CONTROL THERAPY or CONDITIONING.
- Nightmares and SLEEP APNOEA occur during active sleep, whereas NIGHT TERRORS, SOMNAMBULISM, BRUXISM and ENURESIS occur during stage 4 sleep.

Although one third of our lives is spent in sleep, and very many GP consultations concern sleep difficulties, we still do not know why we sleep, or what is its purpose.

Modern sleep research began when the EEG allowed a clear separation of the STAGES OF SLEEP. The fast, irregular, low voltage waking EEG (Fig. 19.1) suggests the summation of many independent electrical activities, which tend to cancel each other out. With relaxation, particularly if the eyes close, the ALPHA RHYTHM (9–13 Hz) appears. The slower BETA RHYTHM (4–8 Hz) appears during STAGE 1 SLEEP, midway in conscious level between sleep and waking. In STAGE 2, the first stage of true sleep, the EEG shows SLEEP SPINDLES, short bursts of 12–16 Hz activity, and K-COMPLEXES, large negative and then positive swings of voltage. STAGES 3 AND 4, together called DEEP SLEEP, show the slow DELTA WAVES (1–4 Hz) which Grey Walter called the 'billowing waves of sleep'. Stages 1 to 4 reflect progressively deeper sleep (meaning that it is more difficult to wake the sleeper).

After a period of stage 4 sleep, a further stage appears, which is very deep but has an EEG pattern similar to waking, except for the presence of SAWTOOTH WAVES. Since RAPID EYE-MOVEMENTS also occur, this

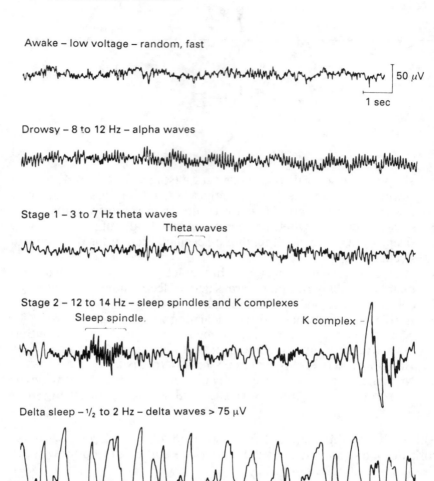

Awake – low voltage – random, fast

50 μV

1 sec

Drowsy – 8 to 12 Hz – alpha waves

Stage 1 – 3 to 7 Hz theta waves

Theta waves

Stage 2 – 12 to 14 Hz – sleep spindles and K complexes

Sleep spindle.

K complex –

Delta sleep – ½ to 2 Hz – delta waves > 75 μV

Fig. 19.1 Typical EEG records of the various stages of sleep. Reproduced with permission of author and publishers from Hauri P (1982), *Current concepts: The Sleep Disorders*, 2nd edn, Michigan, Upjohn Company Press.

stage is known as REM SLEEP, or PARADOXICAL SLEEP, because the waking EEG pattern is at odds with the depth of sleep; it is also known as ACTIVE SLEEP (AS) and DESYNCHRONIZED SLEEP (D), whereas stages 1 to 4 are known as SLOW-WAVE SLEEP (SWS), QUIET SLEEP (QS), and SYNCHRONIZED SLEEP (S). The sleep stages alternate during the night (Fig. 19.2), starting by passing through stages 1, 2 and 3 to stage 4 during the first hour and then entering active sleep for about 15 minutes. The rest of the night consists of 90 minute long cycles (an ULTRADIAN

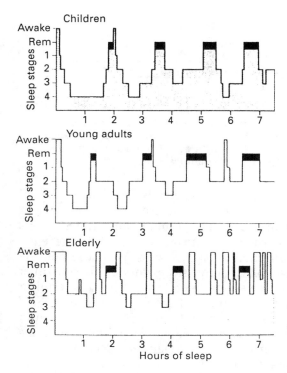

Fig. 19.2 A typical night's sleep in a young child, a young adult, and an elderly person, the ordinate showing the various EEG stages of sleep. Reproduced with permisson from Kales A (1968), Sleep and dreams, *Ann Intern Med,* **68**, 1078–1104

rhythm, faster than the day length), with active sleep increasing and deep sleep lessening through the night.

The sleep–wake cycle is a CIRCADIAN RHYTHM (returning once per day). Although many other biological processes are also circadian (e.g. body temperature falls in the small hours of the night as do serum cortisol levels), they are strictly independent of the sleep–wake cycle, occurring even if one stays awake all night (and perhaps explaining the nadir of performance and the increased weariness at about 4 a.m.). Some endocrine changes are however tightly linked to sleep, the best known being the surge of growth hormone in the first bout of stage 4 sleep (Fig. 19.3); its purpose is not yet known, although it is increased after physical exercise.

Active sleep is very different to quiet sleep. Most obvious are the eye-movements, which are mainly from side-to-side, and appear to be tracking a moving object; by contrast in quiet sleep the eyes gently roll upwards. Persons woken from active sleep report dreams about 80% of the time, compared with after 20% of wakenings from quiet sleep. Active sleep is also associated with flaccid skeletal musculature, erratic respiration and heart-beat, loss of temperature control, and genital engorgement, producing erection in men and clitoral engorgement in women. Quiet sleep shows greater muscle tone, steady respiration, and adequate temperature homeostasis.

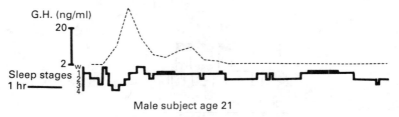

Fig. 19.3 The surge of growth hormone secretion in peripheral blood in relation to slow wave sleep in a young adult. Reproduced with permission from Mendelson W B, Gillin J C and Wyatt R J (1977), *Human sleep and its disorders*, New York, Plenum Press, 68.

Sleep can be manipulated pharmacologically and neurophysiologically. Stimulation of the mainly cholinergic ASCENDING RETICULAR ACTIVATING SYSTEM (ARAS) wakes a sleeping animal, and ARAS lesions induce continuing sleep, as probably occurred in the 1920s epidemic of the viral infection ENCEPHALITIS LETHARGICA. Lesions to the pontine noradrenergic LOCUS COERULEUS affect active sleep without altering quiet sleep, and lesions to the pontine serotoninergic RAPHE NUCLEUS result in permanent cortical desynchronization, and the absence of active *and* quiet sleep. Administration of serotonin, or its precursors, L-tryptophan and 5-hydroxytryptophan, produces increased sleep, and serotonin-depleting drugs such as para-chlorophenylamine, decrease sleep. Cholinergic agonists increase the proportion of active sleep, and shorten the ultradian AS-QS cycle, whereas antagonists have the opposite effect.

The amount and type of sleep varies within individuals, between individuals, and between species. Infants sleep more than adults, due entirely to an increase in active sleep (typically 9 or 10 hours a day at birth, compared with 2 hours in old age), while the proportion of quiet sleep remains much the same from birth to old age, at about 5 hours per night (see Fig. 19.2). Similarly differences between adults who are long, normal or short sleepers are also entirely due to differences in active sleep. Different mammalian species differ enormously both in the amount of active sleep and quiet sleep (Fig. 19.4).

Such differences in amount of sleep suggest they have different functions, and raise the whole question of sleep's purpose. That sleep is *necessary*, and acts as a drive-state, is shown by experimental *sleep deprivation*, in which individuals try harder and harder to sleep (and also suffer many perceptual and other symptoms), particularly after the second night of deprivation, when two or three-second long MICRO-SLEEPS start to interfere with other tasks. After deprivation there is also several days of increased sleep, a REBOUND PHENOMENON. If subjects are connected to an EEG then selective deprivation of active sleep is possible, by waking whenever active sleep starts; subjects are more agitated and impulsive the next day, but otherwise show few symp-

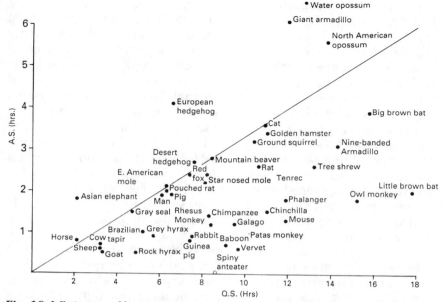

Fig. 19.4 Estimates of hours per day spent in quiet sleep (QS) and active sleep (AS) for a large number of mammalian species. Reproduced with permission from Meddis R (1979), in Oakley D A and Plotkin H C, *Brain, Behaviour and Evolution*, London, Methuen, 99–125.

toms, although the rebound after deprivation suggests a specific need for active sleep. Total quiet sleep deprivation is not technically possible, although *deep* sleep deprivation is possibly by sounding a buzzer whenever stage 3 or 4 sleep is entered; vague physical symptoms are reported, but with little distress, although again post-deprivation rebound occurs.

There are three broad types of theory for sleep's purpose: that it is a PASSIVE or RECUPERATIVE process; that it has a BIOLOGICAL or ETHOLOGICAL function; and that it has a PSYCHOLOGICAL function. These all overlap to some extent.

The oldest theories, which still have much support, are RECUPERATIVE THEORIES, which say that just as after physical activity a period of rest is needed to allow muscle metabolism to return to normal, so after nervous activity the brain also needs to recover. An immediate objection to the theory is that physiological recuperative processes do not take eight hours to occur; and neither does it say why sleep occurs at night, rather than immediately after 'neural exercise'. Partial supportive evidence comes from observations that mitotic rate and protein synthesis are highest during sleep, suggesting that cellular recovery may indeed be occurring, although these activities are linked to circadian rhythms rather than sleep rhythms.

PASSIVE THEORIES suggest that sleep occurs when there is nothing better to do, in particular if there is insufficient sensory input to keep the brain aroused. Two observations dispose of this theory. Firstly during SENSORY DEPRIVATION (in a darkened, silent room immersed in water at body temperature) people do not sleep continuously. Secondly, mid-pontine transection in the cat, just in front of the trigeminal nuclei, restricts sensory input to just that from the first two cranial nerves, and yet the brain shows *increased* amounts of waking.

The second group of theories, of a BIOLOGICAL or ETHOLOGICAL FUNCTION, emphasize the behavioural aspects of sleep. It might be objected that *not doing* anything can hardly be called behaviour, but many important behaviours, such as HABITUATION to a recurring stimulus, or the 'freezing' of a frightened animal, precisely involve doing nothing and are biologically adaptive. Since in active sleep the cortex is apparently as active as during waking, then activity also need not be associated with actual movements.

ETHOLOGICAL THEORIES compare sleep in different species. For this a definition of sleep is necessary: 'a period of prolonged immobility, with raised response thresholds, taking place in a species-specific characteristic site and posture, at a particular phase of the circadian cycle (or in marine animals, the tidal cycle)'. On such a basis, all vertebrates, including fish, show sleep, and sleep can also be found in invertebrates, such as mollusc and insects, and this phylogenetic antiquity emphasizes the biological importance of sleep. Comparative studies (see Fig. 19.4) suggest large inter-species differences in the amount and type of sleep: a horse sleeps for three hours a day while an opossum sleeps nineteen hours each day. The amount of quiet sleep is inversely proportional to the size of an animal, so that a mouse has a lot of quiet sleep and an elephant has only a little. Since metabolic rate and cell turnover is greatest in small animals, this suggests that indeed some cellular recovery process is occurring during quiet sleep. In contrast active sleep is unrelated to body size, but instead relates to an animal's invulnerability to predation, either during the day, while finding food, or at night. One proposed evolutionary function of active sleep is to produce 'active immobility', which increases an organism's chance of survival during times, such as at night, when the risk of predation is greatest, and its best strategy is simply to hide, in a hole in the ground, or in a tree, and keep completely still.

Active and quiet sleep are clearly differentiated in all mammals and birds, but not in reptiles, amphibia and fish. Which is the evolutionary older form of sleep is not clear, since differences in brain structure between genera preclude any direct comparison of EEG wave-forms. Since active sleep is more complex, particularly in its relation to dreaming in man, it has been thought to be evolutionarily more recent, but that view has been challenged on the basis that since active sleep is associated with a loss of temperature regulation, converting the otherwise homoeothermic mammals to poikilotherms, akin to the cold-blooded fish, reptiles and amphibia, then it must be the older form of sleep. Comparative evidence shows that the speed of the AS-QS cycle is inversely proportional to body size (and hence to metabolic rate), elephants having a 124 minute cycle and mice a 12 minute cycle. Since larger animals have a greater thermal capacity they cool less quickly, and therefore can withstand poikilothermy for longer before cooling, and hence have longer bouts of active sleep.

Psychological theories of sleep can be broadly divided into two categories, COGNITIVE THEORIES and PSYCHOANALYTIC THEORIES.

Cognitive theories of sleep derive, like much modern psychological theorizing, from the metaphor of the brain as a computer. Large computer systems with many users accessing many different files from disk and tape commonly used to have a 'down period' during the night when although users could not use the system it was nonetheless very active, carrying out 'housekeeping' functions, such as eliminating unwanted files, checking on users' accounts, cross-referencing between files, etc. By an almost exact analogy, it is suggested that sleep is the time for the brain to carry out housekeeping activities, checking over the day's events and filing memories, cross-referencing events against memories of previous events, etc. On this model, dreaming is explained away as a mere EPIPHENOMENON of cognitive reorganization; an unintended side-effect without functional significance, happening, by accident, to impinge upon consciousness. The theory supposes that cognitive reorganization is occurring during active sleep, since cerebral activity is diminished during quiet sleep. The theory is supported by experimental evidence: rats kept in a boring environment have reduced active sleep (but unchanged amounts of quiet sleep), presumably due to less cognitive organization being needed; LATENT LEARNING (see Chapter 3) in which a rat learns by wandering freely around a novel maze in which it will later be tested, is impaired if active sleep is selectively deprived; and in man long and short sleepers differ primarily in the amount of active sleep, and short-sleepers have been called PRE-PROGRAMMERS, while long-sleepers have been called RE-PROGRAMMERS, the former treating the next day much the same day as the previous one, while the latter analyse and reorganize the previous day's experiences in preparation for the next day. In man, experiments also suggest that sleep deprivation can impair the laying down of permanent memories, and that information learnt late in the day is learnt better, because it is closer in time to sleep and hence to cognitive reorganization and reprocessing.

The greatest psychological theory of sleep must surely be Freud's PSYCHOANALYTIC THEORY (see Chapter 11). However in his theory Freud does not say *why* we sleep. His biological training convinced him that sleep was biologically important, although he did not know why. The

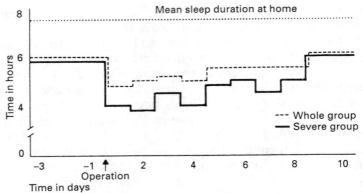

Fig. 19.5 Average duration of sleep in 93 hospitalized patients who were having either major or minor surgery, in comparison with normal average sleep duration when at home. Reproduced with permission from Murphy F, Bentley S, Ellis B W and Dudley H (1977), Sleep deprivation in patients undergoing operation: a factor in the stress of surgery, *Br Med J*, **2**, 1521–2.

role of dreams was to preserve that important sleep: '... the dream is an attempt to put aside the disturbance of sleep by means of a wish fulfilment. The dream is the Guardian of Sleep'. To Freud therefore dreams are not just an epiphenomenon, but neither are they the principal purpose of sleep.

Many patients have sleep problems, 30–40% of the population in surveys reporting problems with sleeping, and about 10% of the population at any one time taking tablets to help them sleep. The commonest problem is INSOMNIA, an inability to get to sleep, often coupled with waking during the night or in the early morning. Sometimes it is secondary to problems such as anxiety or depression (see Chapters 28 & 29), or to side-effects of prescribed drugs (such as rebound effects after using minor tranquillizers), or self-prescribed drugs, typically of caffeine in tea, coffee or cola drinks taken during the evening. Insomnia itself causes tiredness and irritability, and then anxiety and depression, which exacerbate the insomnia. Insomnia is common in hospital patients and is a major complaint about hospital services; partly it is due to a strange place, partly to a natural anxiety about illness, and partly to the very many disturbances that can occur such as noises, lights, conversations, etc. It is particularly problematic for patients on intensive and coronary care-units, where lights are on all night, and staff are continually monitoring, changing drips, and sucking out airways. If sleep does indeed assist in bodily recuperation and repair then deprivation in hospital (see Fig. 19.5), particularly after major surgery, should be of great concern.

Acute insomnia is treated effectively with drugs such as the short-acting benzodiazepines which have little HANG-OVER EFFECT the next day.

Barbiturates should not be used at all, both because they are addictive and abused, and because they specifically reduce active sleep. Tolerance develops rapidly to all hypnotic drugs and they should only be used for a few days or weeks at a time, as an immediate solution to an acute problem. If a continuing mild hypnotic is needed then hot milky drinks, such as Ovaltine or Horlicks, are effective at inducing sleep, presumably because of their tryptophan content, and small (but not large) doses of alcohol can also help relax a patient and encourage sleep.

Psychological treatments of insomnia are effective and of particular benefit in chronic problems where drugs have failed. RELAXATION TRAINING takes as a starting point that poor sleepers cannot sleep because they are over-aroused, perhaps due to anxiety. Patients are given RELAXATION TRAINING, either in groups or with the aid of a tape-recorded commentary, such as successive tensing and relaxing of particular muscle groups. Patients use their relaxation sequence on going to bed, and sleep usually follows. STIMULUS CONTROL THERAPY asks what associations the subject has learned to the stimulus of going to bed. If a patient typically reads in bed, listens to the radio, watches television, or even studies, then an association has been learned between bed and *activity*. Bed must be associated only with sleep, and the patient instructed only to go to bed when sleepy and to carry out no activity other than sleeping in the bedroom (with the exception of sexual activity, which probably also has a direct soporific effect); if sleep does not occur within ten minutes of going to bed, then the patient should get up and do something else. During the day naps must be avoided and getting up should occur at a regular time. Controlled trials show such therapy to be effective and lasting. CONDITIONING has also been attempted, by associating the action of a hypnotic drug (the unconditioned response) with the ticking of a metronome (the conditioned stimulus), so that in the future the playing of the metronome at bedtime will itself induce sleep as a conditioned response.

Several abnormal processes can occur during sleep, usually during particular phases. NIGHTMARES are bad dreams, occurring during active sleep, and waking the sleeper suddenly. They are different from NIGHT TERRORS or PAVOR NOCTURNUS which occur during stage 4 of quiet sleep, particularly in children, and are associated with an overwhelming terror or fear, without any specific recall of dream content, or of reasons for the fear. SOMNAMBULISM, or sleep-walking, also occurs during stage 4 sleep, as do HEAD-BANGING, BRUXISM (continual, noisy teeth grinding), and ENURESIS (bed-wetting), all being more common in children and typically 'grown out of'. Enuresis is well treated by behaviour therapy: a detector under the sheet rings an alarm at the first traces of wetness, waking the child before the bladder empties, and associating the sensation of a full bladder with waking and going to the toilet. Active sleep can show problems of homoeostatic regulation, with irregular respiration and heart-beat: SLEEP APNOEA, when breathing ceases, occurs in adults, particularly if they have chronic obstructive airways disease, and in infants, where it is associated with SUDDEN INFANT DEATH SYNDROME (cot-death).

20

Pain

- Pain is not a simple sensation produced by 'pain receptors' but is an interpretation of the activity of many receptors, which produce the multidimensional perception of pain.
- Signal detection theory can be used for distinguishing true analgesics, which modify d', from placebos and suggestion which modify *beta*.
- The GATE CONTROL THEORY says that pain occurs when the TRANS-MISSION (T) CELLS in lamina 5 of the dorsal horns of the spinal cord are stimulated by small (S) fibre activity. Pain can be stopped by inhibition of the T cells by large (L) fibre activity via the SUBSTANTIA GELATINOSA (SG).
- Anxiety increases pain due to autonomic arousal activating small fibres, whereas stress can reduce pain, as in STRESS ANALGESIA, via opiate mechanisms in the peri-aqueductal grey matter.
- Neurophysiological techniques for pain reduction, such as DORSAL ROOT STIMULATION and TRANSCUTANEOUS NERVE STIMULATION, act by stimulating L fibres and SG cells.
- Psychological techniques for pain reduction act either by reducing S fibre input, as in RELAXATION THERAPY and BIOFEEDBACK, or by producing COGNITIVE COPING SKILLS by IMAGINATIVE INATTENTION or SOMATIZATION.

Pain is probably the commonest of symptoms and analgesics the commonest of treatments. Pain though is a complex phenomenon with physiological and psychological components. It is not a simple sensation, but is better regarded as a perception or an interpretation, and as a response or set of behaviours. Its physiology is complicated, but directly relevant to the psychology. 'Pain receptors', receptors whose activity would cause pain, do not exist, although particular receptors are especially important: there is SPECIALIZATION but not SPECIFICITY.

Pain is difficult to describe. Unlike heat or pressure which vary only in degree, pain conventionally has three dimensions: SENSORY, the particular quality (pricking, scalding, aching, etc.); AFFECTIVE, the emotions produced (sickening, exhausting, frightening, etc.); and EVALUATIVE, assessing its amount (discomfort, distressing, excruciating, etc.). For research these components can be measured by the MCGILL PAIN QUESTIONNAIRE, and hence by appropriate scaling techniques we can say that, say, a STRONG pain is twice as bad as a MODERATE pain, and an EXCRUTIATING pain four times as bad as a strong pain. PAIN THRESHOLD, the mildest stimulus identifiable as pain, is distinguished from PAIN TOLERANCE, the worst stimulus which can be borne for a reasonable amount of time; the threshold is influenced mainly by physiological factors and the tolerance by psychological factors. Pains also vary in time; the acute, fast or phasic component of pain immediately after an injury has a different quality to the slower, chronic, or tonic component, the 'real' pain, which occurs a second or more after the fast pain (so that after hitting a thumb with a hammer there is a moment of detachment and realization before the onset of real pain). Social and cultural influences also affect pain; thus I may report less pain when having blood taken in a venepuncture demonstration in front of several students, than if nervous and on a trolley awaiting an operation. Such measurement problems are avoided in the laboratory by using a signal detection technique (see Chapter 2). Subjects indicate on a standardized scale the amount of pain experienced when infra-red energy is shone on a patch of black India ink painted on the forearm. Statistical analysis separates changes in 'beta' or threshold (a 'stiff upper lip', stoically denying the pain) from changes in d' or pain intensity. Aspirin and Entonox (a mixture of nitrous oxide and oxygen) can be shown to be true analgesics, increasing d' (sensitivity), whereas placebos or suggestion act by changing beta (the criterion for reporting pain), and hence are not true analgesics. The influence of social demands and expectations must make one wary in interpreting results for which such precise analysis is not available.

The philosopher Descartes (1596–1650) produced a common-sensical theory of pain (Fig. 20.1); 'pain receptors' are stimulated (by fire, in this case) and cause alarm bells to ring in the head, which are sensed as pain. However, such a simple model cannot account for many pain phenomena:

i. Pain occurs in the PHANTOM LIMBS that follow amputation.

ii. Paraplegic patients describe pains *below* the level of their spinal transection.

iii. Pain can be the result of damage to spinal cord or brain.

iv. Pain can be relieved by COUNTER-IRRITATION (irritating the skin by blistering or scarification), or by simple procedures such as rubbing.

v. Gross tissue damage need not be accompanied by pain. At the Anzio beach head in the Second World War many severely wounded soldiers reported little or no pain.

vi. Minor stimuli, such as the lightest of touch, can result in an exquisite pain (HYPERAESTHESIA) in CAUSALGIA, which develops after damage to peripheral nerves and neuroma formation.

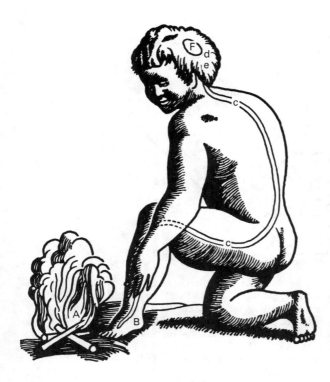

Fig. 20.1 Descartes' original conception of a reflex mechanism for the perception of pain: the fire (A) stimulates a receptor (B), which pulls a thread, and actuates the sense of pain in the brain (F). From Descartes R, (1664), *Traité de l'Homme*, Paris, Angot.

None of these problems should occur if the Cartesian model is correct; either a connection is present or it is not, and the system is activated by tissue damage or it is not. No other condition is possible.

The brain contains no 'pain centre', and no area of cortex is specialized for it (unlike the other sensory modalities). Pain also differs from other senses in having powerful descending influences which modify transmission from the spinal cord; stimulation of peri-aqueductal grey matter produces a deep STIMULATION-INDUCED ANALGESIA, under which surgery is possible without anaesthetic.

In 1965 Melzack and Wall proposed their GATE CONTROL THEORY (Fig. 20.2), which accounts for many troublesome aspects of pain. The TRANSMISSION (T) CELLS (which are probably in lamina 5 of the dorsal horns of the spinal cord) project centrally, and are the input to an ACTION SYSTEM; when stimulated beyond a threshold they produce pain perception and its behavioural manifestations. Small, non-myelinated peripheral nerve fibres have excitatory projections onto the T-cell, and also onto cells in the SUBTANTIA GELATINOSA (SG) of the spinal cord, which in turn activate the T cell. Painful stimuli cause small (S) fibre activity and activate the T cells. Even when S fibre activity has ceased, the T cell continues to be activated by the SG cell, which is 'turned on', and pain therefore lasts longer than the stimulus itself. Large fibre inputs (L) also stimulate the T cell (as when light touch produces

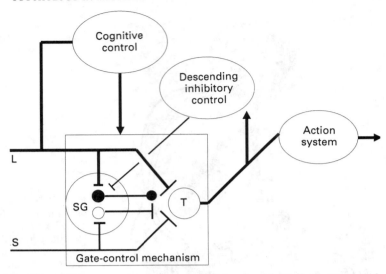

Fig. 20.2 The gate control theory of Melzack and Wall, in its second version. There are both excitatory (white circle) and inhibitory (black circle) links from the substantia gelatinosa cells (SG) to the transmission (T) cells. All connections are excitatory, with the exception of the inhibitory link from SG to T, which may be either pre- or post-synaptic in type. Adapted from Melzack R and Wall P (1982), *The challenge of pain*, Harmondsworth, Penguin Books, 235.

causalgia) but also cause *inhibition* of T cells via the SG cells. L fibre stimulation (as in rubbing, or applying warmth or counter-irritation) therefore decreases T cell activity. T cell activity results from a balance between large and small fibre activity. In causalgia and phantom limb pain, neuroma formation produces excess small fibre activity, and hence pain. The entire gate system, of SG and T cells, can also be controlled from above; direct inhibition from peri-aqueductal grey matter closes the gate, and cognitive control can either close the gate, resulting in lack of pain after severe damage (as in the Anzio soldiers, who were so happy to leave the battlefield alive that their wounds seemed insignificant), or open the gate and produce increased pain sensitivity in anxious or neurotic patients. The model also explains the difference between the fast and slow pains, reflecting the different properties of fast (L) and slow (S) fibres.

The gate control theory is exciting in providing a coherent explanation of diverse phenomena, and in showing how psychological and cognitive influences can directly influence neurophysiology. Such psychological influences are manifold, and only a few examples can be given. Anxiety is a frequent accompaniment to pain, through several mechanisms. Firstly, anxiety increases autonomic arousal, which activates S fibres, and partially opens the gate to the T-cells. Secondly, events normally causing pain, such as punishment or illness, are associated with anxiety, and the learned association of anxiety and pain then causes anticipation of pain, so that cognitive control opens the T-cell gate in expectation of a painful stimulus. Finally, minor symptoms, which occur all the time (a mild ache in the knee, for instance), and for which there is often an immediate explanation ('I banged the knee yesterday') can become exaggerated in the absence of an explanation ('perhaps this is bone cancer'), which produces anxiety, and the dull ache then becomes a mild pain, generating further anxiety, and more support for the sinister interpretation, producing more anxiety, more pain, etc.

Stress appears to have opposite effects to anxiety, reducing pain (STRESS ANALGESIA), probably via the peri-aqueductal grey matter. This makes good biological sense, since in an emergency pain could impair an organism's coping ability. In animals, experimental analgesia can be induced by repeated unavoidable foot shocks. There are at least two mechanisms, one involving the pituitary-adrenal system (probably based on endogenous adrenal medullary opiate-like peptides), and the other involving a non-opiate system. Stress analgesia can also be conditioned, as animals placed in a chamber where previously they have received foot shock analgesia show pain suppression without foot shocks; this suppression depends upon internal opiates, being blocked by naloxone, and showing cross-tolerance with morphine.

Pain control is central to medical practice and many techniques are available. Drugs are discussed at length in textbooks of pharmacology. However, drugs do not always produce adequate pain relief, or else in severe pain can only provide relief at doses that impair consciousness to a degree the patient finds unacceptable. Non-pharmacological techniques are available, many derived from the gate control theory. Surgical techniques, such as TRACTOTOMY, sever the spino-thalamic tract interrupting the T-cell output to the brain. Electrophysiological techniques use implanted electrodes to stimulate directly the dorsal spinal roots, or the dorsal columns, to decrease T-cell activity by stimulating L fibres. Less invasive, but also effective, is TRANSCUTANEOUS NERVE STIMULATION, in which electrical currents stimulate large peripheral nerve fibres directly, producing an immediate and continuing analgesia lasting several hours after stimulation, presumably due to SG cells being 'turned on'.

Effective psychological techniques use two major approaches, reduction of small fibre input and direct cognitive closure of the gate. Pains such as headache are associated with increased frontalis muscle tension producing excessive small fibre input. Tension, and hence autonomic S fibre activity, is reduced indirectly by RELAXATION THERAPY, which reduces all muscle activity, or directly by BIOFEEDBACK, in which electrodes over the muscle provide feedback about muscle tension and the patient learns to reduce activity in the specific muscle. Both techniques are highly effective when used properly. An alternative technique is to encourage COGNITIVE COPING SKILLS, so the patient learns to cope with their pain, to ignore it, and thus for the gate to close and pain actually to diminish. Several methods are used: in IMAGINATIVE INATTENTION, patients are trained to ignore pain by concentrating on other vivid images, such as being at a party, on the beach, or lying in a hot soothing bath; in SOMATIZATION the patient focuses attention on the pain in a remote manner, treating it as external to himself, in academic, intellectual fashion. Such techniques positively exploit defence mechanisms, and are undoubtedly effective. Finally, psychological, drug, and stimulation treatments are combined in MULTIPLE CONVERGENT THERAPY, the combination being more effective than the individual components.

The gate control theory has revolutionized medical approaches to pain, emphasizing that pain is both a perception and a response, and hence under psychological control, albeit within a biological context.

21

Drugs: placebos, addiction and abuse

- Drugs do not only have actions because of their pharmacological effects, but also because of their SYMBOLIC ACTIONS and the EXPECTANCIES associated with them.
- The prescription of a drug is not based only upon strictly medical criteria but is also a response to a social situation.
- PLACEBOS work not mainly because of their size, shape or other physical properties but because of the EXPECTANCIES attached to them, which are acquired by learning, from previous experience, and from social influences.
- PLACEBO RESPONDERS differ from non-responders in many ways, including an ability to produce internal opiates, the action of which can be blocked by naloxone.
- Drug addicts can be classified according to whether they are conformist or unconventional, and whether or not they are part of a DRUG SUBCULTURE, resulting in four types, JUNKIES, STABLES, TWO-WORLDERS and LONERS.
- Opiate addiction occurs rarely after administration for medical purposes because it is not easy for patients to associate the drug's effect with its actual administration.

Drugs are chemicals that alter physiological functioning, and as such are principally the study of pharmacology. However, drugs also exist in a social context, in which they are ascribed properties and powers that transcend pure pharmacology. A majority of GP consultations result in a 'script', a drug prescription. Some of these prescriptions satisfy only the doctors, for 10–20% are never taken to a pharmacist, and must therefore be presumed unwanted by the patients. In other cases, doctors are pressurized by patients to prescribe, despite little likelihood of pharmacological benefit (although benefit may still occur). Many active drugs are also obtained over a chemist's counter without prescription; and patients also use prescription-only drugs prescribed for relatives and friends (particularly skin-creams). Finally, drugs are used illegally, typically opiates or their derivatives or analogues, and psychoactive substances such as amphetamines and

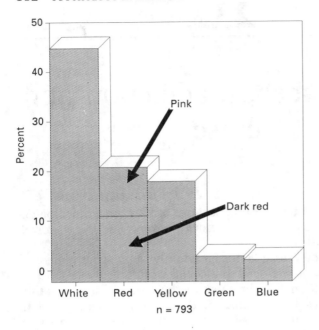

Fig. 21.1 The colours of 793 tablets described in the 1975 edition of the MIMS tablet identification charts.

barbiturates, resulting in a specific DRUG CULTURE, with its own mores and traditions. The term 'drug culture' also reminds us that drugs are a part of general culture, with all its assumptions and inconsistencies, and are not solely the province of pharmacology, but also are part of social science. As an example, drugs have symbolic properties, represented by their colouring and appearance. Although many tablets are 'the little white ones', many are brightly coloured (Fig. 21.1). Since the colours are usually unrelated to the active agent, they must have some other meaning, particularly since colours are not random, certain colours occurring with certain classes of drugs. Drugs for the cardiovascular system (frequently to reduce blood pressure) are often blue, a traditionally calming and soothing colour, and drugs for the genito-urinary system, frequently diuretics, tend to be yellow, perhaps because they are associated with urine. Tablets with nutritional functions are often red, and are mainly iron preparations for pregnant women. However, iron as prescribed is ferrous sulphate (which is green) rather than ferric sulphate (which is red). Nevertheless, iron is commonly associated with red (i.e. rust), thus explaining the mainly red tablets. Drugs acting against infections (mainly antibiotics) are often red (imitating the *calor* and *rubor*, the warmth and inflammation, associated with the body's own healing response to infection); significantly they are *not* green, the colour of putrefaction and gangrene. Finally in the hormone group, of which many are oral contraceptives, almost none are red, perhaps because of an association with menstruation. Such associations are not mere statistical coinci-

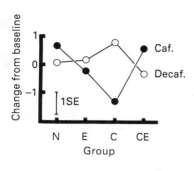

Fig. 21.2 The influence of beliefs about whether or not a drink contains caffeine (Caf) or does not contain caffeine (Decaf), and about whether or not caffeine is likely to be the active agent in coffee (groups N, E, C and CE: see text for details) upon the speed at carrying out a complex psychological task relative to base-line performance (so that negative values indicate faster performance). There is a significant interaction ($p < .025$) between belief about caffeine content and belief about caffeine efficacy. Actual caffeine content had no relation to performance. Unpublished study by Price R and McManus I C (1984), Does a placebo work if you know it's a placebo?

dences, but instead reflect the social and psychological meanings attached to drugs.

The subtle effects of expectations about drug effects are seen in an experiment on the effects of caffeine, in the form of instant coffee, upon a complex cognitive task requiring the simultaneous mental calculation of several running totals. Student subjects repeated the experiment on four successive days in a counter-balanced order, receiving ordinary instant coffee on two days and decaffeinated instant coffee on the other two days. The coffee was made in front of the subject from jars labelled by the manufacturers as caffeinated or decaffeinated, although in half the cases the contents did not correspond with the labels, so that true pharmacological effects of caffeine could therefore be distinguished from expectancies. On day one each subject was given one of four ostensible 'explanations' of why coffee might have effects upon psychological performance. Group C was told it was 'well-known' that performance improved due to caffeine content. Group E was told that actually caffeine was not the active substance in coffee, but recent work had found caffeine had no effect, and performance improved due to endorphin-like substances (and indeed a recent paper in *Nature* had suggested that coffee contained substances binding to morphine receptors). Group CE was told both caffeine *and* endorphins improved psychological performance, and group N was told that scientific research had found there were actually no psychologically active substances in coffee. The results showed that actual caffeine content had no influence on performance, but effects depended instead upon the perceived caffeine content (i.e. the labels) and performance only improved when supposedly caffeinated coffee was drunk *and* the subject believed both that caffeine was the active substance in coffee *and* that it was the only active substance in coffee (Fig. 21.2). In the other cases there was no effect of perceived caffeine content. The effect of the drug therefore depended upon thinking that the substance was pharmacologically active, and

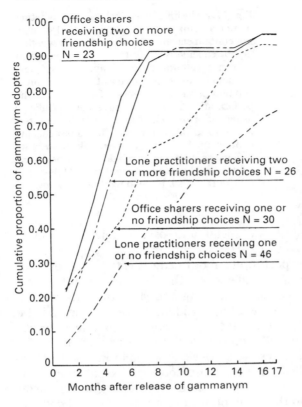

Fig. 21.3 *a*) The proportion of various groups of doctors who had started to prescribe a new drug, gammanym, at various times after its release onto an American market. Doctors were divided according to whether they were in practice on their own (lone) or with others (office sharers) and whether they had extensive social contacts, being named by two or more other doctors as 'friendship choices'.

believing that it was present and also believing no other active substance was present.

Decisions to prescribe drugs also reflect social and psychological factors, and are illustrated by two examples. Nearly 600 GPs were sent case histories of patients with a sore throat, together with a photograph of the tonsils, and were asked if they would prescribe an antibiotic. Minor changes in the history significantly altered the decision; thus 16% of GPs prescribed an antibiotic for the 'Son (aged 12) of the newly appointed district medical officer', whereas 24% prescribed an antibiotic for the 'Son (aged 12) of the newly appointed hospital consultant surgeon': non-medical factors clearly influence apparently pure clinical decisions. The second example is an American study of the prescription, after its release on the market, of a new drug, given the pseudonym 'Gammanym', by different practitioners in an area (Fig. 21.3a). The social conditions under which doctors worked, and their degree of membership of the local medical network, related to speed of uptake. Mathematical modelling (Fig. 21.3b) showed that doctors having frequent social contacts passed the information by word of mouth in a 'chain reaction', whereas more isolated doctors happened upon the new drug by chance.

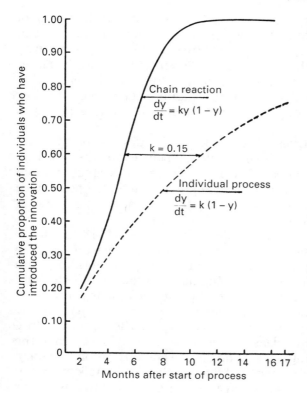

Fig. 21.3 *b*) The theoretical curves expected for two different processes of spread of knowledge about the drug. In the 'individual process' each doctor randomly finds out about the drug, and hence the rate of new adoptions of the drug (dy/dt) is simply proportional to the number of individuals who have as yet not found out about it $(1 - y)$. In the chain reaction process, doctors who do know about the drug (y) pass information on to those who do not know about it $(1 - y)$, so that the rate of change is proportion to $y(1 - y)$, producing a steeper, differently shaped curve. Reproduced with permission from Coleman J S, Katz E and Menzel H (1966), *Medical Innovation: a diffusion study*, Indianapolis, Bobbs-Merrill.

The rest of this chapter considers two psychological aspects of drug behaviour; the action of placebos and the problem of drug abuse and addiction.

PLACEBOS AND THE PLACEBO EFFECT

Placebos are essential for the standard PLACEBO-CONTROLLED CLINICAL TRIAL, in which an active drug is compared with an inert, inactive substance, a placebo. In 1980 the 'Coronary Drug Project Research Group' described a large clinical trial comparing the effects of the hypocholesterolaemic drug, clofibrate, upon coronary artery disease mortality in 1103 men receiving the active drug and 2789 men receiving the placebo. Five-year mortality was the same in both groups (20.0% vs. 20.9%). The authors were worried that not all patients might have taken the drugs regularly, and indeed 33% of patients had taken less than four-fifths of their prescribed tablets. Mortality was higher in the less reliable group (24.9%) than in those who took their tablets reliably (16.2%), the effect being the same in those on active drug

(22.5% *vs* 15.7%) or placebo (25.8% *vs* 16.4%). Either the taking of the tablets had itself conferred benefit by an unknown mechanism, or the people who took tablets reliably were different in some way from non-takers, and had inherently different risks of death. Either way the effect of tablet taking is far greater than any benefit due to pharmacological action. If clinical trials ignore such processes they risk misinterpreting drug actions and missing interesting processes underlying disease.

Placebo-controlled trials often find, to the despair of the trial organizer, that a new drug is of no particular benefit, and the beneficial effect of the placebo compared with no treatment is ignored. Such placebo effects raise many interesting questions, and may possibly be exploited themselves in order to provide therapy (and therapy which is often reassuringly devoid of true side-effects).

The Oxford English Dictionary cites Hooper's Medical Dictionary of 1811 as the first usage in its medical sense of the word PLACEBO: '*placebo*... an epithet given to any medicine adapted more to please than benefit the patient'. This meaning fits with the Latin derivation, 'I shall please', but misses the important point that despite being given only to please, the placebo can actually benefit the patient, by reducing symptoms or modifying physical signs. The PLACEBO, a drug administered merely to please, should be distinguished from the PLACEBO EFFECT, of a therapeutic action despite administration as a mere nostrum. It has also been suggested that we should also talk of NOCEBOS and a NOCEBO EFFECT, treatments given precisely to be unpleasant (as in bitter-tasting tonics) or which result in deleterious effects.

Much has been written on the physical characteristics of the placebo, but most is inconclusive. Blue preparations are said to be better than red, multicoloured better than single-coloured, which are better than colourless, bitter preparations better than sweet, and that 'an extraordinarily large pill impresses by its size, an exceptionally small one by its potency'. In general, there are no adequate studies demonstrating simple effects of the physical nature of the placebo: the patient's or subject's *impression* of the preparation is the crucial factor. In one study, a lactose placebo and phenobarbitone capsules were each without effect because they tasted sweet and the student subjects inferred that each was a placebo; putting them in hard tablets covered in sour-tasting ascorbic acid restored their appropriate actions. Similarly, a GP reported a neurotic patient in whom several placebo preparations had failed until he and his partner acted out a charade in which the GP described one last particularly strong preparation, wherein the partner entered wearing rubber gloves, unscrewed the jar of placebo tablets, removed one with tweezers, and placed it directly in the patient's mouth; the elaborate safety precautions convinced the patient of the placebo's efficacy.

Placebo responding is therefore a *psychological* process determined by our expectations. The old joke about an Englishman *expecting* a pill, an American *expecting* an injection, and a Frenchman *expecting* a suppository, contains a grain of truth.

The three broad psychological theories of placebo responding all involve learning in some form. Humans are often erroneously thought to be the only species showing placebo effects. In an experiment rats were injected with intraperitoneal scopolamine for a number of days. The drug modifies lever-pressing behaviour in a Skinner box, and the effects were clearly observed. After a few days an intraperitoneal injection of a saline placebo was given and produced a similar modification in lever-pressing behaviour. The rats had *learned* the effects of the drug, and therefore 'expected' that yet another injection would also have the same effect. In another study, the probability of a placebo response to amphetamine in rats was directly proportional to the number of active injections, and hence of opportunities for learning. Similar learning is seen in humans. In one experiment subjects were given sublingual glyceryl trinitrate on several occasions, resulting in tachycadia; a similar but inert capsule then resulted also in an increased heart rate, implying that the effects of the drug had been learnt.

A second theory of placebo responding suggests that various SITUATIONAL features of drugs are learnt. If we have a mild pain for which aspirin is usually adequate then a small white tablet may be an adequate placebo. If however our pain is different from those for which we normally use aspirin then a small, white, aspirin-like placebo will not be effective. There is a specific association of symptoms, situation and effectiveness.

A third theory emphasizes social factors in determining placebo responses. If surrounded by people who say a drug has a particular effect, or in whom we have faith, or whom we find threatening, then we are more likely to report drug effects. In one study, side-effects to an inert lactose tablet were proportional to neuroticism when subjects were tested in small groups but were independent of neuroticism when tested individually. Other studies have asked regular cannabis users to rate different 'joints' for their effect; placebo joints were almost as effective as the actual drug, suggesting that the social milieu of cannabis smoking contributes most of the reported psychoactive effects.

Placebos are not equally effective in all conditions. Diseases with the greatest placebo effect are those where symptoms are most under cerebral control, for instance in pain relief, and the relief of migraine, dysmenorrhoea, rheumatic pain and sea-sickness. Similarly in the psychological laboratory the largest placebo effects occur with the most 'cerebral' measures such as speed of response, less occur with measures of accuracy, and least with 'physiological' measures such as flicker fusion frequency or after-image duration.

One of the commonest situations in which placebos are used is pain relief, and there seems little doubt of its effectiveness in clinical practice, even working in situations where morphine would normally be used. However, laboratory studies using controlled stimuli find a much reduced placebo response, and signal detection analysis finds the effect to be entirely a change in *beta* rather than in *d'*. Two separate factors explain this discrepancy. Anxious subjects have repeatedly been found to be placebo responders, and placebos are very effective in reducing anxiety. However, laboratory pain is less associated with anxiety (being less 'real') than clinical pain, and hence responds less to placebos. The second difference is that laboratory studies typically look at pain *threshold*, whereas pain *tolerance* is more relevant in clinical practice. In a recent laboratory study, ischaemic arm pain was produced with an arterial tourniquet, and both pain threshold and tolerance assessed. The anxiety of the subjects was not related to pain threshold or to their placebo response to threshold, whereas anxiety was strongly related to the placebo response to pain tolerance. The implication for clinical work is obvious; if anxiety can be reduced then the vicious circle of anxiety aggravating pain will be broken, and placebos can have precisely that effect.

Studies of placebo response to pain show that some people are stronger placebo responders than others, and many studies have tried to distinguish responders from non-responders. Responders are more neurotic, more introverted, and of lower intelligence. In hospital patients, placebo responders were more impressed with their hospital care, asked for medications less often, were more cooperative with nursing staff, had had less education, and were more frequent church-goers than non-responders. Placebo responders are also more suggestible, acquiesce more easily in the suggestions of others, and are more religious in outlook. Together this suggests that many characteristics of placebo responders are explicable in terms of response or social characteristics, although other aspects are more closely related to personality differences.

Thus far little has been said about the *mechanism* of placebo effects. At present a mechanism is partly understood in only one placebo effect, in dental analgesia. Patients having wisdom teeth removed were all given a placebo injection two hours post-operatively, and then rated their pain on a scale. The patients were divided into two groups, according to whether the injection reduced their pain (placebo responders) or did not alter it (non-responders). One hour later an injection of naloxone, a morphine antagonist, was given. The placebo responders showed *increased* pain after the naloxone, whereas non-responders showed no change in pain levels. Thus naloxone blocked the placebo response in responders, suggesting that they produced an endogenous opiate in response to the placebo, that the opiate had produced analgesia, and its action was blocked by naloxone. The interpretation is compatible with evidence that naloxone does not affect laboratory pain (i.e. threshold rather than tolerance) and it also explains why placebos mainly affect tolerance rather than threshold, since morphine's principal action is not to reduce the actual pain but rather to reduce its motivational and emotional consequences, making it tolerable, albeit still present; presumably endogenous opiates would have a similar effect.

DRUG ABUSE AND ADDICTION

Opiates (morphine, heroin and synthetic analogues such as methodone) and cocaine are the classic drugs of ADDICTION, although addiction also occurs with many other drugs such as amphetamines, barbiturates and benzodiazepines, and ABUSE can occur with almost any chemical, recent examples being the toluene-based glues which have been inhaled from plastic bags (GLUE-SNIFFING). Addiction, or physical dependency in which WITHDRAWAL SYMPTOMS occur on stopping, must be distinguished from PSYCHOLOGICAL DEPENDENCY, where the drug fulfils psychological not physical needs for the person. As well as those physically or psychologically dependent on drugs, there are also many individuals who use drugs occasionally on a 'recreational' basis; thus in America about 45% of high school seniors have used marijuana (cannabis) within the previous year, and about 20% of college students have used cocaine in the past year.

Opiate addiction in Britain has three separate stages in the past half century: relatively constant from 1935 to 1963 with about 500 registered addicts; then a sharp acceleration in the 'swinging sixties', plateauing in the seventies; and then increasing again in the early 1980s, partly in response to increasing youth unemployment. The reasons for addiction have also changed; in 1960, 309 of the 437 known addicts were THERAPEUTIC ADDICTS, who had become addicted after medical treatment with the drug, and a further 63 were MEDICAL ADDICTS, members of the medical profession with easy access to opiates. Such cases have remained constant in number for half a century. The remaining addicts have increased in numbers dramatically, and are the ones now purchasing heroin or other illegal drugs on the streets. It is tempting to assume that this is a homogenous group of 'junkies', but this is not adequate as there are at least four distinct groups, separated along two dimensions. Some opiate addicts are relatively CONFORMIST AND CONVENTIONAL, with regular jobs and a steady income, whereas others are unconventional, often unemployed, and drifting without steady income. The second dimension concerns involvement with the DRUG SUBCULTURE, addicts associating principally with other addicts and eventually spending more and more time with them, and ceasing to be part of a broader culture. The subculture provides three essential needs: the SKILLS for administration of the drug, INFORMATION about drug availability, and an IDEOLOGY, a set of justifications for the addicts' life-style (for as William Burroughs puts it, 'Junk is not a kick. It's a way of life'). Obtaining the several-times daily FIX becomes both the central problem and the purpose of living. That the drug subculture maintains addiction is shown by the 50% of new heroin users who cease using the drug because supplies dry up and they do not know other sources. Of the four types of addicts, the stereotype recognized by the public and media is the JUNKIE, who has little involvement with the conventional world, and high involvement with the subculture; unemployed, and short of money to buy heroin, they resort to criminal activities, involving fraud, burglary, prostitution and drug-dealing to finance purchases from illicit street vendors. In contrast, there is a large group of STABLES, who are involved in the conventional world and not in the subculture, obtaining drugs legally from medical practitioners, being registered as addicts and living lives of apparent normality and respectability, with an income from conventional jobs. These addicts often survive for long periods, as do therapeutic and medical addicts, and are exemplified by an 81 year old woman in one survey who had taken 180 g of morphine daily for 63 years, and who was still alert and well adjusted, implying that chronic opiate usage *per se* does not cause physical or intellectual deterioration. The third group of addicts is the TWO-WORLDERS, who like stables have a regular income but also are involved in the subculture, often dealing and carrying out criminal activities, but basically living two separate lives, each rigidly compartmentalized. Finally, LONERS belong neither to conventional society nor the subculture, and many are psychopathic, unable to form relationships or join ordinary social groups. This differentiation of addicts in relation to conventional society and the subculture also generalizes to other behaviours, such as alcoholism, homosexuality and prostitution, in which subcultures develop, and participants are either part of the 'scene', becoming immersed totally, reject it entirely, or try and live in both worlds at once.

As suggested earlier, chronic opiate usage itself need cause little harm and can be compatible with a normal longevity, without increased risk of psychosis or diminished intellect. However the complications of drug administration, such as transmission of hepatitis and AIDS by sharing syringes and needles, the development of bacterial endocarditis from tap or lavatory water used for preparing injections, and development of abscesses at injection sites, are serious causes of morbidity and mortality, and are particularly common in the subculture, where syringe sharing is common.

The several types of addicts suggest there is unlikely to be a single cause for addiction, and naive attempts to find the ADDICTION-PRONE PERSONALITY are probably misguided, despite a higher incidence of 'personality disorders' in addicts. Similarly, addicts do not all gain the same benefits from their addiction; neurotic personalities report relief of anxiety, psychotic personalities report relief of depression, and psychopathic personalities report elation from their drugs. Nevertheless, some individuals may be genetically more prone to the actions of opiates; in rats selective breeding experiments have obtained strains with a preference for morphine. Recent work suggests some drug addicts might have low levels of self-produced endorphins, which are then provided exogenously by injection.

Heroin injections in normal volunteers are not reported as pleasant, at least for the first few occasions, although a sense of euphoria develops after a while (although it subsequently disappears as TOLERANCE develops). In rats, it is controversial whether pleasure occurs in response to morphine injection, since withdrawal effects are apparent even 24 hours after first administration (particularly if drug action is terminated suddenly with naloxone), and hence further self-adminstration may be to prevent withdrawal rather than to produce positive emotions. In man, opiate withdrawal produces sweating, anorexia, gooseflesh (hence the colloquial term 'cold turkey'), dilated pupils, diarrhoea, restlessness, hypertension, fever and insomnia, and rats show similar symptoms, along with 'wet dog shakes', chattering of the teeth and bulging eyes. Recent work in rats suggests that morphine analgesia is blocked by naloxanazine without altering physical dependence and withdrawal; tolerance and analgesia may therefore use separate brain mechanisms, raising the hope of opiate-like analgesics which are not addictive, and kappa opiate agonists apparently have precisely these actions.

A problem for theories of addiction is that each year several hundred thousand people in Britain receive opiates medically, usually for post-operative analgesia, but only a very few become addicted. One explanation is that addiction requires perception of a precise causal association between drug injection and subsequent effects (be they positive or merely the absence of unpleasant effects). Such perception is easy for the self-injecting addict, but is not so obvious for the post-operative patient who receives many injections, only some of which are opiates, and has many strange physiological responses only some of which are due to opiates, so that the causal association is far from obvious.

A final problem for any explanation of the mechanisms of addiction is that addicts frequently change drugs, often with a cavalier lack of respect for the known facts of psychopharmacology; for instance in the early 1960s when supplies of illicit amphetamine dried up, addicts simply turned to heroin, apparently thereby satisfying their previous needs. The implication is that addicts are not principally addicts for pharmacological reasons.

Sociological theories of addiction emphasize the concept of ANOMIE, a loss of the sense of rules or purpose in society, often occurring when the GOALS prescribed by society are incommensurate with the MEANS provided for attaining them and with the NORMS of behaviour that are allowed. The resulting despair drives addicts into the subculture, where different social rules apply. Although conceived to explain addiction in deprived inner-city areas, especially in association with poor education and high unemployment, the concept also explains the apparently surprising use of drugs amongst conspicuously non-deprived groups such as pop stars and the overly rich but otherwise incompetent and inadequate children of highly successful parents; in each case there are no goals appropriate for means, and the subculture provides new goals.

22

Stress, anxiety and psychosomatic disease

- STRESS and AROUSAL are separate concepts, stress representing a psychological response and arousal a physiological response. The combination is ANXIETY.
- Pre- and post-operative anxiety can be reduced by preparation in which the patient is told the physical and psychological consequences of the operation and is taught strategies for dealing with events such as pain.
- Stress has deleterious physiological consequences via the GENERAL ADAPTATION SYNDROME, which mediates via the adrenal cortex, in contrast to the FIGHT-OR-FLIGHT MECHANISM which mediates via the adrenal medulla.
- High cortisol levels have wide-ranging physiological effects, including a suppression of immune functioning which may be important in the progress of malignant disease.
- LIVE-EVENTS such as death of a spouse, divorce and job loss are associated with illness such as myocardial infarction.
- Individuals with the TYPE A PERSONALITY have higher levels of blood cortisol, glucose and triglycerides, and have a higher rate of coronary artery disease.

STRESS as a psychological concept derives from physics, where it has two meanings: a force *imposed* upon a system, and the effect of a force *upon* the system (which may fatigue or break). Both meanings occur in psychology and are usually clearly delineated, although occasionally STRESSOR is used for the stimulus, and DISTRESS for the response.

Stressors take many forms (overwork, high temperature, loud noises, surgical operations) and if prolonged and severe, they produce a complex, non-specific set of behavioural and physiological changes described by Hans Selye (1907–1982), a Canadian endocrinologist, as the GENERAL ADAPTATION SYNDROME (GAS). In phase I (the ALARM REACTION) there is an initial brief fall in RESISTANCE TO STRESS during the SHOCK, but then the COUNTERSHOCK is followed by phase II (the STAGE OF RESISTANCE), which shows the behavioural changes of increased resistance to stress, until eventually in phase III COLLAPSE, the STAGE OF EXHAUSTION is reached, with FAILURE TO COPE and a precipitous fall in resistance to stress.

AROUSAL is a separate concept from stress, primarily physiological in origin, and reflecting sympathetic activity, with increased heart-rate and raised metabolism. It is produced by many behaviours and need not be at all distressing. The physiology of an athlete crossing the finishing line, of an actor on the stage, or of sexual orgasm, all involve arousal, but it is not stressful, better being described as 'joyous excitement'.

Since arousal and stress are independent, all combinations occur. The separate components are measured easily by simple question-naires. Low stress and low arousal are associated with DROWSINESS, and low arousal and high stress produce UNDERSTIMULATION or BOREDOM. High arousal and low stress is described as EXCITEMENT, whereas high arousal with high stress is a state of overstimulation labelled as ANXIETY, 'a vague, unpleasant emotional state with qualities of apprehension, dread, distress and uneasiness'; it has been described as the archetypal emotion of the twentieth century. Anxiety is often accompanied by autonomic over-arousal (seen particularly as tachycardia, but also tremor, hyperventilation, urinary frequency and diarrhoea, symptoms known to all exam candidates). Objective measurements of stress by recording simple heart-rate are not successful because many other confounding processes also cause tachycardia. However FOURIER ANALY-SIS of heart rate extracts a component varying at about 0.1 Hz (i.e. every ten seconds) which reflects vasomotor control and relates to perceived stress in situations such as driving in heavy traffic (Fig. 22.1).

Anxiety impairs efficiency on many tasks, although not in a straightforward way. The YERKES-DODSON LAW says performance shows an inverted-U relation to anxiety, increasing anxiety improving performance until a maximum is reached, after which performance falls away, being poor at high anxiety levels. A little anxiety can benefit performance, but a lot is harmful, and optimal anxiety decreases as task difficulty increases, probably because otherwise useful cognitive activity is wasted on monitoring the effects of anxiety, leaving less resources available for actual processing.

Anxiety is readily assessed by questionnaires such as Spielberger's STATE-TRAIT ANXIETY INVENTORY (STAI), which measures both STATE and TRAIT ANXIETY (see Chapter 8). As an example, Figure 22.2 shows state anxiety levels in medical students immediately before a preclinical viva examination, and before or after their medical school selection interview, in comparison with age-sex norms for four different situations. Anxiety is slightly greater before the selection interview than after, but in each case is low compared with the very high levels before a viva examination.

Anxiety is common in all hospital patients, and should always be

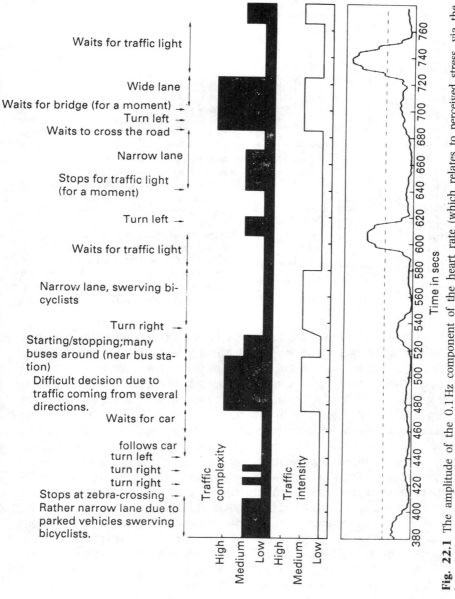

Fig. 22.1 The amplitude of the 0.1 Hz component of the heart rate (which relates to perceived stress, via the hypothalamico-pituitary-adrenal axis) of a person driving in heavy Dutch traffic (and hence turning *left* is a particularly difficult manoeuvre). Note that stress *suppresses* the 0.1 Hz component, so that low levels indicate high stress. Reproduced with permission from Mulder G (1980), *The Heart in mental effort*, unpublished PhD thesis, University of Groningen.

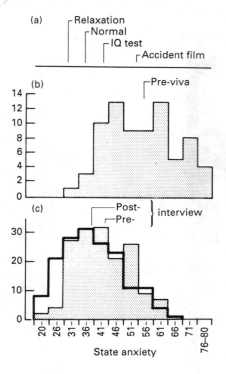

Fig. 22.2 State anxiety levels: *a*) of control subjects while relaxing, when they had just entered the laboratory ('normal'), when they had taken a timed IQ test, and when they had just seen a film of 'gruesome woodworking accidents'. *b*) anxiety levels of preclinical medical students just prior to an important *viva voce* examination. *c*) anxiety levels of medical school applicants just before or after their selection interview. Reproduced with permission from Arndt C B, Guly U M V and McManus I C (1986), Pre-clinical anxiety: the stress associated with a *viva voce* examination, *Medical Education*, **20**, 274–80.

thought about. Figure 22.3 shows anxiety levels before major, minor and dental surgery, showing that anxiety is almost universal before surgery, and extends both before and after the procedure. Careful studies show that pre-operative anxiety is reduced by psychological preparation; giving a clear, realistic description of what to expect physically (will there be drainage tubes? will they be in Intensive Care?) and psychologically (the degree, extent and treatment of pain, etc.). In comparison with controls, reduced post-operative morphine doses are required in patients undergoing intra-abdominal operations who have received pre-operative psychological preparation emphasizing active self-control of pain (e.g. by relaxing abdominal muscles and avoiding tensing muscles while moving) (Fig. 22.4).

Stress is important in medicine because of the recurrent idea, expressed more by patients than doctors, that the stress of daily life causes illness. Stress-induced illness is an example of PSYCHOSOMATIC DISEASE in which instead of the more easily understood sequence of bodily disease affecting the brain and mind ('somatopsychic disease'), the primary event is thought to be behavioural or psychological, which then causes pathological change in the body. Psychosomatic causation for disease is easy to postulate, but difficult to prove convincingly, and several methodological problems are often ignored. Firstly, the mere correlation of two events, A and B, does not prove

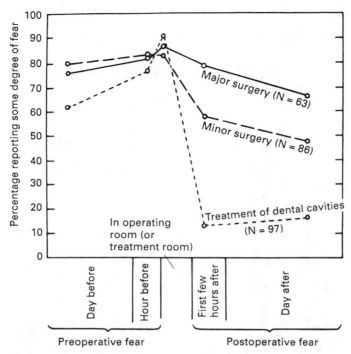

Fig. 22.3 Reported anxiety levels in relation to severity of surgery. Reproduced with permission from Janis I L (1958), *Psychological Stress*, New York, John Wiley, 284.

causation; although A may indeed cause B, B may also cause A, or A and B may be caused by some third event C. Thus it may be that persons regularly attending football matches might be more likely to develop lung cancer, but there is no point in postulating a psychosomatic effect, with the stress of the game *causing* lung cancer, when far more likely is that social class or cigarette smoking correlate with both variables, and create a spurious correlation. A second error is to think that behaviours occur in isolation, whereas in reality they are part of a broader nexus of behaviours. As an example, a recent book claimed that since divorcees had a higher rate of carcinoma of the cervix, then this must be caused by the stress of divorce, and hence cancer of the cervix should be classified as psychosomatic. Divorcees, however, are different from the general population, tending to have had their first sexual intercourse at an earlier age, to have had more sexual partners, more sexually transmitted disease, and married younger. Since strong evidence suggests that carcinoma of the cervix can be caused by infection with *herpes simplex* type II viruses, which are spread like other sexually transmitted diseases, the most parsimonious explanation of the excess of cervical malignancy in divorcees is that they have a higher rate of herpetic infection. Such

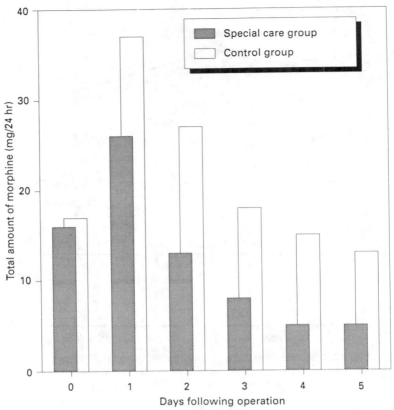

Fig. 22.4 Total daily post-operative morphine requirements of patients who had special psychological preparation for surgery, compared with a control group. Redrawn with permission from Egbert L, Batit G, Welch C and Bartlett M (1964), Reduction of post-operative pain by encouragement and instruction of patients, *New England Journal of Medicine*, **270**, 825–7.

analysis begs the question of *why* these individuals had more sexual behaviour, and it cannot exclude the possibility that the stress of divorce either precipitated disease, prevented its early detection, or enhanced its growth. These possibilities might all be true, but still the original hypothesis of psychosomatic disease causation cannot be supported by the original data. Merely suggesting a psychosomatic aetiology does not dispense with the need for rigorous scientific analysis of cause and effect.

An interesting example of a psychosomatic process that seems beyond serious doubt concerns the simple association of dates of birth and death. Birth dates are known accurately, and are recorded systematically in national statistics. Comparison of dates of birth and death shows individuals are slightly less likely to die in the months before their birthday, and are more likely to die in the months after

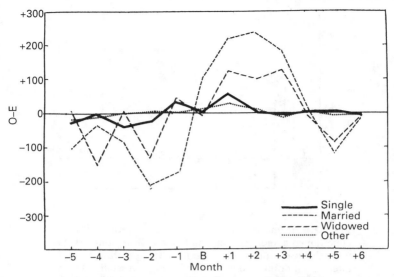

Fig. 22.5 Difference between observed (O) and expected (E) number of deaths of men aged over 74, in England and Wales in 1972, in relation to their birthday (B), according to whether the death was before (minus values) or after (positive values) their birthday. Reproduced with permission from Alderson M (1975), Relationship between month of birth and month of death in the elderly, *British Journal of Preventive and Social Medicine*, **29**, 151–6.

(Fig. 22.5); and the effect is greater over the age of 60, and for the 'important' birthdays, which end in a '5' or a '0'. The simplest explanation is that individuals wish to live until their next birthday, they set this as a goal or challenge, and they successfully strive to achieve it; after the birthday they have less to live for and succumb. The effect is small, affecting only 1% of deaths, but it must be seen as an indubitable triumph of mind over the vicissitudes of body, since basic pathophysiology cannot possibly appreciate the calendar. The converse process, of patients willing themselves to die, and just fading away over days or weeks, is also well documented, and is related to the 'evil eye' phenomenon in primitive tribes in which a person cursed by a witch doctor dies within a matter of days.

Such studies say little of the role of stress in psychosomatic disease, and to understand that we must look at the physiological responses to stressful events that occur. Two separate physiological systems must be distinguished. Cannon's FIGHT-OR-FLIGHT system was discovered first, in which an organism experiences a THREAT TO CONTROL, due to some external event, and there is sympathetic hyperactivity, principally dependent upon adrenaline and noradrenaline from the ADRENAL MEDULLA, although other hormones such as testosterone also increase their levels; corticosteroid levels do not change. The increased arousal

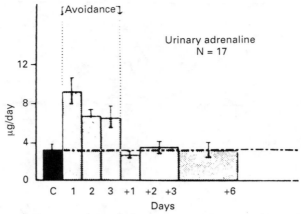

Fig. 22.6 Hormonal responses of monkeys to three days of conditioned avoidance learning (days 1–3) in comparison with the pre-conditioning baseline (C) and the six days after conditioning had ceased. *a*) Urinary adrenaline levels from Mason J W, Tolson W W, Brady J V, Tolliver G A and Gilmore L I (1968), Urinary epinephrine and nore-pinephrine responses to 72-hr avoidance sessions in the monkey, *Psychosomatic Medicine*, **30**, 654–5 and *b*) other hormones, from Mason J W (1968), Organisation of the multiple endocrine responses to avoidance in the monkey, *Psychosomatic Medicine*, **30**, 775.

makes the organism better capable of taking emergency action demanded by the threat. Cannon's system must be contrasted with Selye's General Adaptation Syndrome, which has already been mentioned. LOSS OF CONTROL results in high levels of corticosteroid secretion from the ADRENAL CORTEX, reduction in testosterone levels, and little change in adrenaline or noradrenaline levels. The GAS proceeds through the three stages mentioned earlier, during which RESISTANCE changes (it is measured experimentally by exposing animals to cold or infection, and monitoring survival). Resistance decreases during shock, but then recovers and increases above normal levels in phase II, before falling precipitously during exhaustion and death. The fight-or-flight mechanism is probably controlled by the AMYGDALA and the GAS by the SEPTO-HIPPOCAMPAL SYSTEM. Figure 22.6 shows endocrine responses of monkeys coping for three days with a CONDITIONED AVOIDANCE TASK, in which lever presses helped avoid electric shocks. The fight-or-flight response of increased adrenaline occurred on day 1, but decreased thereafter, whereas GAS responses continued throughout the three days, and in some cases, such as urinary 17-OHCS (17-hydroxycorticosteroid, a principal metabolite of the corticosteroids), thyroxine and growth hormone were still raised several days after the schedule had ceased.

Corticosteroids have a wide range of physiological effects, and

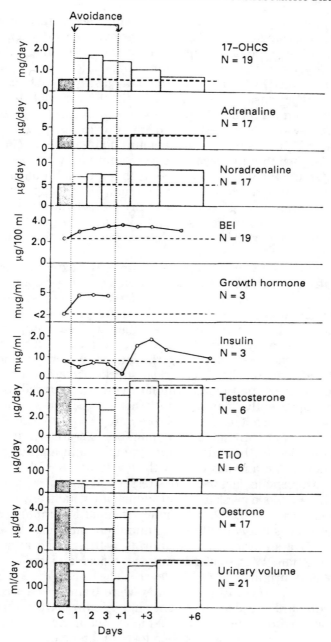

Fig. 22.6 *b) continued*

when administered in large quantities produce peptic ulceration and haemorrhage, diabetes, amenorrhoea, growth retardation, osteoporosis, thinning of the skin, poor wound healing, thrombosis, sodium retention, hypertension and immune suppression. It is therefore possible that the GAS may well underlie diseases such as peptic ulceration, hypertension, rheumatoid arthritis and diabetes, all of which have been claimed to be psychosomatic. Cortisol's effects upon the immune system have resulted in PSYCHONEUROIMMUNOLOGY, which studies the links between brain, behaviour and immune function (and which has argued that the brain views the immune system as another sensory system, which tells it about the internal milieu of the body). Cortisol suppresses immune function, decreasing circulating lymphocytes, and causing a decrease in thymic, splenic and lymphatic tissue. If stress causes cortisol secretion it can then impair immune rejection, as is seen experimentally in mice injected with tumour cells (Fig. 22.7).

The size of the GAS response depends upon the extent of perceived loss of control, and can be assessed biochemically. Figure 22.8 relates urinary hydrocortisone levels in women awaiting breast biopsy for possible malignancy to the degree of failure of psychological defence mechanisms (and these mechanisms are themselves a strong predictor of survival in breast cancer: Fig. 22.9). Perceived control need not be real to be effective, as in experiments in which rats received unpredictable, uncontrollable electrical shocks; isolated rats showed higher ACTH levels than paired animals, which responded to shocks by fighting, apparently 'blaming' the other for the shock, and hence treating it as controllable. Social pressure also produces loss of control; subordinate animals in a dominance hierarchy have higher corticosteroid levels than dominant animals, although eventually levels do fall as the animals cope with low status. Social effects also interact with genetic factors; the stress of living in social groups produces higher blood pressure in rats which are genetically spontaneously hypertensive (Fig. 22.10). Finally it must be emphasized that danger alone does not cause the GAS and there must also be a threat to control. In a study carried out during a threatened attack on a group of Vietnam War soldiers, only the officer and radio-operator had increased urinary 17-OHCS levels. The other men were not suffering a threat to control, since they were trained to act precisely and efficiently under orders, and hence had less threat to control than did the officer, who did not know what to expect in the coming attack, and whose sense of control was therefore threatened.

Stress is also a risk factor in disease in the way individuals respond to life events. Any life, however well-ordered, suffers changes. Some changes, or LIFE-EVENTS, are bad (deaths, financial difficulties, job loss, etc.) and others are good (marriage, children, new job, new house, etc.); however, each requires *change*, and threatens a loss of control,

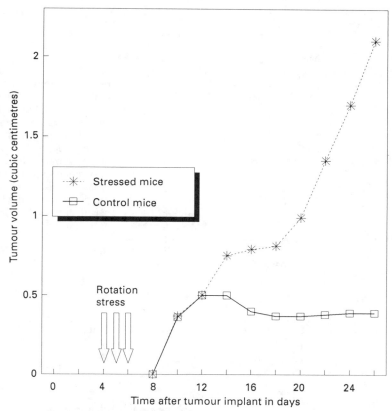

Fig. 22.7 The weight of tumour tissue present in mice which have had the 6C3HED lymphosarcoma implanted subcutaneously on day 0. On days 4, 5 and 6 the experimental group was stressed by spending 10 minutes in each hour in a cage placed on a gramophone turntable rotating at 45 revolutions per minute. Adapted from Riley V (1981), Psychoneuroendocrine influences on immunocompetence and neoplasia, *Science*, **212**, 1100–9.

and hence is stressful. Life-event stress can be measured using a checklist of life-events, the HOLMES-RAHE LIFE CHANGE EVENT INVENTORY (Table 22.1), each of which has been rated for its stress. There is also a special version for students (Table 22.2). Men suffering myocardial infarction have higher life-event scores in the previous six months than controls. That stress comes from *change*, be it good or bad, is seen in studies of death statistics in relation to unemployment and other economic indicators: the death rate rises as unemployment rates rise (as might be predicted) but also rises during rapid economic growth, when increasing wealth and prosperity are accompanied by industrial changes and the need to learn new skills. Following unemployment, death rates rise almost immediately for suicide, after a

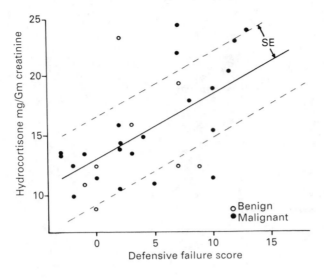

Fig. 22.8 The relation between urinary excretion of hydrocortisone and the failure of defence mechanisms, and development of a sense of loss of social and personal well-being in women undergoing breast biopsy for a lump. Reproduced with permission of author and publishers from Katz J L et al. (1969), *Ann NY Acad Sci,* **164,** 509–15.

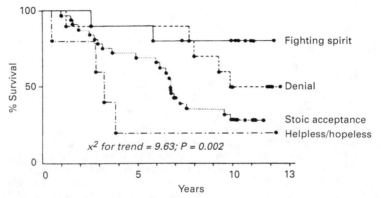

Fig. 22.9 The proportion of women still alive twelve years after breast cancer was diagnosed in relation to the woman's psychological response to the diagnosis (assessed by a psychiatrist within three months of the diagnosis). The difference between groups is not explained by other known predictors of survival such as age, severity at diagnosis, histology, appearance at mammography, or hormonal or immunological measures. Reproduced with permission from Pettingale K W, Morris T, Greer S and Haybittle S L (1985), Mental attitudes to cancer: an additional prognostic factor, *Lancet,* **i**, 750.

lag of two or three years for cardiovascular disease, and after longer lags for chronic diseases, showing the long latencies for psychosomatic effects.

Another source of stress with life-events arises from the person themself. In America, Friedman and Rosenman were studying the diet of patients with myocardial infarctions. The wife of one patient pointed out that she and her husband ate almost identical diets, and

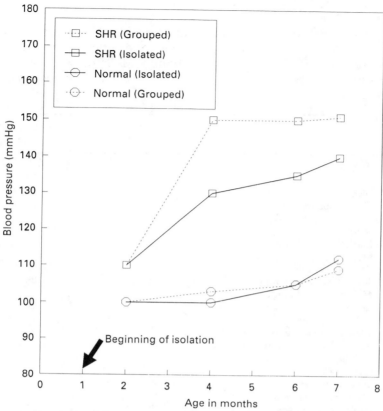

Fig. 22.10 Rats with a genetic tendency to be spontaneously hypertensive (SHR) show a higher blood pressure when kept in social groups than when isolated, whereas no difference is found for normal rats. Redrawn with permission from Hallbaeck M (1975), Interaction between central neurogenic mechanisms and changes in cardiovascular drive in primary hypertension, *Acta Physiol Scand, Suppl 424.*

therefore diet was unlikely to be the problem, and that instead behaviour differences might be the culprit. Spurred on by this, Friedman and Rosenman suggested that the problem might be the TYPE A PERSONALITY, a person aggressively involved in a chronic struggle to achieve too much and to participate in too many events, particularly when under challenge. Many characteristics of type A behaviour, such as a desire to compete, achieve and be successful are particularly prevalent in medical students and doctors, and are also found in 10% or more of the population. Type A behaviour is also associated with higher levels of serum ACTH and cortisol, noradrenaline, blood clotting factors, glucose and triglycerides, and with a higher rate of coronary artery disease, even after smoking, obesity, cholesterol and blood pressure have been taken into account.

Table 22.1

The Holmes-Rahe scale of life change events. The value of 50 was arbitrarily assigned to 'Marriage' and other events rated against it. From Holmes T H and Rahe R H (1967), The social readjustment rating scale, *Journal of Psychosomatic Research,* **11**, 213–18.

	LCU values
Family:	
Death of spouse	100
Divorce	73
Marital separation	65
Death of close family member	63
Marriage	50
Marital reconciliation	45
Major change in health of family	44
Pregnancy	40
Addition of new family member	39
Major change in arguments with wife	35
Son or daughter leaving home	29
In-law troubles	29
Wife starting or ending work	26
Major change in family get-togethers	15
Personal:	
Detention in jail	63
Major personal injury or illness	53
Sexual difficulties	39
Death of a close friend	37
Outstanding personal achievement	28
Start or end of formal schooling	26
Major change in living conditions	25
Major revision of personal habits	24
Changing to a new school	20
Change in residence	20
Major change in recreation	19
Major change in church activities	19
Major change in sleeping habits	16
Major change in eating habits	15
Vacation	13
Christmas	12
Minor violations of the law	11
Work:	
Being fired from work	47
Retirement from work	45
Major business adjustment	39
Changing to different time of work	36
Major change in work responsibilities	29
Trouble with boss	23
Major change in working conditions	20

Table 22.1   *Continued.*

Financial:

Major change in financial state	38
Mortgage or loan over $10 000	31
Mortgage foreclosure	30
Mortgage or loan less than $10 000	17

Table 22.2

Scale of 'Life change events experienced by college students'. College entry was arbitrarily assigned a value of 50, and other items rated against it. From Marx M B, Gavrity T F and Bowers F R (1975), The influence of recent life experience on the health of college freshmen, *Journal of Psychosomatic Research*, **19**, 87–98.

	Unit score
Family	
Death of spouse	87
Marriage	77
Death of close family member	77
Divorce	76
Marital separation	74
Pregnancy or fathered a pregnancy	68
Broke or had broken martial engagement or steady relationship	60
Marital reconciliation	58
Major change in health or behaviour of family member	56
Engagement for marriage	54
Major change in number of arguments with spouse	50
Addition of new family member	50
In-law trouble	42
Spouse began or ceased work outside the home	41
Major change in number of family get-togethers	26
Personal	
Death of close friend	68
Major personal injury or illness	65
Sexual difficulties	58
Major change in self-concept or self-awareness	57
Major change in use of drugs	52
Major conflict or change in values	50
Major change in amount of independence and responsibility	49
Major change in use of alcohol	46
Revision of personal habits	45
Major change in social activities	43
Change in residence or living conditions	42
Change in dating habits	41
Outstanding personal achievement	40
Major change in type and/or amount of recreation	37
Major change in church activities	36
Major change in sleeping habits	34

Table 22.2   *Continued.*

Trip or vacation	33
Make change in eating habits	30
Minor violations of the law	22

Work

Fired from work	62
Entered college	50
Changed to different line of work	50
Changed to new school	50
Major change in responsibilities at work	47
Trouble with school administration	44
Held job while attending school	43
Major change in working hours or conditions	42
Change in or choice of major field of study	41
Trouble with boss	38
Major change in participation in school activities	38

Financial

Major change in financial state	53
Mortgage or loan less than $10 000	52

23

Neuropsychology

- The modern theory of MODULARITY sees some psychological functions such as sensory processing and language as LOCALIZED in particular parts of the cortex, whereas other functions such as intelligence are diffusely organized throughout the cortex.
- The left hemisphere is DOMINANT for language processing in 95% of right-handers and 65% of left-handers. The right hemisphere is specialized principally for visuo-spatial processing.
- LICHTHEIM'S MODEL of APHASIA can explain both BROCA'S and WERNICKE'S aphasias, as well as the DISCONNECTION SYNDROMES of CONDUCTION APHASIA and TRANS-CORTICAL APHASIA.
- The deficits found in Broca's and Wernicke's aphasia may not merely be of speech production and perception, but perhaps of deeper linguistic functions such as syntax and semantics.
- Cases of ACQUIRED DYSLEXIA suggest that normal reading is carried out through two separate processes: a PHONOLOGICAL ROUTE, which uses GRAPHEME-PHONEME TRANSLATION, and a semantic or LEXICOGRAPHIC ROUTE, which can read irregularly spelt words and has access to meanings as well as sounds.
- Right hemisphere lesions typically produce the AGNOSIAS, in which sensation and perception are disconnected, and CONSTRUCTIONAL APRAXIA, in which there is an impaired understanding of three-dimensional space.

Selective damage to the brain, by disease or trauma, can result in psychological deficits which illuminate both brain structure and psychological processes. To be successful, NEUROPSYCHOLOGY has several requirements: a method for locating cerebral lesions; a technique for relating psychological deficits to anatomical deficits; and an adequate theory of normal functioning (mere 'natural history' of syndromes is not sufficient to give a clear understanding of *normal* processing).

The localization of lesions has improved dramatically in the past two decades, before which brain slicing at post-mortem was the only reliable technique. Techniques such as COMPUTERIZED TOMOGRAPHY (CT), and MAGNETIC RESONANCE IMAGING (MRI), can now distinguish abnormal areas in the living brain. Newer techniques, such as POSITRON-EMISSION TOMOGRAPHY (PET) show cerebral metabolism and hence functioning, which is physiology rather than anatomy.

If a patient has a particular brain lesion and a specific functional deficit, does that mean the function is carried out at that site? Surprisingly, the answer is No. The lesion might cause a general deficit (say, in memory or cognition) and the task affected is merely the most vulnerable to the general deficit (a threshold effect). The fallacy can be seen in the apocryphal story of the foolish scientist who amputates the legs of a cockroach, and then, after noticing that the cockroach no longer jumps at loud sounds, concludes that the animal hears through its legs. Psychological functions can only be localized by DOUBLE DISSOCIATION (the previous situation being single dissociation). If patient 1 has a lesion at site X and function A impaired (but B intact), and patient 2 has a lesion at site Y and function B impaired (but A intact) then assuming the brains are organized in the same way, then *either* function A is localized at X *or* function B is localized at Y (but with only two patients, we do not know which). *What* is localized must be interpreted with care. Remember the old anecdote of removing a valve from a radio set, hearing it start to whistle, and falsely assuming the valve's function is to stop the set whistling. Pathological functioning can only be interpreted through an adequate knowledge of *normal* functioning.

Some functional processes may not even be localizable. Since the mid nineteenth century there has been debate between two separate schools of neuropsychology. The LOCALIZATIONISTS, inspired by the successful localization of sensory and motor cortex, and by lesions that specifically damaged language (see below), argued that each psychological ability had its own cerebral location. The alternative view, of MASS ACTION, was put most forcefully by the American psychologist Karl Lashley (1890–1958) in the 1930s; the location of a lesion was unimportant, and what mattered was the *size* of the lesion, larger lesions producing greater deficits. Experiments in rats had shown that the deficit in learning a complex maze related only to the *amount* of cortex damaged and not its location; and in humans a decreased IQ related only to lesion size and not location. These two schools have recently been reconciled in the concept of MODULARITY: input-output processing, concerned with sensory analysis, motor control, and language, is organized as discrete, functionally autonomous MODULES which can be individually impaired by localized lesions, whereas general intellectual activity is diffusely organized, and therefore only affected quantitatively by lesions.

Lesions can have different effects upon the brain. DESTRUCTION of an area completely impairs its functions. DISCONNECTION of the fibres between two areas allows each to function normally but a specific deficit occurs if one area needs to communicate with the other; very specific testing may be needed to detect the problem. ISOLATION occurs when all the connections to and from an area are damaged, leaving the area functioning but unable to communicate; the lesion is functionally equivalent to destruction but there is no actual anatomical damage to the area. Lesions also affect more distant parts of the brain: cerebral shock, or DIASCHISIS, probably due to loss of excitation, can inhibit remote areas and physical effects, such as CEREBRAL OEDEMA, a local swelling of damaged tissue, can compromise blood supplies to other areas. RECOVERY can take place in several ways, perhaps due to lesions being incomplete, or to functional take-over by unaffected areas.

An additional complication in interpreting brain lesions is that although the left and right cerebral hemispheres are almost identical anatomically, functionally they are very different. In mid-nineteenth century France, Marc Dax and Paul Broca (1824–1880) noticed that patients who had lost their speech after cerebral damage had *right*-sided hemiplegias, and hence language must be in the *left* cerebral hemisphere, which was referred to as the DOMINANT or MAJOR HEMISPHERE. The situation was soon seen to be more complicated, with language dominance related to right- and left-handedness, although left-handers were *not* the mirror-image of right-handers; in 95% of right-handers the left hemisphere is dominant, whereas in left-handers, only 65% show left-hemisphere dominance. A majority of both right- and left-handers therefore show left hemisphere dominance, but left-handers show greater variation than right-handers. Left-handedness and language dominance are probably inherited by the same single Mendelian gene which produces FLUCTUATING ASYMMETRY, a random determination of handedness and language dominance, which means that neither right nor left-handers 'breed true', and that monozygotic twins are often discordant for handedness.

Cerebral dominance can be assessed by several techniques. In DICHOTIC LISTENING a subject listens simultaneously through headphones to separate strings of words in each ear, and then recalls the words, those presented to the right ear being remembered better, the RIGHT-EAR ADVANTAGE (REA) reflecting left hemisphere dominance. The technique is useful for assessing dominance in populations, but cannot ascertain dominance in an individual with certainty. TACHISTOSCOPIC VISUAL HALF-FIELD TECHNIQUES require a subject to stare at a fixation spot, and words are then presented briefly to right or left visual half-fields; a right-visual field (RVF) effect demonstrates left hemisphere dominance for language processing, but again cannot be used reliably for assessing individual dominance. Reliable assessments are sometimes necessary before neurosurgery (as when a central brain structure should be approached through the non-dominant rather than the dominant hemisphere, in order to avoid the disaster of post-operative language loss). An effective technique is INTRA-CAROTID SODIUM AMYTAL INJECTION (the WADA TECHNIQUE) in which sodium amytal is injected directly into an internal carotid artery, producing general anaesthesia of the cerebral hemisphere on the same side for three or four minutes, the other hemisphere remaining fully conscious. If speech impairment occurs after the injection then that side is dominant for language.

Dichotic listening and visual half-field studies also show that the right (or so-called 'non-dominant' hemisphere) is superior to the left at processing non-verbal stimuli, such as musical tunes and rhythms, pictures and faces, and it is now accepted that the hemispheres are COMPLEMENTARY, the left preferentially processing material that is verbal, logical, analytic and spread out sequentially in time (as in speech), whereas the right hemisphere processes information in a holistic or intuitive manner, the separate components being analysed simultaneously and in parallel (as in pictures). This functional separation is clearly seen in the syndromes occurring after brain lesions, and which form the rest of this chapter. For simplicity all patients will be assumed to show the archetypal pattern of left-hemisphere dominance for language-related behaviours, and right hemisphere dominance for non-linguistic abilities.

Neuropsychology was founded by Broca when he described a series of patients with what is now known as BROCA'S APHASIA (synonyms: ANTERIOR, NON-FLUENT or MOTOR APHASIA). Aphasia is a specific deficit of language processing, and in Broca's aphasia there is an inability to *produce* spoken language (although perception is unimpaired, the patient can understand commands, and tongue and larynx control is normal; patients can sometimes even sing the very same words of songs that they are unable to speak). The speech that is produced is painfully slow, often being disconnected grunts and noises that individually are similar to those of speech but without integration. Less severe cases show TELEGRAPHIC SPEECH, consisting mainly of nouns, with few verbs or prepositions. Prosody, or intonation, is unimpaired. Classically the lesion occurs in the third left frontal convolution, just anterior to the sensorimotor areas controlling lips, tongue and face. Broca's aphasia is contrasted with WERNICKE'S APHASIA (synonyms: POSTERIOR, FLUENT or SENSORY APHASIA), described two decades later, in which speech is produced fluently, and sounds superficially normal (although produced in such excess as to be called an 'intolerable loquacity'). Detailed speech analysis reveals many pronunciation errors, 'table' being said as 'bable' (a PARAPHONIA), or being compounded with a related word, such as 'chair', to produce 'chable' (a PARAPHASIA). These patients seem unable accurately to monitor their own speech; similar disruption of pronunciation can be produced in normal individuals with DELAYED AUDITORY FEEDBACK, a half second delay between speaking and actually hearing one's own voice through headphones.

The relationship between Broca's and Wernicke's aphasia is well seen in the theoretical model proposed by Lichtheim in 1885 (Fig. 23.1). Sound enters via the ear and is processed firstly by the auditory

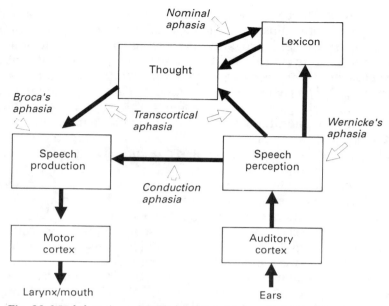

Fig. 23.1 Lichtheim's model of the relationship between speech perception, cognition and speech production. The lexicon is not a part of Lichtheim's original formulation. Open headed arrows indicate the site of lesions producing specific syndromes.

cortex and then by Wernicke's area, which translates speech into the internal code used for 'thought'. The output of Wernicke's area passes to a 'central processor', which processes the information, 'thinks' about it, and sends an output message to Broca's area, which translates the message back from internal code into a speech based code, and then sends its output to the motor cortex and thence to mouth and larynx. In addition, there is a direct link between Wernicke's and Broca's area, which does not require translation into the internal code of thought. Lichtheim's model not only accounts for the deficits of Broca's and Wernicke's aphasias, with their destruction of specific cortical areas, but also explains two DISCONNECTION SYNDROMES. In CONDUCTION APHASIA, patients have only a single, very specific deficit; they are unable to repeat exactly a sentence that is spoken to them. They can understand what is said, they can speak normally, and can speak about the message, even paraphrasing it (e.g. 'The cat sat on the mat' becomes 'the kitten sits on the carpet'), but are simply unable to repeat messages verbatim. The direct route between Wernicke's and Broca's areas is damaged, meaning that an input cannot be copied exactly from input to output and instead must be translated into the internal code and then its meaning translated back into speech, losing accuracy in the process. The lesion is in the ARCUATE FASCICULUS, the bundle of white matter connecting Broca's and Wernicke's areas. The converse syndrome is TRANSCORTICAL APHASIA, which is associated with diffuse brain damage, often due to carbon monoxide poisoning, in which the cognitive processing portions of the brain are disconnected from Broca's and Wernicke's areas; inputs to Wernicke's area pass directly to Broca's area without cognitive processing, so the patient can *only* repeat sentences, without evidence of comprehension, and produces no spontaneous utterances. The only exception to strict repetition is an alteration of grammar, so that sentences refer directly to the speaker, 'How are you today?' becoming 'How am I today?', implying that grammatical analysis occurs in either Broca's or Wernicke's areas.

A further syndrome, ANOMIC APHASIA or ANOMIA, was not described by Lichtheim but can be included in his model. The major defect is in remembering names of objects and people, and it can be regarded as being an amnesia for semantic (not episodic) information. Although superficially normal, patients use circumlocutions to avoid difficult words, often using the words inappropriately (*e.g.* 'I have three children, a son and two females'), and they fail completely when asked directly to name specific objects. The deficit is entirely of *conscious retrieval* from the mental dictionary or LEXICON, since words heard in speech are recognized and interpreted, and the correct names of objects can be recognized as correct.

Although Wernicke's and Broca's aphasias seem to be deficits of speech perception and production respectively, the linguist Roman Jakobson (1896–1982) suggested the deficits may be broader, Broca's aphasia being a deficit of sequencing or syntax, and Wernicke's aphasia a deficit of comprehension or semantics. That interpretation is supported by experiments showing that Broca's aphasics misunderstand the perception of syntax in *spoken* speech (AGRAMMATISM), confusing commands such as 'Put your hand on the book' and 'Put the book on your hand', which differ in syntax; typically the patient guesses at the more likely or more reasonable meaning. Since word order is particularly important in grammar, the speech problem may also be a problem of ordering or *sequencing*, the subtle movements of larynx and mouth in speech not being made at precisely the correct time.

Aphasia is considered in depth because it is common, occurring frequently after cerebrovascular haemorrhage or ischaemia. It must however be emphasized that the most frequent presentation is as GLOBAL APHASIA, with deficits of both speech production and perception. Despite its serious implications for the patient, it is of relatively little neuropsychological interest.

One of neuropsychology's major successes is in discovering and understanding problems of reading after brain-damage in adults (ACQUIRED DYSLEXIA which must not be confused with DEVELOPMENTAL DYSLEXIA, that occurs in childhood and may require very different types

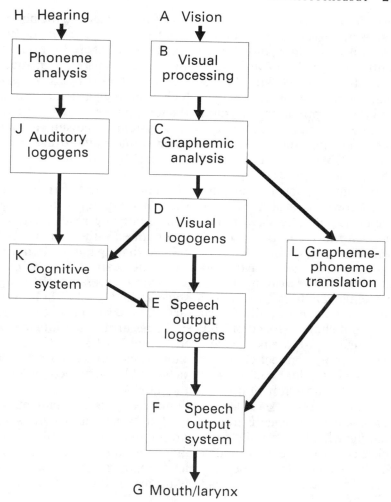

Fig. 23.2 A model of the centres involved in reading words aloud. See text for further details.

of explanation). The dyslexias are rare, but tell us much about normal functioning. Although superficially straightforward, reading is a complex skill (as any illiterate adult will tell you). A visual analysis must first distinguish curves, horizontal and vertical lines, etc. (stage B in Fig. 23.2), before GRAPHEME recognition (stage C in Fig. 23.2) — graphemes being the letters, symbols, etc. of writing; 'A', 'A', 'a' and 'a' all being the same grapheme. Individual graphemes are then combined with other knowledge (such as context, expectations, the visual shape of the word, etc.) by the system known as the VISUAL INPUT LOGOGEN (D). The logogen outputs are understood as meanings by the cognitive system (K), and a speech output can be produced by the SPEECH OUTPUT LOGOGEN (E) that converts meanings into the phonemes of spoken speech, which are then sent to the equivalent of Broca's area (F). In addition direct routes between input and output (as in Lichtheim's model of aphasia) allow simple repetition of material, either by a direct link between D and E, or by a grapheme-phoneme translation system (L), which from any particular grapheme combination produces the standard sound pattern. Such a sequence of analyses would be required by any system processing writing, so that a reading and speaking computer would have to use a similar method. However, it is supported in man by patients with specific deficit syndromes.

The simplest form of acquired dyslexia is LETTER-BY-LETTER READING (also known as PURE ALEXIA and ALEXIA WITHOUT AGRAPHIA), in which reading is painfully slow, individual letters being read slowly aloud, one at a time, and then the word recognized only after it has been spelled out ('H, O, U, S, E, house'). Since these patients do not suffer from AGRAPHIA they can therefore write but cannot read what they may just have written. They are lacking access to the stage of graphemic analysis (a lesion of stage C in Fig. 23.2). Letters are therefore recognized only as arbitrary shapes, so that after the lesion the sound-shape associations have to be relearnt. The route of reading is therefore A-B-Memory-G-Spoken sound-H-I-J-K-E-F-G. A and K therefore only connect via the medium of spoken sounds produced in the outside world. Reading is characterized by slow recognition time, which is a linear function of word length.

PHONOLOGICAL DYSLEXIA is frequently not recognized by patients themselves, since the deficit is in reading aloud NON-WORDS (such as 'bif' or 'kaj', for which most individuals can produce sounds with ease). The deficit is in the direct 'grapheme-phoneme' route (box L); graphemes cannot be converted to sounds unless a logogen already exists for the word. One of the normal reading routes, A-B-C-L-F-G is therefore deficient.

DEEP DYSLECTICS are like phonological dyslectics in being unable to read non-words. However, in addition, they cannot read abstract words lacking in imagability (e.g. 'virtue' or 'sophistication' rather than 'house' or 'curlew'), and find function words (such as verbs and prepositions) more difficult than content words (nouns and adjectives), so that 'ambulance' can be read, but not 'am', or 'bee' can be read but not 'be'. Occasionally there are also semantic errors, so that 'ape' will be read as 'monkey'. This syndrome is the dyslectic equivalent of conduction aphasia, without direct routes between visual logogens and speech output logogens, or a grapheme-phoneme route, so that all information passes through the cognitive system, where meaning is extracted but specifically linguistic information is lost, so that words with diffuse meanings (such as 'be') are lost or distorted. Non-words, which have no meanings, simply cannot be read at all. All reading is therefore through the route A-B-C-D-K-E-F-G, the normal routes D-E and C-L-F being damaged.

SURFACE DYSLEXIA is the inverse of phonological dyslexia, reading being satisfactory for non-words, function words and abstract words, but impaired for longer words (which do not particularly affect the deep dyslectic) and showing an effect of REGULARITY OF SPELLING (which is not shown in deep dyslexia). As any foreigner will affirm, English spelling is eccentric, some words being spelt and pronounced in a regular way, whereas others are ORTHOGRAPHICALLY IRREGULAR, so that, for instance, 'gauge' as normally pronounced should be written 'gage' in regular spelling, or should be pronounced 'gorge' if its spelling were actually regular (as in the regularly spelt 'gaunt'). Surface dyslectics read 'gauge' as 'gorge' (and 'broad' as 'brode' and 'trough' as 'true'). The defect in surface dyslexia is not entirely clear, the difficulty with longer words being similar to that in letter-by-letter reading, but surface dyslectics have the additional problem with irregular words, which suggests that the visual input logogen is working only partially, so that many regular spellings are available but access to the lexicon for unusual and irregular spellings has been lost. The most likely explanation is that the route D-E is damaged, so that reading is either through the routes A-B-C-K-E-F-G, or A-B-C-L-F-G.

Acquired dyslexias often involve the ANGULAR GYRUS, at the junction of the temporal, occipital and parietal areas, a site well placed for auditory-visual integration. Nevertheless, lesions can involve many cortical sites, and in deep dyslexia the lesions are so extensive in the left hemisphere, that it has been hypothesized we are observing the pure reading of the non-dominant right hemisphere.

The left-hemisphere syndromes of aphasia and dyslexia have been described in depth because they illustrate well the methods of neuropsychology. The remaining syndromes will be treated more cursorily, being included principally to illustrate the wide range of neuropsychological deficits.

Two other symptoms are typically associated with the left hemisphere, both involved in motor control. AGRAPHIA, an inability to write, can occur in association with or independently of aphasia and dyslexia, and is classically associated with lesions of EXNER'S AREA, in the frontal lobe adjacent to Broca's area. A more general deficit of motor control is APRAXIA, in which praxis (or action) is impaired at a high intellectual level. Despite no weakness, spasticity, or evidence of upper or motor neurone lesions, apractics are unable to organize movements into a meaningful sequence, as in striking a match or combing hair. Lesions are often at the left angular gyrus, which may store kinaesthetic engrams (or memories); damage not only impairs movements with *either* hand, but also causes difficulty in perceiving and understanding movements made by other people. SYMPATHETIC APRAXIA occurs only in

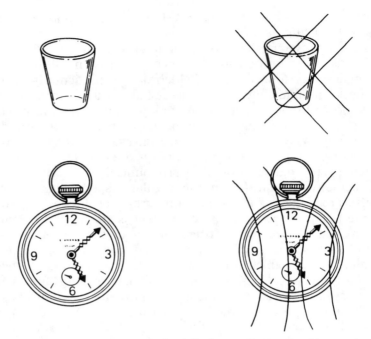

Fig. 23.3 Visual agnosics find it difficult to recognize the objects on the right hand side, in which crossing lines have disrupted the overall outline. The original test was devised by Luria. Reproduced from Kolb B and Whishaw I Q (1985), *Fundamentals of human neuropsychology*, 2nd edn, New York, W H Freeman, 212.

the non-dominant hand, and is a disconnection syndrome, the non-dominant motor cortex having lost contact with the kinaesthetic engrams stored in the dominant angular gyrus, due sometimes to a tiny lesion in the body of the corpus callosum.

The syndromes of the non-dominant hemisphere are well-recognized and described, but have been studied far less, in part because of the greater difficulty of using non-verbal stimuli in experiments.

The AGNOSIAS are syndromes in which sensory processing is complete, but information is not interpreted to form a meaningful whole; SENSATION is present without PERCEPTION (see Chapter 2). The syndromes are modality specific (visual agnosia, auditory agnosia, tactile agnosia, etc.). In visual agnosia, despite being able to identify lines, curves, colours, etc., patients cannot recognize objects, particularly if, as in Fig. 23.3, additional lines confuse the overall outline. Agnosias are often very precise; for instance COLOUR AGNOSIA is an inability to recognize appropriate colours for objects, due to a disconnection of the visual cortex from areas concerned with the memory of colours (Fig. 23.4). PROSOPAGNOSIA, a specific inability to recognize familiar faces, is usually regarded as a right-hemisphere syndrome (and

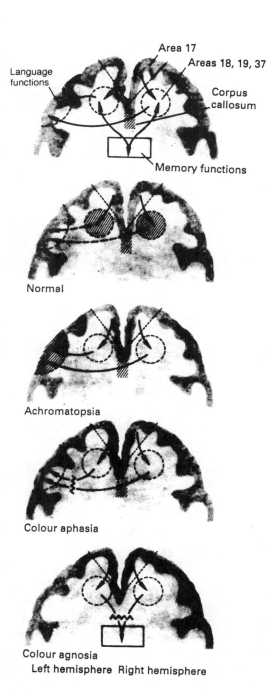

Language
functions

Area 17

Areas 18, 19, 37

Corpus
callosum

Memory functions

Normal

Achromatopsia

Colour aphasia

Colour agnosia

Left hemisphere Right hemisphere

Fig. 23.4 A model for deficits in colour perception. In the normal individual the retinal image is processed by area 17 (primary visual cortex), and then by areas 18, 19 and 37, which access memories of colour information (shown by the square box), before transmitting information about the name of the colour to the language functions of the left hemisphere. ACHROMATOPSIA is a form of cortical colour-blindness, in which colours cannot be distinguished from one another due to bilateral destruction of areas 18, 19 and 37. COLOUR APHASICS show normal differentiation of colours, but are unable to name them, due to disconnection of the language areas from areas concerned with colour perception. In COLOUR AGNOSIA there is normal discrimination of colours but an inability to recognize appropriate associations of colours with objects (e.g. of red with tomatoes) due to disconnection of colour perception areas from memory. Reproduced with permission from Kolb B and Whishaw I Q (1985), *Fundamentals of human neuropsychology*, 2nd edn, New York, W H Freeman, 212. Copyright 1980, 1985 by W H Freeman and Company.

visual half-field studies show a right hemisphere advantage for face recognition), but it is now accepted that bilateral lesions are present in most cases, accounting for the rarity of the syndrome. In UNILATERAL NEGLECT, the patient ignores half of the visual world, simply denying

Model   Patient's copy

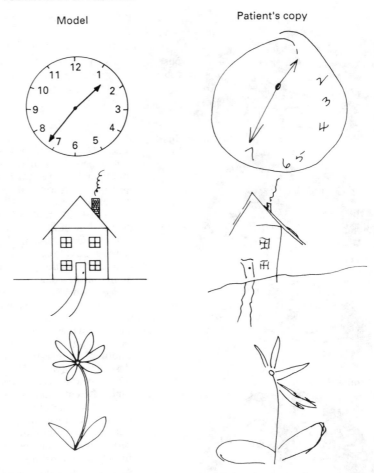

Fig. 23.5 Unilateral neglect in a patient with a lesion in the posterior part of the right hemisphere. The patient was asked to copy the drawings on the left. Reproduced with permission from Springer S P and Deutsch G (1981), *Left brain, right brain*, San Francisco, W H Freeman, 174. Copyright W H Freeman, 1981.

that they see anything there, and drawing only half a clock face (Fig. 23.5), or half a house, and in extreme cases only washing half their body, or only putting on their clothes on one side. A variant of the syndrome is UNILATERAL ASOMATAGNOSIA in which the patient cannot recognize the left half of their own body as belonging to them (asking whose leg or arm it is in the bed with them), or not recognizing that the limb is diseased (ANOSOGNOSIA). Although rare such syndromes give us valuable insights into the nature of normal processes.

The final non-dominant syndrome is CONSTRUCTIONAL APRAXIA, which is an apraxia with an inability to carry out motor actions, but unlike the dominant apraxias the deficit is not in the control of motor

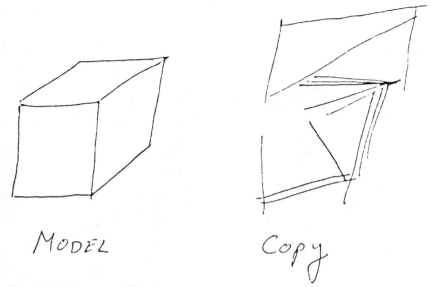

MODEL   Copy

Fig. 23.6 Constructional apraxia after a lesion to the right parietal area. The patient was asked to copy the model on the left. Reproduced with permission of John Wiley and Sons, Inc, all rights reserved, from Hecaen H and Albert M L (1978), *Human neuropsycholo y*, New York, John Wiley.

movements but in the understanding of the three-dimensional space in which movements are made, so a patient cannot draw or copy pictures (Figure 23.6) and, in DRESSING APRAXIA, may be unable to put on clothes because of an inability to understand the apparently baffling topology of a simple garment like a cardigan. Although such defects seem mundane, it is only by observing such problems in the brain-damaged (or the very young) that we appreciate the subtleties and complexities of an everyday action that we take for granted and almost literally carry out 'without [conscious] thinking'.

Specific applications
to medicine

24

Smoking

- The incidence of cigarette smoking has declined dramatically since 1950, when the link with lung cancer was first proposed, although mainly in social classes I, II and III, and particularly in doctors.
- Cigarette smokers are more extravert than non-smokers due to extraverts being more likely to take up smoking.
- Cigarettes do not produce improved performance in smokers, but instead they prevent withdrawal symptoms and return performance to the level found in non-smokers.
- Although nicotine is present in large amounts in cigarette smoke, studies using nicotine injections and chewing gum suggest that it might not be the addictive substance which maintains cigarette smoking.
- Giving up smoking depends both on producing motivation and the reduction of dependence. As yet there are no effective ways of reducing dependence, although drugs acting to reduce craving might have a role to play.
- The advice of a doctor that a patient should give up smoking is cost-effective and would produce a large number of ex-smokers if carried out systematically.

Cigarette smoking is probably the largest single cause of preventable premature death, from diseases such as carcinoma of the bronchus, chronic bronchitis and emphysema, and coronary and cerebrovascular arterial disease. Although the question of causality is not finally settled (and as the geneticist R A Fisher argued, there might be a gene predisposing both to carcinoma of the bronchus *and* to cigarette smoking), it is now indubitable that stopping smoking benefits health. I will take it for granted that cigarette smoking is bad and should be prevented wherever possible. The question is, How? And before answering that, we must ask, Who smokes?, and Why do they smoke?

Since the early 1950s, when a link with lung cancer was first established, the proportion of smokers has fallen steadily. Smoking is now much less common in higher than lower social classes, the rate hardly having changed in social class V since 1950 (Fig. 24.1). Although women smoke less than do men, their rate has also dropped less; in social class I the two sexes now smoke almost equally.

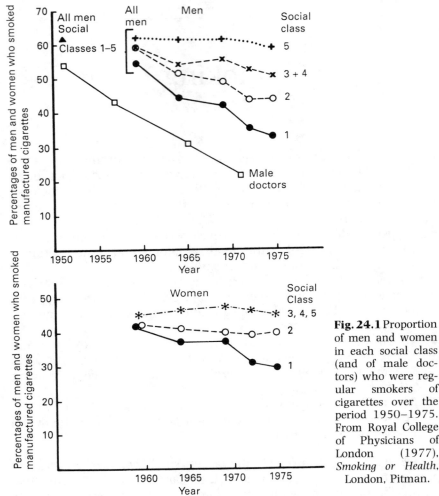

Fig. 24.1 Proportion of men and women in each social class (and of male doctors) who were regular smokers of cigarettes over the period 1950–1975. From Royal College of Physicians of London (1977), *Smoking or Health*, London, Pitman.

Over 30 years, an average cigarette smoker takes about two million puffs, on each of which many physiologically active substances pass from lungs to brain in about eight seconds. The speed of central action (compared with 20–30 seconds for intravenous heroin), and the rate of administration (100 times per day, compared with half a dozen in a heroin addict) produce ideal circumstances for addiction.

Cigarette smokers are more extraverted than non-smokers, the effect being proportional to the number of cigarettes smoked. But do extraverts become smokers, or does smoking make one more extraverted, perhaps by easing sociability? A prospective study of 16-year-old non-smokers who became smokers by age 25 found that subsequent smokers were *already* more extraverted (and more neurotic) by age 16; extraversion therefore causes smoking, rather than vice-versa. Smokers who give up are also less extraverted and less neurotic.

Pipe smokers differ from cigarette smokers in being even more *introverted* than non-smokers. Pipe smokers who have never smoked cigarettes also do not inhale smoke into their lungs and absorb little of the smoke, so that pharmacologically they seem to gain little from smoking; in contrast ex-cigarette smokers who smoke pipes *do* inhale, and hence are still at high risk from their smoking. Psychoanalytic theorists have speculated that pipe-smokers in particular (and smokers in general) are orally fixated (see Chapter 11), and receive oral gratification and reassurance from their habit.

People smoke cigarettes for different reasons, and questionnaire studies have examined the MOTIVES FOR SMOKING. One study found six types of motivation, which could be grouped into two independent dimensions. PHARMACOLOGICAL SMOKERS describe smoking as ADDICTIVE (with a strong desire for more cigarettes and smoking in bed in the morning), AUTOMATIC (forgetting they are smoking or lighting a cigarette while another is still alight), or STIMULANT (smoking when working hard, concentrating, tired, or for cheering up). Subjects scoring high on one factor tend to score high on the others. Uncorrelated with pharmacological motives are NON-PHARMACOLOGICAL MOTIVES, these smokers being INDULGENT (smoking after meals or when relaxed), PSYCHOSOCIAL (feeling confident in company or appearing mature, relaxed or attractive to the opposite sex), or SENSORIMOTOR (enjoying the sensations of the cigarette, the taste, the blowing of smoke, and the rituals of lighting up). Although it was originally hoped that a classification of motives would allow specific therapies for different types of smoker, that hope has yet to be fulfilled.

Like all centrally active drugs, cigarettes modify behaviour. In smokers, concurrent cigarette smoking improves performance in tasks involving rapid reactions, vigilance, or the processing of conflicting or rapid information, and it also alleviates alcohol's depressive effect upon reaction time and mental arithmetic (although exacerbating the body sway and motor incoordination caused by alcohol). Cigarettes also increase heart rate and blood pressure. Although these latter physiological effects occur both in habitual smokers and in non-smokers, the apparently beneficial cognitive effects occur only in regular smokers. Closer examination shows that cigarettes in regular smokers act only to restore performance to the normal level of non-smokers. As Schacter cynically put it, 'The heavy smoker gets nothing out of smoking. He smokes only to prevent withdrawal'. An analogy is with a heroin addict, who indeed performs tasks better on the drug than without, but the drug is not actually beneficial, only acting to prevent withdrawal and thereby produce performance equivalent to that in the non-addict.

Most doctors, most of the lay public, and probably the producers of the government tar and nicotine tables, tacitly assume that people smoke primarily in order to obtain nicotine. Amongst a myriad of physiologically active substances, nicotine is indeed present in the largest quantities. However, in contrast to alcohol and opiates, it is very difficult to produce nicotine addiction in laboratory animals or to get them to self-administer nicotine. The evidence is also poor that humans smoke specifically to obtain nicotine. Something in cigarettes is indeed addictive, since subjects will increase consumption when given weak cigarettes, and decrease consumption with strong cigarettes, SELF-TITRATION or AUTO-REGULATION, and smoke dilution by ventilation holes in the cigarette's side produces more frequent and deeper puffs. But these changes alter *all* the smoke's constituents at the same time. In an experiment altering just nicotine intake, smokers were injected intravenously with nicotine or placebo; the nicotine, equivalent to a day's cigarette intake, only decreased average consumption from 24 to 22 cigarettes per day. Nicotine chewing gum has a similarly small effect, which although statistically significant, is of little practical importance. Cigarette smokers also say that nicotine chewing gum alone does not give the same satisfaction as a cigarette. Experimental subjects smoking lettuce-leaf cigarettes (which contain no nicotine) complain they are less good than ordinary cigarettes, but continue to smoke them; more importantly, adding nicotine does not render lettuce-leaf cigarettes more acceptable. Finally, although ordinary smokers alter puff size and depth from puff to puff, following small puffs with larger ones, indicating auto-regulation on a minute-to-minute basis, this control is not affected by injecting nicotine intravenously. Taking these results together it seems very unlikely that the addictive substance in cigarettes is nicotine, although the real addictive substance is not clear. It is unlikely to be carbon monoxide as snuff takers and tobacco chewers also appear to be addicted, and for similar reasons it is unlikely to be any of the pyrolysed products of partial tobacco combustion.

Most people find their first cigarette disgusting and frequently are nauseous or vomit (the side-effects of a large dose of nicotine). Most regular smokers start before the age of 20, and a third or so have started by nine years of age. Although addictive, cigarettes are disgusting to the non-addict. Something must therefore bridge the gap between first cigarette and habit acquisition. The extra motivation is due to social pressure, peer group influence and modelling of relatives and friends. Children who smoke at age 12 are recognized by their non-smoking contemporaries as doing it to show off and to appear grown up. These 12-year-old smokers also tend to have parents or siblings who smoke. Adolescents must gain something from smoking, and measures of lower self-esteem and higher trait anxiety suggest cigarettes are used to manage a sense of personal inadequacy or ineffectiveness. Prevention of childhood smoking is not simple as

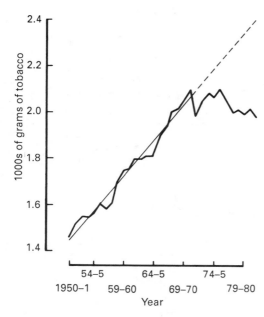

Fig. 24.2 Cigarette consumption per capita per annum in Norway from 1950 to 1980. In 1970, a ban on cigarette advertising was first discussed, and in 1975 all advertising was banned. From Royal College of Physicians (1983), *Health or Smoking?*, London, Pitman.

neither anti-smoking teaching at school nor punishment have much influence, although in one study a concerted educational campaign by schools did result in a 50% reduction in childhood smoking. Undoubtedly advertising by cigarette companies increases smoking (see Fig. 24.2), and many advertisers now direct their campaigns directly at young people, by emphasizing links with sports, such as motor racing.

Three quarters of smokers attempt to stop at some time, and 10% of a random sample of smokers at a GP's surgery have tried to stop *in the previous month*. As with other aspects of smoking there is a paradox: most smokers *want* to give up and yet few succeed. Most smokers know they want to give up, they know they have chronic coughs and bronchitis, and they know smoking causes lung cancer, heart disease and chronic bronchitis. And for those who are not impressed by such correlations, or discount them as being thirty years in the future, other adverse effects can also be used for propaganda, such as an earlier menopause, premature and excessive facial skin-wrinkling, decreased intelligence of children following smoking in pregnancy, and increased respiratory illness in early childhood from passive smoking. The problem is that while smokers know they *should* stop, they do not know *how to*; it is like a drowning man, who knows his mouth must be kept shut until he breaks the surface of the water but knows no way of fighting the strong reflexes forcing him to inhale. Cigarettes are physiologically addictive (and are as difficult to give up as heroin or alcohol – see Fig. 24.3). Smoking cessation therefore requires both a high motivation *and* a way of reducing dependence.

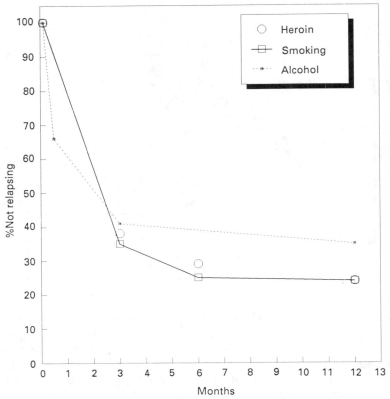

Fig. 24.3 Relapse rates in patients giving up smoking, alcohol or heroin. Similar curves also apply to exercise, dietary modification and preventive dental care. Reproduced with permission from Hunt W A, Barnett L W and Ranch L G (1971), Relapse rates in addiction programs, *J Clin Psychol*, **27**, 455–6.

Anti-smoking campaigns are good at producing motivation, and are the first step in cessation. But they do not stop smoking and can be counter-productive if cognitive dissonance ('I should stop smoking; I can't') (see Chapter 12) produces rationalizations which work against the propaganda ('Experts aren't always right'; 'I smoke because I like it, not because I'm addicted'; etc.). The problem is finding ways of reducing dependency. Until the addictive basis of smoking becomes clear there can be no *rational* approach to alleviating dependency, and high dependency smokers are unlikely to be helped much. A possible solution considers the pharmacology of CRAVING, the intense desire for a cigarette in the first 24 hours of cessation. Craving occurs in withdrawal from all addictions, be they cigarettes, alcohol or opiates, and in opiate withdrawal is helped by clonidine, an alpha-2-noradrenergic agonist, whose action (like enkephalins and opiates) probably reduces activity in the LOCUS COERULEUS, which produces most

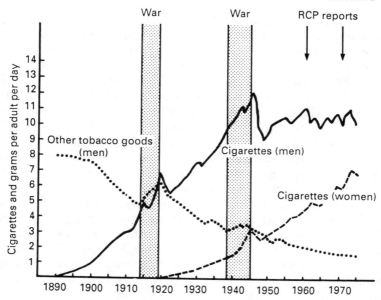

Fig. 24.4 Tobacco consumption in the United Kingdom from 1890 to 1981, in terms of average cigarettes per adult per day (both smokers and non-smokers being included in the calculation). Dates of the two previous Royal College of Physicians (RCP) reports on ill-effects of smoking are indicated, and are followed by falls in tobacco consumption. From Royal College of Physicians (1983), *Health or Smoking?*, London, Pitman.

of the cerebral noradrenaline that accentuates craving. Clonidine also reduces craving in cigarette withdrawal and may help treatment in the early stages of cessation. It might also explain the links between smoking and stress, when central noradrenergic levels are raised, thereby increasing craving, and the cross-tolerance between smoking and opiates; opiate addicts find that smoking reduces their opiate craving.

Propaganda in successful anti-smoking campaigns probably increases motivation in low dependency smokers, as shown by the decreases in tobacco consumption after each edition of the Royal College of Physician's reports on smoking (Figure 24.4), the relatively low proportion of smokers amongst doctors in recent years (Fig. 24.1), and the lower incidence of smoking among medical students than other students. However, the high incidence of smoking among nurses, particularly on intensive care and coronary-care units, suggests that propaganda and knowledge are far from completely successful at reducing smoking.

Specific treatments for smoking are numerous and have been extensively studied. Tranquillizers and anti-nicotine drugs; aversive therapy, using either electric shocks or 'rapid smoking' (which induces nausea); self-control involving timers, diaries and other feedback devices; hypnosis; role-play; psychoanalysis; and sensory deprivation all have been tried and none are convincingly superior to placebo. The poor response in anti-smoking campaigns is easily illustrated by an example: 30 976 questionnaires were distributed to a population of which 21 553 were returned, 11 477 by smokers, of whom 4755 said that they would like to stop smoking and were invited to attend a withdrawal clinic. Only 150 smokers actually attended the clinic, of whom 64 stopped smoking, and only 35 were still not smoking at the end of the year; just 0.3% of the original smokers.

That placebos are effective, in that *any* anti-smoking treatment is beneficial, suggests the placebo effect itself might be exploited in helping patients to give up smoking. A controlled trial of personal advice to stop smoking from a patient's own general practitioner found that by the end of a year nearly 8% of patients were not smoking compared with 3% of controls. Although the effect does not appear large, if every GP in the United Kingdom used the procedure there would be about half a million ex-smokers within a year, which would be the equivalent of setting up 10 000 specialist anti-smoking clinics.

25

Alcohol

- *Alcohol abuse* and *alcoholism* are common, especially in doctors, who have three times the general population rate.
- The effects of alcohol in impairing intellectual and motor function and increasing aggression are due to the drug itself, whereas the effects upon antisocial behaviour, increased consumption and sexual arousal are due to LEARNED EXPECTANCIES.
- Alcoholism results from operant conditioning, classical conditioning and imitation, and in addition there may be genetic predispositions.
- Cross-tolerance between alcohol and opiates suggests that alcohol may have its effects upon central endorphin-mediated mechanisms.
- Total alcohol consumption in society is directly related to the real price of alcohol, taxation and the amount spent on advertising.

Alcohol is perhaps the only drug of addiction which is sometimes used by most of the adult population. That many individuals become physically addicted, or suffer serious acute or chronic side effects is therefore hardly surprising. Table 25.1 shows the risks associated with different levels of alcohol consumption measured in STANDARD UNITS.

Alcohol use must be distinguished from ALCOHOLISM, which is a true addiction. Although most of us use alcohol, and most are not alcoholics, a clear dividing line is not obvious. Certainly the old joke that 'an alcoholic is a person who drinks more than their doctor' is inappropriate, since doctors have three times the general rate of alcoholism and alcohol-related diseases. Probably a suitable definition is that of the World Health Organization: 'Alcoholics are those excessive drinkers whose dependence on alcohol has attained such a degree that it shows a noticeable mental disturbance or interference with their bodily health, their interpersonal relations, and their smooth social and economic functions, or who show the prodromal signs of such development. They therefore require treatment'.

The acute effects of alcohol are well-known: a decrease in sensory and motor abilities, proportional to the dose; increased sociability and decreased social inhibition, the 'ice-melting effect' at parties; and a

Table 25.1

Units of alcohol ('standard drinks') in commonly dispensed measures of different drinks. Men drinking less than 36 units per week (women 24 units) are unlikely to suffer health problems. Men drinking between 36 and 50 units per week (women 24–36) are probably drinking too much, and are likely either to become dependent or to risk their health. Men drinking over 50 units per week (women 36) are probably suffering ill health as a result of their drinking, and men drinking over 96 units per week (women 64) are almost certainly dependent upon alcohol and feeling the consequences. Reproduced with permission from Health Education Council (1989), *That's the limit*, London.

		STANDARD DRINKS
BEERS AND LAGER		
Ordinary strength beer or lager	$\frac{1}{2}$ pint	1
	1 pint	2
	1 can	$1\frac{1}{2}$
Export beer	1 pint	$2\frac{1}{2}$
	1 can	2
Strong ale or lager	$\frac{1}{2}$ pint	2
	1 pint	4
	1 can	3
Extra strength beer or lager	$\frac{1}{2}$ pint	$2\frac{1}{2}$
	1 pint	5
	1 can	4
CIDERS		
Average cider	$\frac{1}{2}$ pint	$1\frac{1}{2}$
	1 pint	3
	quart bottle	6
Strong cider	$\frac{1}{2}$ pint	2
	1 pint	4
	quart bottle	8
SPIRITS		
	1 standard single measure in most of England and Wales ($\frac{1}{6}$ gill)	1
	1 standard single measure in Northern Ireland ($\frac{1}{4}$ gill)	$1\frac{1}{2}$
	$\frac{1}{5}$ gill measure	$1\frac{1}{4}$
	$\frac{1}{4}$ gill measure served in some parts of Scotland	$1\frac{1}{2}$
	1 bottle	30
TABLE WINE		
(including cider wine and barley wine)	1 standard glass	1
	1 bottle	7
	1 litre bottle	10
SHERRY AND FORTIFIED WINE		
	1 standard small measure	1
	1 bottle	12
These figures are approximate.		

lowered threshold for antisocial or unsociable acts, so that, as Oliver Zangwill (1914–1987) put it, 'the super-ego is that part of the mind which is soluble in alcohol'. Although most psychomotor tasks deteriorate with alcohol, two are interesting as they are unexpected. Slowly moving objects are tracked visually by SMOOTH TRACKING MOVEMENTS, which as objects speed up eventually break down into SACCADES or jumps; the threshold at which smooth tracking changes to saccades is directly proportional to blood alcohol concentrations, effects being seen even at 20 mg%, well below 80 mg%, the legal maximum for driving. Alcohol also diminishes ability to recover from sudden bright lights ('glare'), the effect being cortical not retinal in origin. The implications for the most serious social consequence of acute alcohol intoxication, road traffic accidents, are obvious, and it is beyond doubt that many road traffic accidents result from alcohol consumption. Less well known is that alcohol levels are raised in pedestrians involved in road accidents, in persons injured in non-traffic accidents, be they industrial or domestic, and in drowning accidents. The final effect of alcohol is that upon sexual function, described well by the porter in *Macbeth*, 'Lechery, sir, it provokes and unprovokes; it provokes the desire, but it takes away the performance'.

Not all alcohol's effects are pharmacological, some being due to LEARNED EXPECTANCY. Placebo studies using alcohol (usually vodka in dilute orange juice) or placebo (orange juice only, in a glass with vodka smeared around the rim to give the smell of alcohol) find many effects are produced as strongly by the placebo as by alcohol; they are produced in expectation, presumably from previous experience. Deviant antisocial behaviour, including excessive consumption itself, illicit behaviour and sexual arousal are mainly a result of expectancy, whereas impaired intellectual and motor performance, and increased aggression are truly a result of alcohol consumption rather than expectancy.

Alcohol apparently does not affect people equally, although many differences reflect difference in usage of words describing states of intoxication. Whereas some people describe themselves as 'drunk' when feeling slightly impaired, others only 'feel drunk' when losing gross bodily control of walking, or perhaps only on being unable to remember the night before do they conclude retrospectively that they were 'drunk'. Given such perceptions, one can understand how individuals can both agree that 'drunken driving is wrong', and then drive after six whiskies because they do not perceive themselves as being 'drunk'. In taking a drinking history, doctors must also be careful, particularly as many patients will underestimate consumption by as much as 50%; this is mainly a response to implied criticism by the doctor, since more accurate responses are given to an interactive computer program.

Alcoholism transcends normal alcohol use, even with its temporary excesses, and becomes a state of DEPENDENCE, in which it is 'normal' to have alcohol in the blood stream (or 'blood in the alcohol stream'). Dependent behaviours revolve around alcohol, often rather than alcohol being a small part of daily life; often there is LOSS OF CONTROL, in which a single drink initiates a 'bender', when the patient is unable to stop drinking. Dependent drinkers also consume alcohol at unusual times (before or instead of breakfast, or at work) or in places where alcohol is normally unacceptable (and alcohol on a patient's breath in a GP's surgery is said to be a good indicator of dependent drinking).

Dependent drinkers narrow their drinking repertoire, drinking regularly, day in, day out, rather than in relation to social events. Although CRAVING is conventionally said to be a separate symptom of dependence, both placebo and alcohol in abstinent alcoholics have equivalent effects upon craving suggesting that it is merely a re-description of the alcoholic's other symptoms. Alcoholics also show personality changes, and changed relationships with spouse and friends, becoming argumentative and uncaring, particularly when drinking is frustrated; the drinking itself is blamed upon the uncontrollable actions of inexorable fate, or else, by the defence mechanism of paranoid projection, upon the faults of family, employer, etc.

What makes some people become alcoholic? An immediate explanation is that it is learnt, and in a trivial sense this is true, since alcohol, like cigarettes, is unpleasant at first. Learning theories take three forms. OPERANT CONDITIONING says alcohol consumption is rewarded by reduction in anxiety or stress, or the easing of social relationships, and as each glass of alcohol is rewarding, so the operant response, drinking, will increase in frequency. Certainly in animals alcohol reduces stress reactions, and stressed animals work to drink alcohol rather than water. Alcohol *in vitro* acts like a benzodiazepine and *in vivo* can have an anxiolytic action. The CLASSICAL CONDITIONING theory says that as in operant conditioning, alcohol reduces anxiety, but that eventually the unconditioned response (anxiety reduction) produced by the unconditioned stimulus (alcohol consumption) becomes conditioned to other stimuli occurring concurrently (such as the bar or pub, or the people one drinks with), and those objects themselves become anxiety reducing; however when in a bar the obvious thing to do is to have a drink, and so drinking behaviour increases in frequency. IMITATION is the third form of learning and takes two forms. Parental drinking can provide a model of appropriate behaviour for their children and be imitated; of especial interest is that heavy drinking men often have heavy drinking fathers (but not mothers) and vice-versa in heavy drinking women. Reaction formation can also occur to parental role-models, and TEETOTALLERS (total abstainers from alcohol) also report *higher* incidences of alcoholic parents than do moderate drinkers. Imitation can also involve social modelling. Society regards drinking as normal and allows advertisers to use all the subtle forms of persuasion in their armamentarium to imply that alcohol is 'good', makes one appear 'masculine' or 'feminine', produces success with the opposite sex, etc., in the same way that cigarette advertising promotes similar ends (and heavy drinkers tend to be heavy smokers). Alcohol advertising undoubtedly works; a 10% reduction in advertising results in a 1.3% reduction in alcohol consumption, so that a total ban on advertising could decrease consumption by 13%.

Alcoholism differs in frequency between societies and between groups within a society; for instance Jewish, Chinese and Italians in America have low rates, whereas Irish Americans have high rates of alcoholism. Cross-cultural studies by anthropologists suggest that alcoholism relates to lax social organization, tightly organized groups with strong social hierarchies having low rates. Similar factors are probably important within social groups, and perhaps even within families in our society.

Another explanation of alcohol use and abuse is genetic or constitutional. Alcohol use and alcoholism are more similar in monozygotic than dizygotic twins, and although this might reflect more similar environments, studies also show that drinking habits and alcoholism are more similar to those of biological than adoptive parents in adopted children. Studies in experimental animals show that alcohol preference and rate of alcohol metabolism are highly heritable, being readily selected for. Some individuals may therefore have a genetic predisposition to consume alcohol heavily or to become alcoholic; nevertheless such individuals must first be exposed to readily available alcohol before the gene could manifest.

A neurobiological theory of alcohol action says its effects are due to stimulation of normally inhibitory GABA receptors, which are also stimulated by barbiturates and benzodiazepines, resulting in cross-tolerance between these drugs and alcohol. Recent work shows that Ro15-4513, a specific competitive inhibitor of GABA, can block alcohol's behavioural effects in rats (general stupor, staggering gait and impaired righting reflex), supporting the idea that alcohol acts on these receptors. Ro15-4513 cannot treat the life-threatening complications of alcohol, such as respiratory depression and coma, which are mediated by direct effects upon cell membranes; it is also unlikely to prevent the long term metabolic effects of abuse.

Learning theories of alcoholism are only partly able to account for the final stage of DEPENDENCE when the consequences of drinking become more and more unpleasant. Although the alcoholic may still be drinking for learned reasons, physical dependence means that drinking is also the operant behaviour which avoids the punishing effects of the unpleasant consequences of withdrawal. Acute alcohol withdrawal produces DELIRIUM TREMENS with its tremor, hallucinations, fits and delirium, starting eight hours or so after the last drink, lasting several days and producing reduced serum magnesium (causing the fits), hyperventilation, respiratory alkalosis and hypoglycaemia. Opiate addicts have long known that opiates reduce the symptoms of alcohol withdrawal, and alcohol reduces the symptoms of opiate withdrawal, resulting in a theory that physical dependence upon alcohol is endorphin mediated. Injection of naloxone into mice during acquisition of alcohol dependence prevents subsequent alcohol withdrawal symptoms. In man alcohol is metabolized to acetaldehydes, which are precursors of the tetrahydroisoquinolines, addictive opiate-like substances. Both alcoholics and their relatives have more efficient systems for converting alcohol to acetaldehyde, suggesting a possible genetic mechanism.

This account has mostly asked why individuals become alcoholic. Treatment and prevention may be considered more quickly, since their state is far less satisfactory. Many treatments are entirely empirical, without theoretical rationale. An exception is disulfiram ('Antabuse'), which produces a toxic reaction with alcohol, producing discomfort, due to nausea, vomiting and tachycardia. The drug therefore acts by producing a LEARNED AVERSION, the response (alcohol) producing punishment (nausea), and thus decreasing the rate of responding, and inducing abstinence. Although not as effective as might be hoped, this is partly due to a lack of compliance in taking the drug. With little doubt the most effective treatment for alcoholism is provided by *Alcoholics Anonymous* (AA), and emphasizes the need for individuals to be responsible for their own drinking, and assists this with substantial social support, particularly from ex-alcoholics who have themselves been through the process.

The most important medical role in treating alcoholism is in *recognizing* alcoholics. Each GP is estimated to know only 1 or 2 of the 15 alcoholics in their practice, most of whom are not 'skid row' down-and-outs, but ordinary, respectable individuals with a problem. Effective screening methods include questionnaires (which work well if the patient is co-operative), detection of alcohol on the breath, measurement in serum of alcohol or of raised levels of the liver enzymes, gamma-glutamyl transpeptidase (GGTP) and aspartate transaminase (AspT), and the finding of macrocytosis without anaemia. Alcoholism has been called the great imitator (displacing syphilis and tuberculosis from that role), and undoubtedly in accident and emergency departments, psychiatric units, and general medical and surgical units many cases are misdiagnosed.

Prevention of alcoholism and alcohol abuse is not principally a medical or psychological problem, but instead a case for political action. Alcoholism needs alcohol and ready availability increases alcohol consumption (as for instance in Finland where allowing general stores to sell alcohol produced a sudden and sustained increase in consumption). Alcohol consumption closely follows the price in

Alcoholic drink consumption by volume 1963–87

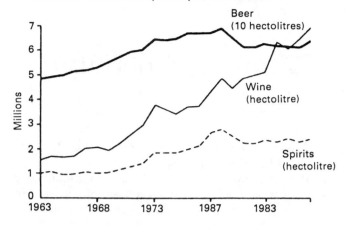

Real prices of beer, wine and spirits

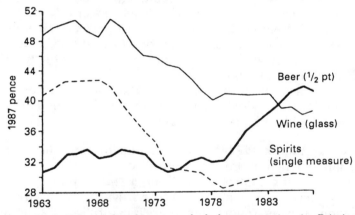

Fig. 25.1 Relationship between alcohol consumption in Britain, 1963–1987, and the real price of beer, wine and spirits. Reproduced with permission from Smith R (1989), *Br Med J*, **298**, 701.

real terms (Fig. 25.1). Advertising undoubtedly increases alcohol intake; and alcohol consumption is directly related to alcoholism rates. Alcohol consumption is reduced by increased taxation, a 10% price increase reducing consumption by 2.5%. The *prevention* of alcoholism and alcohol abuse is thus primarily in the hands of government.

26

Eating and obesity

- Eating and body weight control are not due to the simple homoeostasis of blood glucose levels.
- Lesions to the VENTRO-MEDIAL NUCLEUS of the hypothalamus produce overeating, massive obesity and increased metabolic efficiency, whereas lesions to the LATERAL HYPOTHALAMIC AREA produce APHAGIA.
- Eating may well be controlled by monitoring the relative levels of anabolism and catabolism by measuring either portal blood glucose or blood glucagon levels.
- Mild obesity may be due to a failure to interpret INTEROCEPTIVE STIMULI, and hence a need to use EXTERNAL CUES for initiating eating.
- Behavioural treatments of obesity, using CONDITIONED AVERSION, COVERT OPERANT CONTROL, SELF-CONTROL or GROUP TREATMENTS are more effective than drug therapies, and maintain weight loss longer after treatment has ended.
- Specific food dislikes and CANCER ANOREXIA are both due to food becoming associated with illness by one-trial learning. They can be treated with SYSTEMATIC DESENSITIZATION.

Eating is essential for life but it can be impaired in illness, or even produce illness when improperly controlled.

Theories of eating control divide into PERIPHERAL and CENTRAL, each of which is 'thermostatic' in type, with NEGATIVE FEEDBACK as the means of regulation (as when room temperature is controlled by a thermostat connected to a heater). Monitoring is by the mouth, stomach or bowels in peripheral theories, and directly by the brain in central theories. The oldest peripheral theories, such as of Erasmus Darwin (1731–1802), said hunger was caused by the rugae of the empty stomach rubbing together. Gastric activity is indeed greater in hunger than in satiation but such activity cannot explain eating control, since gastrectomy or vagotomy do not produce chronic hunger or obesity (and vagotomy is sometimes used to treat gross obesity). Similarly, taste is unimportant in weight control since rats not only learn to push a lever to inject bland liquid food into the stomach but also maintain accurate weight control if the food is diluted or the schedule of injections is altered, confirming it is the nutrient effect controlling intake.

HUMORAL THEORIES propose that eating maintains a constant level of some substance in the blood. The oldest theory, and the one with the most lay (and often medical) support, is that falling blood glucose causes eating, which increases blood glucose and food intake ceases. The theory fails for several reasons. Undoubtedly intravenous glucose injection causes cessation of eating, and insulin-induced hypogly-caemia causes both hunger and eating. However, continuous glucose monitoring shows blood levels do not fall before meals (which is hardly surprising given the elaborate control mechanisms involving insulin, glucagon, cortisol and growth hormone, whose function is precisely to maintain a constant glucose level); and to encourage eating by removing the brain's principal nutrient is a dubious survival strategy. The non-specific role of glucose is shown by hypoglycaemic eating also being inhibited by non-carbohydrate nutrients such as amino acids. Also problematic is that maturity onset diabetics show chronic *hyper*glycaemia (raised blood glucose) and yet also over-eat and are obese. The final nail in the coffin of simple glucose homoeostasis is that after a meal, hunger and eating cease long before blood glucose levels have risen significantly.

Clinical cases have long suggested that hypothalamic lesions, as in FROHLICH'S SYNDROME, could cause gross obesity (and also hypogonad-ism). In 1939, Hetherington and Ranson showed that bilateral ventro-medial nucleus (VMN) lesions in the rat hypothalamus produced massive obesity, animals weighing two or three times their normal body weight. Immediately after operation (Fig. 26.1) the animals become HYPERPHAGIC (eating more), and rapidly gain weight (the DYNAMIC PHASE) after which food intake decreases, but still remains above normal, and a new steady weight is attained (the STATIC PHASE). What is wrong with VMN animals? Certainly they eat more food, which partly explains the obesity. However when pair-fed with a normal rat, so that the VMN rat eats identical amounts to the normal rat, the VMN rat *still* gains more weight than the control rat, implying a more efficient metabolism (Fig. 26.2); this hypothesis is confirmed by the increased lipogenesis found *in vitro* in liver removed 48 hours after VMN lesioning in rats, before weight gain has occurred, confirming that metabolic change is not a *consequence* of weight gain.

If a VMN animal eats more then is it hungrier? Surprisingly the answer is, no. A hungrier animal should be more willing to eat quinine-adulterated food which tastes bitter; VMN rats actually eat *less* adulterated food than normals. Hungrier rats should also work harder to get food; but VMN rats work *less* hard than normal rats. Counter-intuitively, we must conclude that the VMN rat is actually less hungry than a normal rat.

One theory of the VMN rat which failed was that the VMN contained gluco-receptors which the lesion destroyed, resulting in an absence of control, causing weight to rise inexorably because satiation could

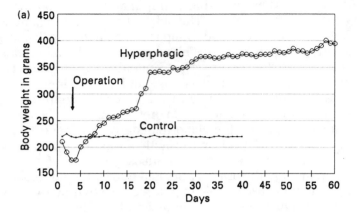

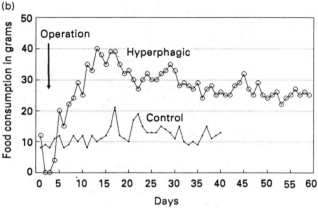

Fig. 26.1 The dynamic (early) and static (late) phases of the development of obesity in a rat following bilateral lesions of the ventro-medial nucleus of the hypothalamus, showing both increased food intake (bottom) and increased body weight (top), compared with a control animal. The dynamic phase lasts until about day 20. Adapted from Teitelbaum P (1961), in Jones M R, Ed, *Nebraska symposium on motivation*, Lincoln, University of Nebraska Press.

never occur. However if VMN-lesioned rats are force-fed to become even fatter (Fig. 26.3) they then decrease intake and return to their new 'ideal' weight (albeit three times normal) which is 'defended'; the control mechanism is still present, but reset to a higher value than normal.

Bilateral LATERAL HYPOTHALAMIC AREA (LH) lesions have opposite effects to VMN lesions, producing APHAGIA (absence of eating) and ADIPSIA (absence of drinking). Death rapidly ensues due to dehydration, but if tube-fed then eventually there is a very brittle 'recovery' with spontaneous eating. A second, more extensive, lesion causes further

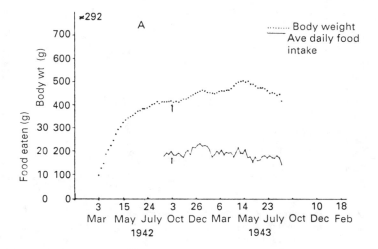

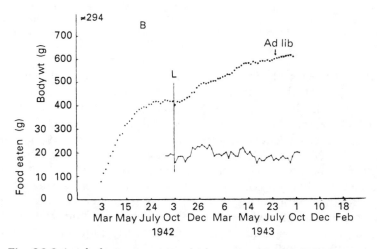

Fig. 26.2 A yoked experiment in which rat B received a VMN lesion at time L, while rat A, a litter-mate of B, acted as a control. Rat A was allowed to eat freely, *ad libitum*, and rat B was given food exactly in the same amounts as eaten by rat A. Reproduced with permission from Brooks C M and Lambert E F (1946). A study of the effect of limitation of food intake and the method of feeding on the rate of weight gain during hypothalamic obesity in the albino rat, *Am J Physiol*, **147**, 695–707.

aphagia and adipsia, confirming that previous 'recovery' was due to an incomplete first lesion. Chemical stimulation of the LH with adrenaline produces eating whereas acetylcholine produces drinking, implying separate control mechanisms at the same site.

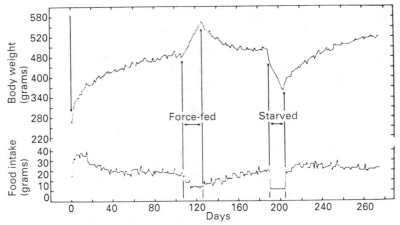

Fig. 26.3 Figure showing that even in VMN rats who are forcibly overfed or are starved, there is still a particular weight which is 'defended'. The upper line shows body weight and lower shows food intake. The animals were lesioned on day 0. Between days 108 and 126 the animals were force-fed, increasing their weight yet further; immediately after this their weight returned to its previous level. Reproduced with permission from Hoebel R G and Teitelbaum P (1966), Weight regulation in normal and hypothalamic hyperphagic rats, *Journal of Comparative and Physiological Psychology*, **61**, 189–93.

Modern theories of eating in animals are less dogmatically 'peripheral' or 'central'. Although the hypothalamus is important in eating control, the idea of 'eating centres' or 'satiety centres' is unsatisfactory, partly because many and varied lesions can affect eating, and partly because lesions may destroy fibres of passage rather than specific centres. The brain must monitor something which tells it about food balance, and a popular recent suggestion is that hepatic anabolism/catabolism is monitored, since the liver is the focus of energy balance. Monitoring is either by sensory nerves in the vagus, measuring portal glucose levels, or by measuring glucagon levels in blood (and eating is inhibited by glucagon injection and stimulated by glucagon antibodies).

Eating is induced by many environmental manipulations, such as lowering ambient temperature, which requires higher calorific intake. Mild stress, produced by gently pinching a rat's tail, also induces overeating; in man, life-stress, assessed by the Holmes-Rahe scale, correlates with food consumption by the obese (but not by normals). Tail-pinch induced eating is probably mediated via opioid peptides, and opiates in general induce eating (particularly of high-calorie food stuffs) whereas naloxone inhibits eating; opiates apparently act not by initiating more bouts of eating, but by delaying satiation, probably by making food more rewarding. Intriguingly, some food stuffs contain opiate-like substances (EXORPHINS) which, it is postulated, may themselves induce further eating by stimulating opiate receptors, perhaps causing some types of extreme obesity. Many drugs or physiologically active substaces stimulate eating (e.g. barbiturates, benzodiazepines, phenothiazines, lithium, and amitriptyline, all of which are sometimes used in patients *complaining* of obesity), and others inhibit eating (e.g. amphetamine, cocaine, prostaglandins, calcitonin, and thyrotrophin and corticotrophin releasing factors). Currently, no theoretical integration of these disaparate effects is available, although a massive research effort continues.

Initiation and termination of eating (SATIATION) are carried out by separate processes, since the effects of food are not physiologically apparent until some time after adequate quantities of food are ingested. The principal cue for cessation of eating is distention of the stomach, although gastrin release may also help in stopping eating.

After considering control of eating in normal individuals we must consider problems of eating control, of which the commonest is OBESITY; we can only really discuss human obesity since spontaneous 'natural' obesity in animals is rare, although genetic mutations such as the *ob/ob* and *fa/fa* genotypes in mice and rats do cause obesity.

Obesity is usually defined relative to height, either as PERCENTAGE OF IDEAL BODY WEIGHT or DESIRABLE WEIGHT, which has been assessed by life insurance companies, or as indices such as the PONDERAL INDEX, BODY MASS INDEX or QUETELET'S INDEX defined as weight/(height)^2. If weight is measured in kilograms, and height in metres, then ponderal indices greater than 25 are regarded as obese (Fig. 26.4): grade I obesity is clinically minor but causes psychological morbidity; grade II is clinically important, with a doubled mortality; and grade III is almost incompatible with a normal life-style.

Obesity is associated with increased mortality and morbidity from many conditions, particularly in association with smoking and hypertension. There is also substantial psychological morbidity, due to negative social attitudes to the obese; thus 6-year-old children describe the obese as 'cheats, forgets, lazy, sloppy, naughty, dirty, stupid' and even educated adults found them 'unattractive, weak, unsuccessful, not like a wife, old, not like a sister, a follower and uninfluential'. Actual discrimination is suggested from evidence that the obese are downwardly socially mobile, and less likely to enter university, even after taking differences in IQ, attainment and school record into account. Not surprisingly the obese have a NEGATIVE SELF-IMAGE and suffer much anxiety about their problem.

Obesity is common. In the UK 27%, 51% and 71% of 15–29, 30–49, and 50–65 year olds weighed more than 20% of ideal body weight, obesity being slightly more common in females than males. Some evidence suggests there may be two separate types of human obesity, mild and severe, the border-line between the two being at about 150% of ideal body weight.

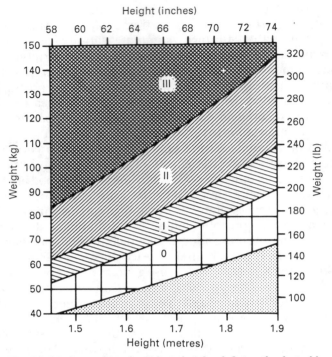

Fig. 26.4 Relationship of weight to height, defining the desirable range (0), and grades I, II and III obesity. Reproduced with permission from Garrow J S (1981), *Treat obesity seriously: a clinical manual*, Edinburgh, Churchill Livingstone.

The obese do not generally eat more food than normals, but do eat more quickly, prefer sweet foods, eat larger meals, and eat *less* meals (due to DIETARY RESTRAINT, which often takes the form of missing one meal, usually breakfast). They are, however, more likely to snack frequently between meals, and to ignore or repress this fact when recalling their daily consumption. As in VMN rats, the obese may be metabolically more efficient, although they have a higher basal metabolic rate than normals, and after correction for total body size (or when measured in obese individuals who have dieted to normal weight), it is *lower* than normals. An obese person who has slimmed to normal weight requires *less* food to maintain that weight than a normal person (and hence, in part, the problem of *staying* slim once dieted). In animals, increased metabolic efficiency, the so-called THRIFTY GENOTYPE, is genetically transmitted, and even in non-obese heterozygotes produces increased resistance to starvation, and hence a HETEROZYGOTE ADVANTAGE which maintains the gene in the gene-pool. Human obesity undoubtedly runs in families, and adoption studies strongly suggest that there is a genetic component.

Metabolic problems and hypothalamic damage account for a minority of the grossly obese and do not account for the mildly obese at all. In America, young adults have increased in body weight by about fourteen pounds in the past two decades, a change that is not due to genetic or neurological problems. The most influential psychological explanation for mild obesity is by the American psychologist Stanley Schacter, who is concerned with how individuals infer hunger from sensory data. Sensory inputs are either INTEROCEPTIVE (monitoring the state of the viscera) or EXTEROCEPTIVE (monitoring the outside world by touch, sight, smell and hearing). Schacter suggests the mildly obese cannot interpret internal signals and instead therefore use exteroceptive stimuli to control eating. Following a suggestion by the psychoanalyst Hilde Bruch that parents of obese children fundamentally reject their children and then compensate for a lack of love by over-feeding the child, Schacter argued that such infants had not had appropriate opportunities for understanding their interoceptions. Infants cry not only for hunger, but also if they are thirsty, cold, in pain, needing winding, requiring a nappy change, etc. If parents respond to all these forms of crying with feeding then the child cannot learn to discriminate those bodily states that mean hunger, but will learn to associate eating with any relief of distress. Schachter suggests that the obese depend upon EXTERNAL CUES to signal hunger, rather than internal cues related to metabolic needs. To encapsulate Schacter's theory, normal subjects eat at 6.00 pm because they *are* hungry, but the obese eat at 6.00 pm because it is 6.00 pm and they *should* be hungry. A range of ingenious experiments support this theory. In one experiment subjects reported when they had hunger pangs, while gastric contractions were monitored; in normal subjects the hunger pangs correlated with stomach contractions, but the obese showed no relation, because they were not monitoring their internal state. In another experiment while subjects carried out a range of cognitive tests (the apparent purpose of the study) they were allowed to eat freely from biscuits left on a table. The only furniture in the bare room was a clock which could be speeded up or slowed down by the experimenter. Obese subjects ate more food when they thought it was late (the clock was fast) than when they thought it was early (the clock was slow); normal subjects showed no such relationship.

Schacter's theory also predicts the obese will find fasting *easier* if there are no external cues to eating, and more difficult if there are many external cues; normals should show no such differences. Schacter studied New York Jews fasting for Yom Kippur. Obese Jews attending synagogue all day found fasting easy (there being no food-related cues) while those staying at home found fasting difficult (being surrounded by the food-associated cues of everyday life); normal weight Jews found fasting equally difficult at home or at synagogue.

Many treatments are available for obesity. Some, such as intestinal bypass surgery for the massively obese, are of little psychological interest. Psychological treatments generally try to reduce cues which might suggest eating, to neutralize cues which do occur, to provide strategies for coping with them, and to negate the positive consequences of overeating and reduce food consumption. Three main strategies are used. CONDITIONED FOOD AVERSION produces bad associations by presenting food (real or photographs) with aversive stimuli such as electric shocks, foul smells, cigarette smoke, pictures of the obese subject themself in swimming costume or underwear, or induced nausea or vomiting. Future presentations of food (the conditioned stimulus) produce revulsion (the conditioned response), and food is avoided. In controlled trials weight loss is significantly better than with a placebo condition. COVERT OPERANT CONTROL TECHNIQUES use the principle that cognitive behaviours (i.e. thoughts) are reinforced just as actual behaviours. The patient is encouraged to think about the unpleasant consequences of being fat, or the advantages of being slim, before common, everyday, rewarding activity, such as reading the newspaper or watching television, so that each occurrence of the activity results in secondary reinforcement of the thought, and encouragement of weight control behaviour. Once again controlled trials show an advantage over placebo treatments. SELF-CONTROL PACK-AGES modify deleterious behaviours associated with eating, patients learning to eat at particular times, to pause between bites, to chew food well, to avoid temptation with high calorie foods, to eat moderately in company, and to monitor food intake. Again results are better than placebo treatments. SOCIAL or GROUP TREATMENTS such as SELF-HELP GROUPS use social pressure as their main weapon. Patients meet weekly (as in *Weight Watchers* or similar groups), are weighed publicly, and mutual encouragement and support provided by discussion of problems and difficulties. The groups produce very good results. EXERCISE is also used, either alone or with other treatments, since the obese are certainly less active than normals, and although a slow treatment, it not only produces a well-maintained weight loss but also has other health advantages as well as enhancing well-being. Exercise is effective only if aerobic for half an hour or more per day, and works not only because of calorie consumption during exercise but also due to an increased metabolic rate lasting 24 hours or more (Fig. 26.5), resulting from enzymatic FUTILE CYCLING. ANORECTIC DRUGS, usually amphetamine derivatives such as fenfluramine, do produce weight loss, but it is typically small (often because patients believe that with the tablets they can eat *anything*), ceases when treatment ends, and there is a serious risk of dependence or abuse.

RECIDIVISM, the tendency to regress when treatment finishes, is a problem with treatment for all behavioural disorders, such as obesity, smoking, alcoholism and drug addiction (see Fig. 24.3 in Chapter 24). Although a particular problem with drug treatments, behaviour

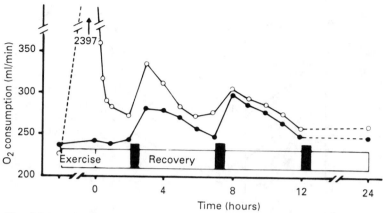

Fig. 26.5 Oxygen consumption over a 24-hour period with (open circles) and without (closed circles) exercise. The shaded areas indicate meals. Reproduced with permission from Newsholme E A (1983), Exercise and obesity, in *Exercise, health and medicine*, London, The Sports Council, 41–2.

therapies maintain results even after specific treatment has finished (Fig. 26.6), suggesting long-term behavioural change has resulted; consequently behaviour therapy is now the treatment of choice for mild to moderate obesity. Recidivism is a particular problem in treating grade III obesity by JAW WIRING, where weight is rapidly regained despite losing 35 kg from an initial average weight of 111 kg (Fig. 26.7). The simple device of an unstretchable welded nylon cord around the waist provides immediate, unpleasant feedback as weight increases unduly and prevents weight regain.

Although overeating is the commonest eating problem other disorders have undereating as the major problem.

SPECIFIC FOOD DISLIKES are produced by classical conditioning when food ingestion is associated with illness (see Chapter 3). It is well-recognized in wild rats that do not eat poisoned bait after previously nibbling a tiny quantity resulting in illness. In laboratory rats, a novel food (the conditioned stimulus) is given with a lithium chloride injection (the unconditioned stimulus) which induces gastro-intestinal distress and nausea (the conditioned response); future food presentations produce nausea and food avoidance. The procedure works even if illness occurs 24 hours after food ingestion. Undoubtedly, many human dislikes of specific foods are due to similar mechanisms; the psychologist Seligman described cooking a *sauce béarnaise*, developing 'flu 24 hours later, and subsequently disliking the sauce, even though in no sense did the food *cause* the illness. The same mechanism causes CANCER ANOREXIA in which patients on treatment for malignancies develop a lack of interest in food, it should not be confused with CACHEXIA, the massive weight loss caused by the malignancy. Radi-

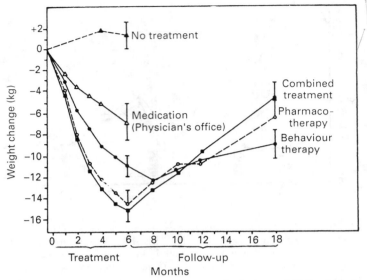

Fig. 26.6 Treatment of 145 obese individuals (over 160% of ideal body weight). Patients were randomized to three main treatments: behaviour therapy carried out in groups; pharmacotherapy (fenflura-mine) also carried out in groups; and both behaviour and pharmaco-therapy. The two control groups received either no treatment or just medication ('doctor's office') where fenfluramine and dietary advice were dispensed from the doctor's office (to control for the group meetings in the main treatment conditions). Active treatment ceased after 6 months and patients were followed for a further 12 months. Reproduced with permission from Craighead L W, Stunkard A J and O'Brien R (1981), Behaviour therapy and pharmacotherapy for obesity, *Arch Gen Psychiat*, **38**, 763–8; copyright 1981, American Medical Association.

otherapy and antineoplastic drugs used in cancer therapy produce nausea and vomiting as side-effects; any food ingested in the previous 24 hours therefore becomes associated with illness and becomes disliked. Conditioned food aversion is readily treated by SYSTEMATIC DESENSITIZATION, the relaxed patient gradually being exposed to more potent food stimuli.

ANOREXIA NERVOSA is a psychiatric condition, particularly common in adolescent women (about one in every hundred), in which a morbid fear of becoming excessively fat results in persistent food refusal, and a very low body weight; menstruation ceases, and infectious disease becomes a serious risk. Some patients also show BINGE-EATING, disposing of excess food by self-induced vomiting and purging, BULIMIA NERVOSA. Anorectics have a DISTORTED BODY-IMAGE, measured by asking the patient to adjust the proportions of a computer-generated photograph until it accurately reflects true bodily proportions, seeing themselves as fatter than they really are, so their own excessive slimness is perceived

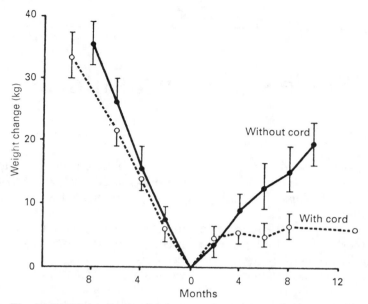

Fig. 26.7 Weight change after jaw wiring in massively obese women. Jaw wires were removed at time 0. Half the women had a nylon cord placed around the waist when the desired result had been achieved. Reproduced with permission from Garrow J S and Gardiner G T (1981), Maintenance of weight loss in obese patients after jaw wiring, *Br Med J*, **282**, 858–60.

as normal. The cause of anorexia is not clear. Social pressure is important, the incidence of disease rising as slimness is emphasized more in sexual attractivity. However, an unconscious rejection of femininity, and an attempt to suppress menstruation and cause breast atrophy, are also important. Pituitary axis abnormalities occur, although they might be primary or secondary. Treatment of anorexia nervosa is by a combination of psychotherapy, behaviour therapy and drugs such as tricyclic antidepressants.

27

Models of mental illness

- The definition of ABNORMALITY, both in psychology and medicine, is fraught with difficulties and cannot be based solely on statistical criteria, biological maladaptivity, or personal awareness by the patient.
- As they pass through medical school, students change their perceptions of whether particular conditions are 'diseases', becoming less ESSENTIALIST and more NOMINALIST.
- The MEDICAL MODEL and the BEHAVIOURAL MODEL of psychiatric illness differ in most of their implicit assumptions about the nature of psychiatric illness and its appropriate treatment. Many practising psychiatrists are ECLECTIC, utilizing features from both in the BIO-PSYCHO-SOCIAL MODEL.
- Psychological models, such as LEARNING THEORY, PERSONAL CONSTRUCT THEORY and PSYCHOANALYTIC THEORY differ to a large extent in the time-scale over which they try to produce explanations of behaviour.

Mental illness is common. At some time in their life, 1% of the population develop schizophrenia, one in ten are admitted to a mental hospital, and a much higher proportion receive psychoactive medication. Yet even the term 'mental *illness*' is controversial, and the role of psychiatry and psychology in dealing with abnormal behaviour is not clear. Here I will consider the problems of defining and classifying abnormal behaviour and disease, and will compare the MEDICAL MODEL with other models of psychological disorder. The difficulties described are not unique to psychological problems, being seen in all aspects of medicine, but are especially acute for behavioural conditions.

ABNORMALITY is impossible to define precisely and all straightforward definitions have problems. A statistical perspective might say that if unusual enough (more than two standard deviations from the mean) then symptoms or behaviour are abnormal; but this would classify as 'abnormal' those with an IQ of over 130 (including most medical students), and would also ascribe 'normality' to those in populations such as the Pima Indians where a majority show symptoms of diabetes. An alternative view sees abnormality as *biologically* maladaptive, and classifies behaviours such as suicide as abnormal (although lemmings may provide a problem), but also has to say that chastity is 'abnormal'. More problematic is that many homozygous genes, such as sickle-cell anaemia, are disadvantageous for individuals but nevertheless selected for due to their beneficial effects in heterozygotes; should therefore biological maladaptation be considered for the individual or the population? An alternative defines abnormality as being antisocial, and although including the arsonist's fire-raising, the definition also includes minor offences like parking on a yellow line, or over-consumption of garlic. Yet another approach defines abnormality as a person seeing themselves as abnormal, so that symptoms are defined by the patient's decision to attend a doctor. Unfortunately a defining characteristic of psychoses is an absence of insight (see Chapter 28), as also in temporal-lobe fugues and sleep-walking, where even conscious awareness of the behaviour is absent. One possibly acceptable definition of abnormality asks whether the behaviour is maladaptive for the individual (although not perhaps seen as such by the individual). The definition does not imply that treatment should or must be given, and does circumvent many obvious problems, such as whether homosexuality is 'abnormal'; the answer is *No* if the individual is satisfied with their condition, but *Yes* if they find it repellent, have become obsessed, or it is putting their livelihood at risk, and request help.

The difficulty of knowing whether behaviour is abnormal can be seen in an example. A few years ago the Deans of British and American medical schools each received a short letter:

'Dear Dr.,
Please be advised of my opinion that Medical Students should be instructed in the Physiology of Fear.
Thank you,
Yours sincerely,
————— MB ChB (Edin), MRCPath(UK), FRCP(C)'

Checking in the Medical Directory showed the sender's qualifications were valid. Although clearly eccentric, the letter could, with special pleading, be seen as within the bounds of normality. A second letter, shown below, was more eccentric still, and the *combination* of the letters makes one suspect a more disordered psyche meriting the term *abnormal*.

'Dear Dr.,
Please be advised of my opinion that if you contemplate the concept of your own demise with reasonable equanimity then you may well be as psychologically mature as you are going to be.
Thank you,
Yours sincerely,
————— MB ChB(Edin), MRCPath(UK), FRCP(C)'

Abnormal behaviour alone does not indicate mental illness, any more than one cough indicates physical disease. As a concept, DISEASE is broader and more difficult to define, despite it being obvious that, say, leukaemia, pneumonia or scurvy are diseases. But what about spina bifida, colour-blindness or other congenital abnormalities? Or barbiturate overdose or drowning? There is a large 'grey area', many items being better labelled as 'conditions' rather than 'diseases'. When asked to indicate which of a long list of conditions are diseases, individuals disagree, although doctors usually classify more items as diseases then do laymen, a process sociologists call MEDICALIZATION. Medical students shift between these positions (see Fig. 27.1), and also become more precise at differentiating disease from non-disease (i.e. in Figure 27.1 the slopes of the line becomes steeper). Doctors and laymen also differ in their philosophical views about disease. The lay public is ESSENTIALIST, saying diseases exist, and medicine's role is to discover, understand, and treat them, whereas doctors are NOMINALISTS, seeing the definition of disease as mainly a matter of convenience and utility, and arbitrary to a large extent. Doctors typically see conditions as disease if caused by external agents, particularly if infectious or toxic, or if amenable to specifically medical treatments. Conditions therefore change their status as our knowledge of them changes.

Even in physical medicine, diagnosis and classification of disease is often not clear. Diagnosis of some diseases such as malaria is straightforward (are there malarial parasites in the blood?), but others do not have a single criterion which alone confirms the diagnosis. Thus rheumatoid arthritis is 'classical' if seven or more of 11 specific symptoms or signs is present, 'definite' if five features are present, and 'probable' if three features are present, although no single feature is either necessary or sufficient for the diagnosis. Such POLYMORPHOUS CONCEPTS are peculiarly difficult to manipulate psychologically, even though common in practice. Diagnosis of other diseases such as septicaemia seems straightforward (fever and bacterial growth from blood cultures), but what if a patient is asymptomatic and grows a few bacteria from the blood? Gilbert's syndrome, of a marginally raised serum bilirubin, familial in origin, and without symptoms or long-term consequences is marginal in its status as a disease and must be contrasted with hypertension, which also is asymptomatic and familial, but has serious adverse consequences if untreated; and as a further difficulty no clear threshold separates high from normal blood pressure. Such problems are particularly pertinent in psychiatry and psychology and for research purposes are avoided by strict assessment of well-defined and codified symptoms in such protocols as the PRESENT-STATE EXAMINATION and DSM-IV (the fourth revision of the DIAGNOSTIC AND STATISTICAL MANUAL OF THE AMERICAN PSYCHIATRIC ASSOCIATION).

LABELLING a person as having disease can modify their response to their own health. In an American study which screened factory

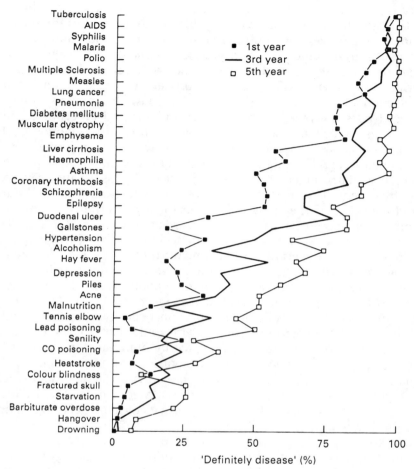

Fig. 27.1 Shows the proportion of first year (preclinical), third year (first clinical) and fifth year (final clinical) medical students who feel that particular conditions (shown vertically) are 'diseases', the conditions being placed in order from most disease-like to least disease-like (averaged across all years). Reproduced with permission from Stefan M D and McManus I C, The concept of disease: its evaluation in medical students, *Social Science and Medicine*, **29**, 791–2.

workers for hypertension, individuals who were told about their raised blood pressure subsequently showed more absenteeism for minor illness than did hypertensives unaware of their raised blood pressure. Labelling as 'hypertensive' explained symptoms that otherwise would be ignored or dismissed as part of everyday life, and these symptoms then legitimized an absence from work as an appropriate response to an 'illness'.

The concept of disease does not exist in isolation, but also implies other assumptions in what is now described as the MEDICAL MODEL OF DISEASE, which is contrasted with other models such as the psychoanalytical and moral models. With psychiatric abnormalities the medical model emphasizes the central role of a clear, specific and accurate DIAGNOSIS, from which comes a precise treatment and prognosis. The AETIOLOGY (cause) of a disease may not actually be known but in principle is always knowable. SYMPTOMS are regarded as an inexact reflection of the disease process, which may be better assessed by special tests. TREATMENT is by medical and surgical procedures, such as drugs, which are specific and depend upon the diagnosis. The PROGNOSIS is also specific, but may always be transformed by a therapeutic breakthrough. Attempted SUICIDE is an especial problem with psychiatric illness, and must be predicted if possible and prevented by treatment. The FUNCTION OF THE HOSPITAL is to care, treat and cure, and HOSPITALIZATION ends when the doctor decides that the patient is cured. The appropriate PERSONNEL for care are doctors and nurses. The PATIENT'S RIGHTS AND DUTIES are a right to knowledge of the diagnosis and a duty to cooperate with treatment; that is, the SICK ROLE should be adopted. The FAMILYS' RIGHTS AND DUTIES are a duty to bring sick relatives to doctors, and a right to know about their relative's illness and to expect appropriate treatment. SOCIETY'S RIGHTS AND DUTIES are a duty to treat the mentally ill and to protect society from them, and a right to expect cooperation from patients and society. The medical (or BIO-MEDICAL) model is implicitly accepted by many doctors, at least for physical illness, and by many psychiatrists for mental illness. By making its assumptions explicit it can be contrasted with other models, of which the PSYCHOANALYTIC MODEL (or BEHAVIOURAL MODEL) is the most important. The central difference from the medical model is in denying the utility of a diagnosis, since all individuals differ; naming will not help the patient, and may harm them as society uses labelling pejoratively to prevent treatment as an individual. Aetiology is specific to each patient, arising from experiences in earlier life, which will never be the same in any two patients. Symptoms are the most precise guide as to the patient's condition and to the effects of treatment, which is carried out by those experienced with psychological problems, and is behavioural in form, being tailored to the specific needs of the patient. A prognosis is given only with difficulty. Attempted suicide should be interpreted as would any other symptom. The hospital provides a refuge, removing an environment that may have precipitated the patient's problems, and is a convenient place for patient and therapist to meet. Hospitalization ends when the patient has insight into their problems, and accepts that behaviour and symptoms have improved.

In their pure form these models differ substantially. In practice many psychiatrists and psychologists are ECLECTIC, extracting features from these and other models in the so-called BIO-PSYCHO-SOCIAL MODEL.

Other models of mental illness often contribute components; for instance the MORAL MODEL is concerned entirely with behaviour which is regarded as bad or sinful and sees treatment as simply to prevent deviant behaviour; and the FAMILY INTERACTION MODEL emphasizes that it is not individuals who are sick but rather entire families can be abnormal, externalizing problems through an individual who acts as scape-goat; and the SOCIETAL MODEL extends that argument by saying that society itself is sick, the illness of individuals being its symptoms.

It must be emphasized that these models are not merely right or wrong, for they transcend ordinary empirical data, and determine all actions of which they are a part. Stepping outside their implicit assumptions is as difficult as thinking in other languages or in conceptualizing mathematical worlds with five dimensions or non-Euclidean geometries; possible but very difficult. Their importance is in making explicit the hidden assumptions that often hide behind apparently objective descriptions of problems.

In the following chapters the word 'model' will be applied in a slightly different sense of PSYCHOLOGICAL MODELS, to the three most important types of mental illness: the neuroses, depression, and schizophrenia. A psychological model is a theory which explains the phenomena of a condition, says what it must be like to experience that condition, explains its origins, and makes predictions about the condition. For each major condition, I will describe the LEARNING THEORY MODEL, the PERSONAL CONSTRUCT THEORY MODEL and the PSYCHOANALYTIC MODEL, with additional models in some cases. Different models are not competing hypotheses of which one only is correct; rather they are different perspectives on the same object, just as the plan and the elevation of a building describe the same building. Figure 27.2 might illustrate the relationship of the models. Dots indicate individual behaviours, which are inter-related by links. Learning theory emphasizes the precise linkage of two behaviours as shown by ring A. Personal construct theory takes a broader view, of all the behaviours and cognitive processes at time t, as shown by ring B. And to some extent learning theory and personal construct theory both consider how behaviour at time t was caused by previous behaviour at time $t - 1$. Standing further back, psychoanalytic models ask how the behaviours at time t developed from the undifferentiated psyche present at birth (time 0), and consider the evolution or development of behaviour within the individual (ring C). The models differ therefore in scale, or perspective. Although it is tempting to see only the learning theory model as 'really' explaining a patient's condition, the limitations of its microscopic analysis may be seen by analogy with a physical illness. A patient presents with a range of symptoms, which after investigation are diagnosed as hepatic cirrhosis, caused by excessive alcohol consumption, and is confirmed by liver biopsy, which demonstrates fibrosis, distortion of cellular architecture and nodular hyper-

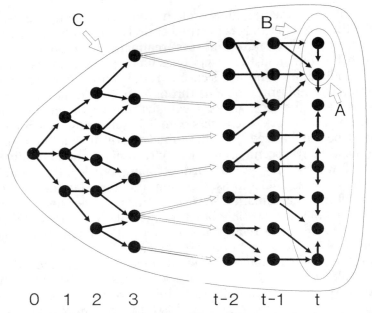

Fig. 27.2 A diagrammatic representation of the levels of explanation of learning theory (A), personal construct theory (B), and psychoanalytic theory (C). See text for further details.

plasia. This observation, equivalent to level A in Figure 27.2, might seem a complete explanation to a reductionist. The astute physician will however ask how it explains the patient's spider naevi, the flapping tremor of the hands, the gynaecomastia, and the mental confusion. *Merely* knowing hepatic histology does not explain the symptoms, but only says that an abnormality is present. Symptoms must be interpreted at the level of the entire patient, integrating the histology into a dynamic and responsive physiology (level B in Fig. 27.2). But describing the patient as they are *at this moment* does not explain how they became like it; why did alcohol have this effect, and why did they consume so much alcohol? For answers to such questions, and to the particularly important question of the best treatment for the patient, we must consider the evolution of the disease in the context of the patient's metabolism, life, and social conditions (level C in Fig. 27.2). When seeing this patient with cirrhosis a good physician will simultaneously consider their biochemistry, histology, pathophysiology, and the evolution of their disease in its social and behavioural context. No single level of analysis alone is correct, and nor do the levels compete; they are different parts of the same story. Similarly in the next three chapters, conditions will be described from several view-points, all of which make unique contributions to understanding the total picture of the patient and their problem. Since however this book's purpose is principally to describe psychology, treatment will not be considered in depth, except in so far as it illuminates *psychological* processes; therapy is primarily the province of psychiatry and of clinical psychology, and you must go elsewhere for a detailed discussion of those matters.

28

The neuroses

- NEUROSES, such as FREE-FLOATING ANXIETY, PHOBIAS and OBSESSIVE-COM-PULSIVE DISORDERS are characterized by the emotion of ANXIETY, and are distinguished from the PSYCHOSES by the presence of INSIGHT.
- The TWO-STAGE THEORY of phobias says that they are initiated by classical conditioning of fear to a stimulus and are maintained by operant conditioning, which produces avoidance of the stimulus, thereby preventing extinction.
- Behavioural treatment of phobias uses either SYSTEMATIC DESENSITIZATION or FLOODING, to extinguish the association between the stimulus and fear.
- The personal construct system of a phobic is MONOLITHIC, with a single construct against which all events are evaluated. PERSONAL CONSTRUCT PSYCHOTHERAPY loosens such TIGHT CONSTRUCTS by means of FIXED-ROLE THERAPY.
- In psychoanalytic theory, neuroses arise from FIXATION earlier in psychosexual development, late or early phallic fixation resulting in a predisposition to hysteria or agoraphobia, and anal fixation resulting in obsessive-compulsive disorder.
- Psychoanalytic treatment of neuroses requires a detailed interpretation of the specific events and their appropriate symbolic meanings for the patient, who then works through and eventually accepts those meanings.

NEUROSES must be distinguished from PSYCHOSES, more serious disorders that severely disrupt mental functioning. Although sometimes called MINOR REACTIONS, neuroses can utterly disrupt the life of both patient and family. They are characterized by a single behavioural problem in an otherwise intact personality, with normal perception of the world, normal emotional responses, and normal social sensitivity. Neurotics have INSIGHT, being aware of their problem and asking for help with it. In contrast, the psychotic's more profound problem is a MAJOR REACTION, with personality disorganization or disintegration, which makes it difficult to accept one is dealing with the same person as before the illness. Internal and external events (subjective and objective) become confused, altering the sense of personal identity (EGO DISINTEGRATION). Emotions either flatten or are wildly inappropriate, social interaction is impaired, and despite the severe problem, insight is absent.

The characteristic emotion of neurosis is ANXIETY, manifested psychologically by needless worrying, particularly about minutiae, intolerance of strong stimuli (shown by wearing sun-glasses on dull days), psychological exhaustion (once called NEURASTHENIA), difficulty in falling asleep, nightmares, and unrealistic fear of physical disease (HYPOCHONDRIASIS); physical symptoms are sweating, goose-pimples, dry mouth, pupillary dilatation, frequency of micturition, diarrhoea, tachycardia, and hyperventilation, sometimes leading to tetany.

Anxiety can be DIFFUSE or FREE-FLOATING, unconnected with specific events, and occasionally causing a PANIC ATTACK. SPECIFIC ANXIETY typically occurs in the PHOBIAS, where anxiety is caused by a particular object (as in the MONOPHOBIAS of spiders, cats, snakes, blood, or syringe needles) or situation (the DIFFUSE PHOBIAS, of CLAUSTROPHOBIA, a fear of enclosed spaces, and AGORAPHOBIA, a fear of open spaces, or more precisely, of *public* places). Fears can GENERALIZE from the original object so that a spider phobic might fear even to go upstairs, because a spider might be in the bathroom, and an agoraphobic might be unable even to leave their house. Specific anxiety also occurs in OBSESSIVE-COMPULSIVE DISORDERS; the OBSESSION is a recurrent mental preoccupation about particular actions (the COMPULSION). The actions are often repetitive and RITUALIZED, as before bed checking each lock, gas tap and electric socket a specific number of times in a particular order, the ritual taking several hours, with any interruption requiring restarting from the beginning. In obessive cleanliness and hygiene, compulsory hand washing can occur so often that it produces excoriation. Anxiety is not central to the rituals, but occurs when their completion is frustrated.

In phobias and obsessive-compulsive disorder, the symptoms are separate from other mental activities, which are normal, and the patient can hold a job and have ordinary social relationships. The patient recognizes the irrationality of the behaviour, but simply cannot stop it.

Other, less common, neurotic disorders such as CONVERSION HYSTERIA (see Chapter 11) will not be considered here, as phobias and obsessive-compulsive disorders are adequate examples of the application of psychological models.

THE LEARNING THEORY MODEL OF NEUROSIS

Learning theory says phobias result from classical conditioning. Some innocuous stimulus, such as a spider, occurs in association (perhaps accidentally) with an event producing anxiety or fear, so that in future the stimulus also induces fear. This was shown experimentally by the founder of behaviourism, J B Watson (1878–1958), with a 9-month-old boy called 'Little Albert'. A white rat (the conditioned stimulus), which previously was not a phobic object, was presented to the boy just as fear (the unconditioned response) was induced by a loud noise (the unconditioned stimulus). Subsequently, the boy showed a phobic response to the rat, which induced fear (the conditioned response). Although attractive, this simple theory of phobias has two problems. Firstly, extinction should be rapid when the child subsequently sees the rat without a concurrent noise. It does not occur because of secondary operant conditioning by which phobics avoid the stimulus associated with fear, thereby reducing their anxiety, reinforcing an AVOIDANCE RESPONSE and preventing extinction. In the TWO STAGE THEORY, the phobia is initiated by classical conditioning but maintained by operant conditioning. A second problem is that many stimuli are associated with fearful events, but few produce phobias. Certain objects, such as rats or snakes, induce phobias far more often than do others, such as teddy bears or kittens. BIOLOGICAL PREPAREDNESS is suggested to make certain stimuli more easily conditioned, and more resistant to extinction, this being evolutionarily of selective value.

Learning theory suggests two distinct forms of treatment for phobias. In SYSTEMATIC DESENSITIZATION the patient learns to relax, and then is presented with a graded series of stimuli, from very mildly phobic (a picture of a very small spider), to very fear provoking (a live tarantula). The patient relaxes with each stimulus, and moves to the next only when able to cope with the present one. Two processes are occurring: relaxation is associated with the stimulus, and the association between fear and the stimulus is extinguished. The technique is applicable to a broad range of problems and is widely used (for instance in deconditioning fears of social events). The second technique, FLOODING, appears the exact opposite of systematic desensitization. The patient is placed where they cannot avoid the phobic stimulus, as in a small room with several large spiders. The two stage theory says extinction of classical conditioning does not occur because of avoidance responses. Flooding prevents avoidance and allows extinction of the stimulus-fear association. Exposure may be quite lengthy, perhaps for several hours, but is then very successful.

Learning theory in obsessive-compulsive disorder says that the primary problem is anxiety, either induced by specific objects (such as gas taps) or by specific thoughts (as of disease). The anxiety originates from operant conditioning, the patient discovering, perhaps by accident, that some specific action reduces anxiety, and the anxiety reduction therefore reinforces the action, which then increases in frequency because each production results in further transient decreases in anxiety. In a laboratory demonstration, a hungry pigeon in a Skinner box can be given food automatically at random intervals, independently of any specific behaviour by the pigeon. If food delivery coincides with a particular action (such as standing on one leg), then this action is effectively rewarded, and subsequently is performed more often. Eventually the animals spends much of its time carrying out SUPERSTITIOUS or RITUALIZED behaviour, mistakenly assuming that the behaviour actually *caused* the reinforcement.

Behavioural treatment of obsessive-compulsive disorder also takes several forms. SYSTEMATIC DESENSITIZATION can reduce the association between an object or thought and subsequent anxiety, although it is not very successful in long established cases. A second approach reduces the association between ritualistic behaviour and anxiety reduction, by associating the behaviour with aversive stimuli, such as mild electric shocks. Although successful, it only treats the compulsion and not the obsession, and therefore is not desirable. The third approach, which is the treatment of choice, is FLOODING combined with RESPONSE PREVENTION. The patient is put in the anxiety provoking situation, is prevented from making the obsessive response (physically if necessary), and learns that the obsessional thought is not genuinely anxiety provoking, and hence can be coped with.

PERSONAL CONSTRUCT THEORY OF NEUROSIS

Personal construct theory sees anxiety as the predominant emotion of the neuroses, the anxiety reflecting failure of the construct system adequately to predict the world. However, construct systems often fail in daily life (and indeed that is essential, for otherwise they could not improve). The neurotic differs in their response to failure of the construct system from normal individuals, who alter constructs to make them more successful. Phobics adopt a different approach. Since the construct system failed to cope with a particular event a solution is to inhabit a world in which the event does not occur, or is not allowed to occur. This 'cooking the books' does not allow events which might invalidate the system. However, phobic objects, by their nature, can occur at any time, and progressively more and more of the construct system is devoted to anticipating the possible occurrence of the object, and avoiding it. Hence the phobic develops a MONOLITHIC or 'one-track' construct system, in which the usual three or four independent clusters of constructs are replaced with a single, massive construct system, with each construct simply implying 'good' or 'bad' in relation to the likely occurrence or not of the phobic object; so-called TIGHT CONSTRUING.

The obsessive-compulsive is slightly different. Once again the construct system is failing, but not because of uncontrollable external events, but due to being very LOOSE, with very many independent constructs, which do not inter-relate to each other. Such a construct system should be tightened; however that, of course, would be anxiety provoking. The obsessive-compulsive therefore prefers not to tighten the entire system but instead concentrates on a small portion (see Fig. 30.3 in Chapter 30). The obsessional therefore, as it were, lives in one corner of the construct system, choosing a construct such as safety or health with which to interpret all events.

PERSONAL CONSTRUCT PSYCHOTHERAPY has a range of treatments which try to change the construct system, in the case of neurotic disorders by loosening overly tight systems, by an interactive process between therapist and patient. Kelly said that if an appropriate model of man was of a scientist trying to understand the world, then the appropriate model for therapist and client was that of research student and supervisor; one, the patient, is well-informed about the specifics of their own condition whereas the other, the therapist, has general experience of the problems of patients. Completion and interpretation of a repertory grid can itself be therapeutic for a patient, forcing them to see the limitations of their thought processes and the room for expansion of the construct system. A useful way to promote change is FIXED-ROLE THERAPY; the patient first produces a SELF-CHARACTERIZATION, a description of themself as written by a friend. Patient and therapist then negotiate a FIXED-ROLE SKETCH describing a person with many opposite attributes to the patient themself, and the therapist then helps the patient explore what it would mean to *be* such a person. The patient then acts such a role, and thereby realizes the viability of other views of the world and incorporates some into their own construct system. Thus the patient not only explores their own personality but also realizes its mutability, being under their own control, and that other options can be tried and incorporated if beneficial. The 'suspension of disbelief' that occurs when watching a play or film, or reading a book, allows precisely the same acting out and exploration of different ways of being in the world, as we watch and identify with the various characters.

THE PSYCHOANALYTIC MODEL OF NEUROSIS

If the learning theory of neuroses considers a simple association of stimulus and response, and personal construct theory assesses the impact of that association upon the entire adult construct system, psychoanalysis steps further back and views neurosis in relation to the patient's whole life, especially in relation to infancy.

As in other models of neurosis, psychoanalytic theory sees anxiety as the predominant emotion, in this case arising from a CONFLICT between the demands of the ego and the unconscious. The anxiety can be partly reduced by EGO-DEFENCE MECHANISMS (see Chapter 11), but these also restrict the character of the individual and exacerbate problems. Present conflicts arise out of failure of resolution of conflicts occurring earlier in psychosexual life, causing FIXATION at oral, anal or phallic stages, the type of neurosis depending upon the time of fixation: the late phallic stage causes concern with sexual fulfilment and a predisposition to hysteria; the early phallic stage causes avoidance of sexual relations and a predisposition to agoraphobia (and hence avoidance of temptation); and the anal stage causes a concern with MASTERY, with a sadistic or masochistic component and a predisposition to obsessive-compulsive disorder. In each case, fixation produces a *predisposition*, or increased likelihood of problems, not a *certainty*. Fixations leave the psyche weakened and vulnerable to subsequent traumas. Freud also emphasized the similarities between obsessive-compulsive rituals and the formal ritual of religion, and argued not only that QUASI-RELIGIOUS CEREMONIALS in obsessionals are an individualized religion, but also, and more controversially, that religion itself is a UNIVERSAL OBSESSIONAL NEUROSIS, with fixation at a societal level.

Psychoanalytic understanding of a patient's neurosis requires detailed analysis of their specific problems. The strengths and weaknesses of the analytic approach are best seen in a case history described by Freud in his *Introductory Lectures on Psychoanalysis*. The patient was a 19-year-old girl who was the only child of parents of lesser education and lower intellectual ability than herself. In her childhood she had been wild and high-spirited, and over the previous three or four years had become progressively affected by her neurosis. The principal symptoms were irritability, particularly expressed at the mother, and a continual sense of dissatisfaction and 'depression'. She had problems in being unable to walk by herself across squares, wide streets or other public places; an agoraphobia. She also had an obsessive-compulsive disorder, involving an elaborate 'sleep ceremonial', taking one or two hours each night, and seriously disrupting her and her parent's life. The rest of this account will consider the sleep ceremonial, and use the general psychoanalytic principle that symptoms are not random but have specific meanings, which might require interpretation, the symbolic value not being apparent at first. Successful treatment will require the patient's insight into those underlying meanings, and hence resolution of the conflicts.

The sleep ceremonial is typical of the rituals seen in such patients. Their ostensible purpose was to produce quiet, so the patient could sleep better, all sources of noise being removed. Specifically:

i. the big clock in the bedroom was stopped.

ii. all small clocks and watches were removed.

iii. the flower pots and vases were put on the writing table 'so that they might not fall over and break', and hence disturb sleep.

iv. the connecting door with the parents' bedroom was wedged in the *half-open* position (even though this would clearly *not* prevent disturbing noise).

v. the large pillow on the continental bed was placed so that it did not touch the wooden bedstead.

vi. the small square pillow was placed in a diamond shape on the long, lower pillow.

vii. the duvet was first shaken so that all the feathers were in a bulge at the bottom, and were then ritualistically smoothed out.

Using psychoanalytic techniques, Freud explored the symbolic meaning of the various components of the ceremonial. Clocks and watches frequently symbolize the female genitals through their periodicity (and many women describe their menstruation as 'regular as clockwork'). However, the girl associated the ticking of the large clock with the throbbing sensation found in the clitoris during sexual excitement. Flower pots and vases are also female symbols, and the breaking of a pot is symbolic of a loss of virginity (and at some Mediterranean weddings, men smash vases or plates to show renunciation of the bride as a possible sexual partner). The soft, yielding pillows are also female symbols, whereas the firm, upright bedstead is a male phallic symbol.

By now the elements of the ceremonial are seen not to be just random but to have a systematic meaning, with a recurrent theme of prevention of sexual activity (stopping the clocks and watches), and with protection of virginity (symbolized not only by the unbroken vases, but being supported by a childhood recollection when she had fallen, dropped a vase she was carrying, and cut her finger which bled profusely, and which she associated with the metaphorical falling of loss of virginity and haemorrhage). The male and female symbols, pillow and bedstead, were kept apart, and these symbolized the parents who were also kept apart, not least by the girl keeping open the door to their bedroom. As a girl she recalled simulating nocturnal fears in order to be taken into her parents' bed, and when older had slept in the parental bed with the father, while her mother occupied the daughter's bed. The girl was an only child, and had been frightened of her parents having another child, and that fear was still seen in· the ruffling of the duvet to produce a pregnancy-like swelling, followed by its smoothing away and thus the abolition of her fears. The large and small pillows represented mother and daughter, and placing the small pillow over the large represented an Oedipal wish to replace the mother in the father's affections. The sexuality of this wish was seen by the diamond-shape placing of the pillow, the diamond being a well-known, if crude, graffito for the female genitals (as can be verified in many public toilets). The ceremonial ended with the girl's head being placed on the pillow (i.e. over her own symbolic genitals) rather than against the male bedstead, to demonstrate the ego-defence mechanisms which had produced the elaborate ritual. Freud interpreted the case as representing an unresolved Oedipal conflict at the phallic stage, resulting in the girl developing an erotic fascination with her own father.

At this point you may well feel that the case has been heavily over-interpreted, and is highly unlikely, perhaps even impossible, for a young girl in late nineteenth century Vienna. Perhaps so, and Freud himself was aware of such criticism. Nevertheless the story has a unity and a completeness which would be difficult to derive from, say, a learning theory account of the patient. Freud concluded his own description of the case thus:

'Wild thoughts, you will say, to be running through an unmarried girl's head. I admit that this is so. But you must not forget that I did not make these things but only interpreted them. A sleep-ceremonial like this is a strange thing too, and you will not fail to see how the ceremonial corresponds to the phantasies which are revealed by the interpretation.' Freud, S, *Introductory Lectures in Psychoanalysis*, Standard edition, **16**, 268–9.

29

Depression

- REACTIVE or NEUROTIC depression and ENDOGENOUS or PSYCHOTIC depression differ in their symptoms. BIOLOGICAL SYMPTOMS are more frequent in psychotic depression, whereas CAUSAL INSIGHT expressed by the patient into the origin of the depressive attack is more common in neurotic depression.
- If dogs are exposed to unavoidable shocks they develop the syndrome of LEARNED HELPLESSNESS, which shows many of the features of human depression, including decreased cerebral noradrenaline levels, which must be seen as *caused* by the depression rather than *causing* the depression.
- Depressive cognitions are marked by a diminished SELF-ESTEEM and NEGATIVE thoughts about the world, coupled with GUILT that the self-image is not as it should be.
- Melanie Klein described the early stages of attachment in which the child develops hatred and then AMBIVALENCE towards loved objects which have temporarily frustrated it by separation. Permanent loss can result in INTROJECTION of self-hatred, and vulnerability to depression.
- Brown and Harris' model of depression emphasizes the causal role of serious RECENT PROVOKING EVENTS in causing depression, modulated by VULNERABILITY and PROTECTIVE FACTORS. Early loss of a parent is a SYMPTOM-MODIFICATION FACTOR, loss by death producing psychotic symptoms and loss by separation producing neurotic symptoms.

Depressive symptoms occur in most of the population at some time during their lives. The principal abnormalities are of MOOD or AFFECT, with pervasive feelings of SADNESS, accompanied by TEARFULNESS or WEEPING, and varying from mild despondency ('the blues'), to utter DESPAIR, with SUICIDE a real possibility. Thought processes are slowed, and inability to concentrate or make decisions often show early as loss of interest in hobbies or activities; intellectual slowing down is accompanied by a more general RETARDATION, with slowed motor actions and speech, which shows long pauses, absent spontaneous utterances, and mono-syllabic replies to questions. Those thoughts that do occur are self-concerned, inward-looking and described by patients as 'painful', and concerned only with problems and difficulties, and are self-deprecatory and self-accusatory, the individual taking upon themself the burdens and the responsibilities of the world. The NEGATIVE SELF-IMAGE is often associated with HYPOCHONDRIASIS, an unrealistic fear of serious physical illness, which can be precipitated by the so-called BIOLOGICAL SYMPTOMS of depression, which can be seen as physiological retardation, with loss of appetite and weight, reduced libido, and constipation (often misinterpreted as a symptom of bowel cancer), and disturbed sleep, in particular showing early morning wakening. Mood often varies during the course of the day, DIURNAL VARIATION.

Depression is classified in several ways. MANIA is the opposite of depression with excessive elevation of mood, an overwhelming sense of well-being and ability to carry out any task (without actually completing any), pressure of ideas, and flights of fancy. In BIPOLAR DEPRESSION or MANIC-DEPRESSIVE PSYCHOSIS, mood swings from mania to depression and back again, over days or weeks, passing through relative normality *en route*. Bipolar depression is relatively rare, and is probably genetic with a specific biochemical defect. It will not be considered further here. The more usual UNIPOLAR DEPRESSION shows mood changes between normality and depression, without a manic phase. Unipolar depressives can be divided into REACTIVE and ENDOGENOUS, each with several synonyms. REACTIVE, EXOGENOUS or NEUROTIC DEPRESSION apparently arises from a specific event in a patient's life, a loss or a failure, whereas in ENDOGENOUS or PSYCHOTIC DEPRESSION the patient is unaware of a precipitating factor, and lacks insight into the aetiology, the illness apparently arising from within without cause. Biological symptoms are more common in endogenous depression, and diurnal variation differs, moods being worst in the morning and improving during the day in endogenous depression, whereas in reactive depression mood becomes worse towards evening. Whether these are two separate conditions, or are merely extremes on a continuum, is still controversial.

This chapter will consider learning theory, personal construct theory, and psychoanalytic models of depression, and will also consider a sociologically based model to broaden the perspective.

LEARNING THEORY MODEL OF DEPRESSION

When a dog is placed in a SHUTTLE BOX, a cage with a low barrier down the middle, and is given mild electric shocks through the floor of one side, preceded by a warning bell or light, then it rapidly learns to escape shock by jumping the barrier. If, previously, the animal has been given a series of UNAVOIDABLE SHOCKS, against which at first it struggles but then accepts passively, then in the shuttle box it does not try to avoid the shocks but instead sits meekly in one corner and accepts them. Such animals also perform poorly in other learning conditions, and in many ways appear to be depressed, showing no spontaneous activity, impaired sleeping, etc. The animals suffer from LEARNED HELPLESSNESS, the unavoidable shocks having taught them that their actions have no effect upon the world, and hence all action is without effect and not worth making. The learning has generalized to the nature of learning itself. Of especial interest is that human depressives, especially suicides, have decreased cerebral noradrenaline levels; since the brains of animals with learned helplessness also show decreased noradrenaline levels, the implication is that biochemical changes are *secondary* to the depressed mood which followed behavioural events, rather than the biochemistry *causing* the depressed behaviour.

The theory of learned helplessness is similar to cognitive theories which say that depression results from diminished SELF-ESTEEM, an inability to see one's own actions as responsible for change in the world, an emphasis upon FAILURE rather than ACHIEVEMENT, a stressing of negative connotations of events, and ATTRIBUTION of success to external agencies rather than to the person themself.

Therapies derived from learned helplessness and cognitive models make the subject aware of controlling their own actions, and seeing the consequences of those actions. A dog with learned helplessness can be treated behaviourally by dragging it over the barrier while being shocked, demonstrating that its action will stop the punishment. (Interestingly the dog is also helped by electro-convulsive therapy and by antidepressant drugs, which are used in human depression.) Cognitive therapies aim to restrict depressed, negative thoughts, by identifying depressive cognitions, which are often AUTOMATIC THOUGHTS, reflex responses to particular situations (e.g. a friend in a hurry rushes off; the depressive thinks 'They are bored. Everyone finds me boring'), and consciously replacing them with alternatives ('Well they were in a hurry, I'll ring later and invite them to the cinema'). The treatment is coupled with EXPERIENCE OF SUCCESS; small easy tasks are successfully accomplished and rewarded, helping to show the fallacy of self-fulfilling cognitions such as 'What's the point in trying, I'm bound to fail?'

PERSONAL CONSTRUCT THEORY OF DEPRESSION

In depression the predominant emotion is GUILT, which arises from an awareness of contradictions or separation between the core constructs of 'actual self' and 'self as ought to be'; the separation is inversely related to SELF-ESTEEM, which is least in depressives and highest in manics, with normals in between. Consider the problem of depression in students. The construct of 'Student – not student' has other constructs in parallel, perhaps:

Student	—	*Not student*
Active	—	Inactive
Interesting	—	Boring
Thinking	—	Unthinking
Vivacious	—	Inactive
Living for today	—	Living only for the future
Stimulating	—	Tedious
Always out at theatres, concerts, etc.	—	Sit at home working all the time

And if the construct 'Self as should be – self as really am' is also put on this system then it will appear as:

Student	—	*Not student*
Self as should be	—	Self as really am

Although the *image* of students is one thing, *reality* is different. If the terms on the left-hand side are also those associated with core constructs for important aspects of living, then guilt emerges. That guilt can be removed in several ways. The construct system could be rebuilt in a way that accepts that stereotypes often don't correspond to realities, and that one can live a life with components of stereotype and reality; such a change would however induce anxiety, and be threatening, particularly if imposed from outside, by problems with social life or exams. Alternatively, the number of constructs can be reduced so that contradictions disappear; but that is the route to the monolithic construct system of neurosis. The depressive response does not alter the structure of the system but instead reverses the components associated with the self, accepting that 'self as should be' is the same as 'self as really am', and hence concentrates only on work, perhaps seeing it principally as a way of getting on in life, etc. The problem with that solution is that the self is construed almost entirely in *negative* terms (uninteresting, boring, etc.), which makes further contradictions emerge, with further guilt; and so on. Contradictions can be minimized by construing less elements (by having less interests, meeting fewer people, doing less things, etc.) but that also exacerbates the problem.

THE PSYCHOANALYTIC MODEL OF DEPRESSION

In 1917, in his *Mourning and Melancholia*, Freud noted the similarities between grief and melancholia (an old-fashioned name for depression), and discussed the processes of ATTACHMENT and LOSS. Freud said that attachment involves a discharge of emotion (the LIBIDO) on to an external object (a person or thing) and the creation of a mental image

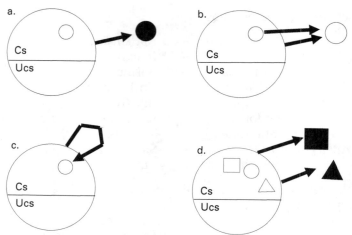

Fig. 29.1 The process of attachment and loss in adults. *a*) The object (solid circle) has emotions projected on to it, and a mental image (open circle) is formed in the conscious mind (Cs). *b*) After loss the mental image of the object firstly causes an hallucinatory external image of the object (large open circle) to occur in the outside world. *c*) The normally outward directed emotions directed inwards to the mental image of the object. *d*) The emotions are transferred to other objects, for which mental images are formed. The mental image of the original object still continues to exist.

of that object (Fig. 29.1a). After loss we firstly hallucinate an object on to which we discharge the emotion (Fig. 29.1b), but then the ego's REALITY TESTING confirms the object does not exist, and the emotions are directed inward to the mental image of the object (Fig. 29.1c). Finally CATHEXIS occurs when the emotion discharges onto new objects, albeit while retaining the mental image of the old object, which perpetually remains a part of us (Fig. 29.1d).

Freud gave no detailed account of how this process resulted in depression, and for that we must look at the work of the British psychoanalyst Melanie Klein (1882–1960) who undertook psycho-analytic explorations of infancy and childhood, and formulated a theory of OBJECT RELATIONS, of early attachment. In earliest infancy, the child relates to objects (either people or things) by expressing love; the archetypical object is the mother's breast, the fount of all good things. The love initially is expressed just onto the object (Fig. 29.2a) but then with INTROJECTION a portion of the object is taken into oneself as a mental image, and love is directed at the image as well as the object (Fig. 29.2b), and the object thereby acquires new properties by PROJECTION. Inevitably temporary SEPARATION from the object occurs, as also do frustrations when the object does not reciprocate love; then hate is directed both at the object (or its absence) and at the mental image (Fig. 29.2c). The child learns not only to direct love but also

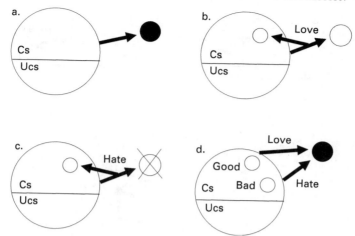

Fig. 29.2 Development of the paranoid-schizoid and depressive positions in infants. *a*) Emotions are projected outwards onto the object. *b*) A mental image of the object is formed and the emotion of love is projected both outwards onto the object itself and inwards onto the mental image of the object. *c*) The image outside either disappears temporarily or otherwise frustrates the infant so that the emotion of hate is directed both outwards onto the object and inwards onto the mental image of the object. *d*) The infant accepts that the same object has both good and bad aspects, towards which love and hate can both be directed, and separate good and bad mental images of the object are formed.

to direct hatred. At times that hatred is directed at the same object that previously had been loved (SPLITTING), resulting in the PARANOID-SCHIZOID POSITION.

At first a child fails to integrate the separate parts of an object, so the mother's breast, face, arms, etc., are different PART OBJECTS, and separate emotions are directed at them. As the child understands that one object has several facets, so GUILT develops at the hatred, directed at different parts of the now complete object, especially the mother, resulting in the Kleinian DEPRESSIVE POSITION; it is realized that loved and hated objects are the same, having both good and bad aspects, to which love and hate are separately directed (AMBIVALENCE), and two separate internal images develop, one good and one bad (the 'good breast' and the 'bad breast' in Kleinian terminology).

Early LOSS (i.e. a permanent loss, rather than normal, inevitable temporary separations) produces a situation in which after the expression of love (Fig. 29.3a), hate is then expressed at the object and its mental image (Fig. 29.3b). However, the child cannot explain the object's disappearance, and therefore blames itself for the loss, and introjects hatred against both the object and itself (Fig. 29.3c), the self-hatred being unconscious, and associated with GUILT at driving away the loved object. This vulnerability means that subsequent losses

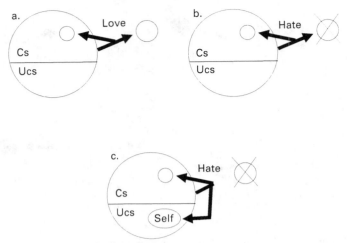

Fig. 29.3 The effects of loss in infancy. *a*) As in Figure 29.2, the infant projects love onto both the external object and also onto its own internal representation of it. *b*) The object disappears permanently (rather than temporarily as in Figure 29.2), and at first the infant acts as in the case of temporary separation, projecting hate onto the object and its image. *c*) The object fails to reappear and infant blames itself for the loss, directing the hate inwards onto both the conscious representation of the object and onto the unconscious (Ucs) representation of the self, which was felt to be responsible for the loss.

in adult life produce a reversion to infantile self-hatred resulting from guilt at responsibility for the loss, particularly when the adult loss involves ambivalence, with feelings of love and hate towards the lost object. Although the precipitating loss in adulthood may be fairly trivial it can result in a severe depressive attack in a vulnerable psyche.

A SOCIOLOGICAL MODEL OF DEPRESSION

The previous models have suggested that depression is a response to events in the immediate world, which affect the way that world is construed and are greater if the psyche is already damaged by loss at an early age. The British sociologists, Brown and Harris, have integrated those ideas into a comprehensive model, which is impressive in its elucidation and its testing against empirical data, and provides a general model for the influence of social phenomena upon disease, physical or psychological. The hypothesis (Fig. 29.4) says the immediate cause of depression is RECENT PROVOKING EVENTS, which produce the condition. However, since provoking events do not *always* cause disease, some individuals must have VULNERABILITY FACTORS, which

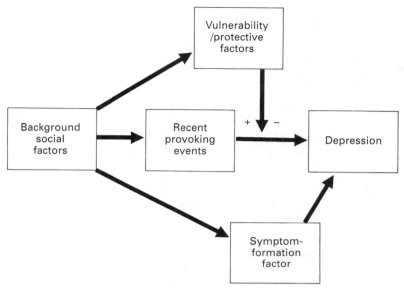

Fig. 29.4 Brown and Harris' model of the aetiology of depression. Adapted from Brown G W and Harris T (1978), *Social origins of depression*, London, Tavistock, 48.

exaggerate the provoking events, or PROTECTIVE FACTORS, which immunize against provoking events. Not all individuals who develop the condition have identical symptoms, and SYMPTOM-FORMATION FACTORS determine the precise nature of the disease, without necessarily affecting the likelihood of disease itself. Finally each factor, be it provoking event, vulnerability or protective factor, or symptom-formation factor, is influenced by background factors, such as social class, early experience, etc.

The core of the model says that recent provoking events *cause* depression; proof requires two steps, demonstration of a correlation and evidence that the relation is causal rather than mere association. Brown and Harris took careful systematic histories from a large population of women to assess 'events' in their lives over the previous year. Severity of events was assessed by independent judges. Depressed women had more *severe* events during the previous year, but *non-severe* events were as frequent in controls as in depressives. Therefore, not all events cause depression, only those perceived as severe. Severe events occurred throughout the previous year, but particularly in the six weeks prior to the illness (Fig. 29.5). Correlation had therefore been demonstrated. Causation is more difficult. Either events may be FORMATIVE, the event causing the depression (e.g. husband leaves and woman then becomes depressed) or TRIGGERING, in which depression occurs spontaneously and then causes the event (e.g. woman becomes depressed and husband leaves *because* she is depressed). These situ-

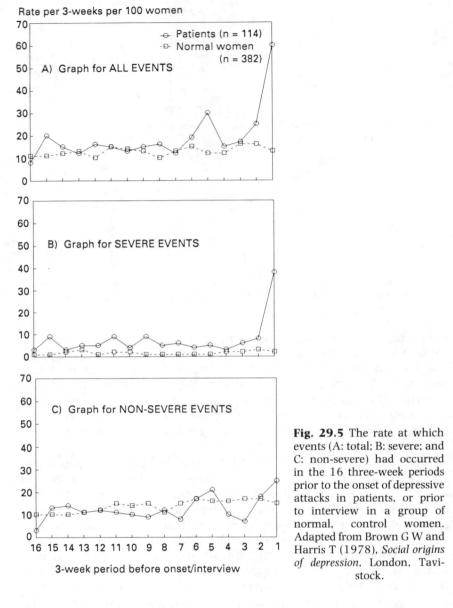

Rate per 3-weeks per 100 women

A) Graph for ALL EVENTS

-○- Patients (n = 114)
-□- Normal women (n = 382)

B) Graph for SEVERE EVENTS

C) Graph for NON-SEVERE EVENTS

3-week period before onset/interview

Fig. 29.5 The rate at which events (A: total; B: severe; and C: non-severe) had occurred in the 16 three-week periods prior to the onset of depressive attacks in patients, or prior to interview in a group of normal, control women. Adapted from Brown G W and Harris T (1978), *Social origins of depression*, London, Tavistock.

ations are distinguishable by the TIME BROUGHT FORWARD INDEX. Imagine a clock that strikes the hours. If an event occurs at random then there will be a certain delay until the clock next strikes. Some events occur just before the hour, and others long before, with an average delay of 30 minutes before the clock struck. If an event (such as a finger inside the works) *caused* the clock to strike then the delay before the next strike would be less than if event and strike were independent. If striking was caused by events then they should occur sooner than expected, and the strikes are said to be brought forward in time as compared with chance expectations. It is measured by the TIME BROUGHT FORWARD INDEX, which if short indicates triggering, whereas if long indicates formative influences. Attacks of depression are brought forward nearly two years by severe events, indicating a formative or causal influence. Non-severe events bring forward attacks by only ten weeks or so, suggesting triggering, with illness causing event. When applied to acute schizophrenic attacks, where previous work had suggested social events were unlikely to be causal, the time brought forward index for severe events was only ten weeks, indicating triggering, and providing a 'control' for depression, where events are formative.

Vulnerability and protective factors manifest not simply by correlating with depression, but by modulating the relationship between events and depression. Considering *only* individuals experiencing severe events in the past year, 10% of those with high psychological intimacy with their husband became depressed, compared with 26% with medium intimacy and 41% with low intimacy. Intimacy, the ability to express feelings freely, without self-consciousness, with trust, effective understanding, and ready access, is therefore a protective factor. Intimacy was less common in women of lower social classes, showing the pervasive role of background factors and partly explaining the social distribution of depression. Husband's employment, lack of employment for the woman outside the home, having three or more children at home, and loss of a mother before the age of 11 were all vulnerability factors. The latter is particularly important in relation to psychoanalysis, especially as loss of a mother only made women more vulnerable when it occurred before 11 years of age in conjunction with severe events; loss of mother was unrelated to depression after non-severe events, and loss of a *father* (before or after age 11) did not alter vulnerability.

On becoming depressed it is symptom-formation factors that determine the degree and type of the symptoms. The SEVERITY of a depressive attack related to the number of severe events suffered (but not their type), and was greater in those experiencing loss of mother or sibling before age 11. Loss of mother is therefore *both* a vulnerability factor *and* a symptom-formation factor. Depressions also vary in symptom type, some having a neurotic pattern, with a specific cause apparent to the patient, and others are psychotic, without causal insight and with 'biological' symptoms. Depression type did not relate to the number, severity or type of provoking events, but was related to age (older patients having more psychotic symptomatology) and to experience of loss. Not only was previous loss more common in psychotic depression, but the manner of loss related to depression

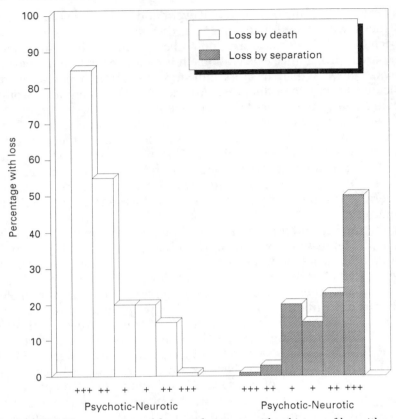

Fig. 29.6 The proportion of depressed patients with a history of loss either by separation or by death, according to the type of depression (psychotic or neurotic), and its severity (low, medium or high). Adapted from Brown G W and Harris T (1978), *Social origins of depression*, London, Tavistock.

type; loss of parent or sibling before age 11 by DEATH was associated with psychotic symptoms, whereas loss by SEPARATION (e.g. divorce, etc.) was related to neurotic symptoms (Fig. 29.6). Childhood loss therefore affected the symptoms seen in adult depression two, three or four decades later. The child's implicit explanation of family loss subsequently related to understanding of their adult illness, either being explicable and comprehensible in the case of separation, particularly if associated with prior arguments and discord, or being inexplicable, arbitrary and the blows of incomprehensible fate in the case of death due to illness or accident. The Brown and Harris model therefore says that the distinction between endogenous and reactive depression is aetiologically inappropriate (for they propose *all* depressions are causally reactive on prior severe events) but is important symptomatically, indicating differing cognitive explanations of illness in relation to early experience.

This chapter has tried to emphasize how depression can be analysed at many levels, from the behavioural model in laboratory animals, to the interpretations of the analyst's couch, and to large-scale sociological models, with each having common components in its emphasis upon *loss*, its explanation and understanding, and the subsequent generalization to future losses. No single model can be correct; rather all emphasize different aspects of a common problem.

30

Schizophrenia

- Schizophrenia is characterized by HALLUCINATIONS, DELUSIONAL PERCEPTIONS and DELUSIONAL EXPERIENCES, as well as by THOUGHT DISORDER, in which thinking is illogical, language is disordered, and thought is concrete rather than abstract.
- Schizophrenia probably has a genetic component, although this is probably not primarily an abnormality of neurotransmission, but may instead be a deficit of ATTENTION or HABITUATION, which manifests early in childhood.
- Many of the abnormal behaviours shown by schizophrenics are the result of INSTITUTIONALIZATION and inappropriate reinforcement of behaviour.
- LOOSE CONSTRUING can be induced by SERIAL INVALIDATION, a process akin to the DOUBLE-BIND, early invalidation resulting in non-paranoid schizophrenia and late invalidation in paranoid schizophrenia.
- Psychoses cannot be treated by psychoanalysis due to a failure to form a TRANSFERENCE relationship with the analyst. This may reflect fixation at the PARANOID-SCHIZOID position and the inability to form proper OBJECT RELATIONS.

Schizophrenia is the most difficult of all the mental disorders. The clearest and most serious example of a psychosis, it is difficult to treat, difficult for families and relatives to cope with, and difficult for an outsider to understand, the utter lack of insight by the patient being complemented by an absence of empathy by outsiders for the patient's mental state; unlike neurosis or depression, where we all have suffered minor forms of the conditions, in schizophrenia we can draw on almost no personal experience that will help us to see the world through the patient's eyes.

Schizophrenia was first described systematically in 1896 by the German psychiatrist Kraepelin (1856–1926), who called it by the inappropriate name of DEMENTIA PRAECOX (precocious or premature dementia), inappropriate because there is no dementia as intelligence and memory are unimpaired. In 1911, Bleuler (1857–1939) coined the modern term SCHIZOPHRENIA, from the Greek *schizos* (a split) and *phrenos* (mind). Despite recurrent misusage in the popular press, schizophrenia is *not* a split mind or DUAL PERSONALITY (a 'Jekyll-and-

Hyde syndrome', an entirely separate condition which does occur, albeit rarely); rather the split is both between thought, feelings and activities, which no longer act in harmony, and also in the normal differentiation in space and time between self and not-self.

Clinical diagnosis looks for Schneider's FIRST-RANK SYMPTOMS of hallucinations, delusional experiences and delusional perceptions, any of which, in the absence of organic lesions, are sufficient for a presumptive diagnosis of schizophrenia. HALLUCINATIONS are experiences indistinguishable from sensory events that occur in the absence of sensations; they must not be confused with ILLUSIONS, which are distortions of sensation or perception, or DELUSIONS in which a *belief* is erroneous. Schizophrenic hallucinations are auditory (and other modalities indicate other conditions, typically being visual in *delirium tremens*, olfactory in temporal lobe epilepsy, and cutaneous in cocaine overdosage), and are either audible thoughts, voices arguing or voices commenting on the patient's actions (when they are grammatically in the third person, unlike the rare auditory hallucinations of severe depression which are in the first person). Auditory hallucinations while falling asleep or when waking, HYPNAGOGIC and HYPNOPOMPIC HALLUCINATIONS, are common and regarded as entirely normal. DELUSIONAL EXPERIENCES are disorders of the EGO BOUNDARY. Normally we have a precise sense of the extent of our own body which we control, compared with the rest of the world which is beyond direct control. If I put my hand on a table I know the fingers are mine, and I can move them and feel things touching them, whereas the table, only a micron beneath my fingers is not me, and I neither control it nor derive sensation from it. In schizophrenia the ego boundary shifts, patients either believing their body controlled by others (PASSIVITY), or that thoughts are inserted in their mind, or wishes, instincts or emotions are controlled externally, or that their thoughts are broadcast and affect other people directly. DELUSIONAL PERCEPTIONS (or just DELUSIONS or PRIMARY DELUSIONS) are abnormal beliefs about the world, often with a bizarre content involving ideas or threat or persecution (PARANOID DELUSIONS) or in DELUSIONS OF GRANDEUR of being a person of importance (e.g. Napoleon or Jesus Christ). Delusions are incomprehensible to an outsider and are characterized by:

i. Being held with absolute conviction.

ii. Being experienced as self-evident truths, typically of great personal significance.

iii. Not being amenable to reason or modifiable by experience.

iv. The content being fantastic or at best inherently unlikely.

v. Not being shared by those of a common social or cultural background.

Such criteria ensure that simple values or beliefs (for instance concerning political or religious questions) are not interpreted as delusions (although delusions often have religious or political content). Leonard Woolf described a typical delusion when his wife Virginia, during a psychotic attack, believed the birds in the garden were singing in Greek; and he gave eloquent testimony to the folly of attempting to reason with the holders of such delusions.

Psychologically schizophrenia is characterized by THOUGHT DISORDER, a disorder of cognitive processing. Language is used unsystematically, with distorted grammar. Sentences are incomplete and rambling, phrases or sentences are not logically connected, and there are sudden changes of direction and irrelevancies. Thinking is illogical, with OVER-INCLUSION, conceptual and semantic boundaries being ignored, resulting in CLANG ASSOCIATIONS, where similar word sounds imply similar meanings, and the creation of NEOLOGISMS, words or phrases newly created from parts of other words or phrases (e.g. 'cosmetic neurosurgery', or 'placebionic' from 'placebo' and 'bionic'). Thought disorder can be demonstrated experimentally by sorting playing cards, schizophrenics being idiosyncratic in their placing, and ignoring conventional distinctions of suit and value. Thought is also CONCRETE, abstract ideas not being processed properly, as is shown clinically by asking a patient to explain a proverb such as 'A rolling stone gathers no moss'; they talk at length about moss being unable to stick, or grow, and ignore the metaphorical meaning of the proverb. Similarly, descriptions of pictures are concrete rather than abstract, emphasizing the physical objects present and ignoring the relationships between individuals or their motives. Schizophrenic thought can have a poetic flavour (as when a patient was asked the difference between a wall and a fence: 'A fence you can see through but a wall has ears'), and it is suggested that a milder variant, called the SCHIZOID PERSONALITY, is associated with artistic creativity.

Schizophrenia can be subdivided in several ways. Two particular distinctions are useful in practice. Paranoid patients typically present in middle age with mainly paranoid delusions of slow insidious onset, and little thought disorder; non-paranoid patients present between 15 and 35 years of age with an acute attack and relatively minor delusions but extensive thought disorder. Auditory hallucinations occur in both types, and in both types remission can occur, especially if treated with major tranquillizers such as chlorpromazine. Relapse can then follow, resulting in the chronic or 'burnt out' form of the disease found in patients institutionalized for many years. Recently, TYPE I schizophrenia, marked by 'positive' symptoms, such as hallucinations, delusions and thought disorders, which occur acutely and respond well to neuroleptics, has been distinguished from TYPE II schizophrenia, the chronic condition where symptoms are mainly 'negative', with cognitive impairment, poor response to neuroleptics, and increased ventricular size and reduced cortical substance seen on cerebral tomography. The different types of schizophrenia may have different aetiologies, implying a heterogeneous disorder.

An idea of the peculiar and special flavour of schizophrenic thought can be given in a letter written by Ivor Gurney, a talented composer and First World War poet, who from the age of 33 spent the last fifteen years of his life in an asylum. He developed auditory hallucinations, and delusions that he was tortured by wireless waves and could converse with the great composers and had in fact written much of their music. This letter was written when aged 43, as if from Siegfried Wagner, the son of the composer:

'This is Franz Schubert's death day and enough for Kent Reach to think of — whose chimneys smoked grandly, but Nature said 'W.E. Henley Prague 1731' — So light dies down — But after saying that Europe should not stand war for its thought, by 137 degrees —

Barnet won I think/especially about the South, most likely — but perhaps about the going North, where may Italy (North) and Rochester book-sellers flourish.

The weeks and battles forgotten — (terrible to remember) need all the good of Artois and Picardy's poetry —

Meanwhile the regrets and hopes of Highnam Manor float about the world — now vast in great victory, and as urgently as Sidgwick & Jackson cry out for the honour of provinces.

Virgil is running 2/3, and is the master of business — music is at last in a very healthy state/and Rutland Boughton's group is announced — Rudford and Minster, that accepts such news, now forgets its threats and terrible fears, St. Maur gives news of pride every day, and seems to enjoy Welsh local poetry.

It seems true that Anton Dvorak and Rochester Cathedral have truly the salvation of music and poetry — and one might want for Spring with 137 hopes — But desperate is Hebbel's need for Frankfort's urgencies.

'Lyrik, lyrik' in Schiller's name ever demanding, and let London lose its regrets and clear its history there with the brutality of Eaglefield-Hull, and as the name of Thames flows steadily to honour.

Nature, now sombre, sometimes says tremendous things, and sometimes lightly, as of the biographer of F. P. Schubert, and waits for Florence City's reasons and reason —

That London may honour St. Crispin — a saint glorious enough for Aquitaine/and to please William Cartwright, magister artis.

I ask for some more money, please, and a small poetry book if there is one (modern if it can be got). It is painful and hard to write about modern anthologies though – and so better to rejoice (theoretically) about Max Reger —/ England is a South Place story . . .

The glory of 1913 and 1914 is here remembered/as always worth the imagination of Petrograd and Moscow. (140–183); later

with the surpassing interest of men's music — like our hopes of
Novgorod's earth.
with best wishes
(yours very sincerely)
Ivor Gurney
Oct 23 1933   Dartford. Kent.'

Reproduced with permission from
Hurd M, *The ordeal of Ivor Gurney* (1978)
Oxford University Press, 165

The letter shows clear signs of thought disorder, with disordered
grammar, and incomplete rambling sentence structure; nonetheless
it is clearly not just 'noise', but has a deep and complex meaning,
albeit obscure, and at times its beautiful imagery is replete with
associations, particularly for those who can perceive the musical,
military and literary motifs.

Many models have been proposed for a disease as serious and
complex as schizophrenia. As previously we will consider the learning,
personal construct and psychoanalytic models, and will also consider
the biochemical-genetic model as well.

THE BIOCHEMICAL-GENETIC MODEL OF SCHIZOPHRENIA

This model is not only extremely popular but also has several inherent
fallacies of particular interest.

Schizophrenia undoubtedly has a genetic component. The life-time
prevalence is 1% in the general population compared with 35% if one
parent is schizophrenic, or 70% if both parents are schizophrenic. If
both parents are normal then the risk is 10% with an affected sibling,
15% with an affected dizygotic twin, and 50–80% with an affected
monozygotic twin. That these familial trends are genetic rather than
environmental is shown in adoption studies, a child being more
like biological than adoptive parents. Nevertheless, neither a single
Mendelian gene nor polygenes explain the pattern of inheritance.

Genes produce proteins, particularly enzymes, and since enzymes
metabolize neurotransmitters, schizophrenia has been argued to be
due to abnormal neurotransmission. But which neurotransmitter?
During the past four decades many candidates have been proposed:
acetylcholine, noradrenaline, serotonin, GABA, dopamine, prostaglandins, and endorphins. Each has had its heyday, usually following
an improved measurement technique, rather than strict argument.
The most convincing hypothesis implicates abnormal dopamine transmission, and the logic of that specific argument will be considered
here.

The 'dopamine theory of schizophrenia' originated in the discovery that major tranquillizers, or NEUROLEPTICS, such as CHLORPROMAZINE, not only alleviate the symptoms of schizophrenia but also block dopamine transmission, both *in vivo* and *in vitro*; hence it was argued that the antipsychotic effect occurred *because* of blocking dopamine transmission. That, however, is still controversial: degree of dopamine blocking and neuroleptic antipsychotic action are only moderately correlated; dopamine blocking occurs within minutes *in vivo* and yet antipsychotic action takes several weeks to occur; and those behavioural effects of neuroleptics related to dopamine blockade show TOLERANCE after several weeks, whereas no tolerance is shown in antipsychotic action. Nevertheless, despite such difficulties, 'the dopamine hypothesis of neuroleptic action' is generally felt to be correct. But that does not prove the 'dopamine hypothesis of the *cause* of schizophrenia'. Consider some clear counter-examples: Parkinson's disease is alleviated by anticholinergics, but is due to a dopamine deficit; and Huntington's chorea is treated with dopamine blockers but is due to a GABA deficiency. To push the argument to its logical absurdity, pneumonia is treated with penicillin, but in no sense is due to low levels of penicillin in the lungs or serum. More direct evidence is needed that excess dopamine is the cause of schizophrenia, but such evidence has not been forthcoming, dopamine levels not being convincingly raised in the brains of schizophrenics. A variant of the model therefore argues for increased receptor sensitivity to normal levels of dopamine, and that seemed to have been found in some post-mortem studies. However, most schizophrenics now receive treatment with dopamine blockers, which could actually be causing the receptor differences; and post-mortem examination of the rare brains of schizophrenics who are not on medication indeed suggests receptor sensitivity is normal.

I wish to argue that the biochemical model is overly simplistic, ignoring the inherent complexity of mental illness, and the interaction between brain function and environment. The simple model (Fig. 30.1a) is inadequate for the reasons given above. A more complex model (Fig. 30.1b) argues for a PRIMARY COGNITIVE DISABILITY caused partly by genetic factors; certainly longitudinal studies show that children subsequently developing schizophrenia were passive babies, had short attention spans, difficulties at school, poor control of emotions, and were disruptive in class. By age 15 they showed signs of early thought disorder. Such behaviour is not itself psychotic, but eventually results in a PRIMARY PSYCHOTIC DEFECT, which as a result of other disruptive factors such as social processes, or even environmental factors such as viral infections, results in the florid symptoms of schizophrenia, the SECONDARY PSYCHOTIC DEFECT, which then further impairs social interactions, and exacerbates the problem further. Treatment by neuroleptics diminishes the primary psychotic defect, but this alone is insufficient to alter the secondary defect, which is

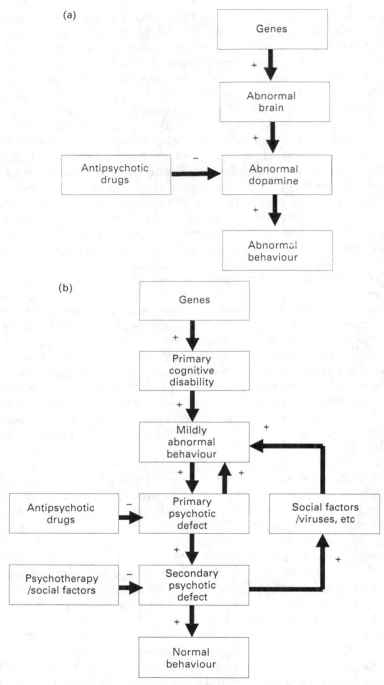

Fig. 30.1 *a*) A simple biochemical model; *b*) a more complex biochemical model. See text for further details.

maintained by social factors; however psychotherapy and social therapy, in combination with drugs, help remove the secondary defect, albeit after some time, and relatively normal behaviour is restored, leaving a system still vulnerable to future problems.

Such a model pre-supposes a primary cognitive disability present in early life, which might be a defect in ATTENTION. Normally we are bombarded by sensory inputs, most of which are consciously ignored until something interesting occurs, when consciousness is directed at them; thus as you read this you were probably unaware of the pressure of the chair upon your buttocks until it was mentioned, when suddenly it impinged upon consciousness. Much evidence suggests an ATTENTIONAL DEFICIT in schizophrenics, who are continually bombarded with sensations they are unable to ignore, both from external events, and from internal processes, such as memories, etc.; this partly explains the pressure of ideas and the clang associations in thought disorder. The other side of attention is HABITUATION, ignoring a frequently presented stimulus. In normal individuals, the GALVANIC SKIN RESPONSE (GSR) to a repeated stimulus shows a sudden rise in skin conductance at presentation followed by a return to normal levels. A slow return to normal indicates lessened habituation. Children of schizophrenic parents, who are at higher risk of becoming schizophrenic, show decreased habituation and less attention than controls. Chlorpromazine, in man and animals, decreases distractibility, and hence increases attention and habituation, perhaps explaining its role in treating the primary psychotic disorder of schizophrenia. Of interest is that hippocampal lesions in monkeys not only produce decreased attention and GSR habituation, but these can be treated by chlorpromazine. There is now growing evidence that human schizophrenics show structural abnormalities in the temporal lobe, particularly in the left hemisphere.

The biochemical-genetic model has been examined in detail because it is a popular model of the aetiology and pharmacotherapy of schizophrenia. However, it tells us little of the *experience* of schizophrenia, and ignores many aspects of the disease, for which we must look to specifically psychological models.

THE LEARNING THEORY MODEL OF SCHIZOPHRENIA

Learning theory has no specific model for the *cause* of schizophrenia, but nonetheless explains many of the strange behaviours of schizophrenics. Being schizophrenic does not make one incapable of learning, and of responding to events in the world. If that world is bizarre, then bizarre behaviours can result. The world of a chronic schizophrenic, the long-stay mental hospital, is indeed strange and many behaviours result from that social environment due to inadvertent reinforcement

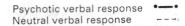

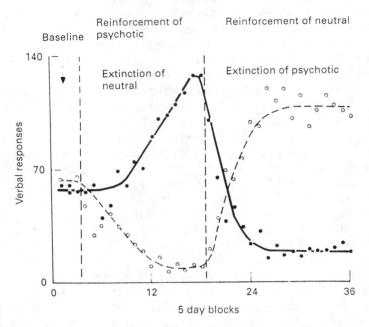

Fig. 30.2 The influence of differential reinforcement of 'psychotic' or 'normal' types of speech on the verbal behaviour of psychotic patients. Reproduced with permission from Allyn T and Houghton E (1964), Modification of symptomatic verbal behaviour of mental patients, *Behaviour Research and Therapy*, **2**, 87–97.

by staff and patients, and as a result of INSTITUTIONALIZATION. If patients are ignored by staff or told to be quiet then some will learn to be taciturn and uncommunicative; and if a well-meaning person listens to a patient's paranoid delusions, nodding their head repeatedly, but ignoring the content, then such speech and ideas are reinforced (see Fig. 30.2). Head-banging and tantrums are also examples of ATTENTION SEEKING behaviours, which are rewarded by attention from staff. Learning is itself exploited in TOKEN ECONOMIES; beneficial social behaviours such as self-care, good appearance and voluntary activities are rewarded with tokens which are exchanged for privileges or goods (see Chapter 31).

Some theorists argue that schizophrenia itself is a learned response to the social environment of the family. Bateson's DOUBLE-BIND THEORY suggested that parents place their children in situations where they cannot possibly do right. A mother might complain that the child hasn't kissed her, but withdraw and show dislike when kissed; whether affection is shown or not the mother's behaviour shows dislike, and since the situation is inescapable, the child learns that all behaviours result in punishment, and instead the child withdraws into itself and learns to ignore the outside world. Although poorly supported by empirical evidence, the theory is popular and the phrase SCHIZOPHRENO-GENIC MOTHER is now a part of psychiatric terminology. The theory influenced ANTI-PSYCHIATRISTS, such as R D Laing, who said schizophrenic symptoms were meaningful responses to an intolerable situation in which the entire family was abnormal. Although also not supported by adequate data, such family studies have inspired specific studies on the problems of relapse in schizophrenic patients discharged home on neuroleptic medication, which show unequivocally that high levels of EXPRESSED EMOTION in the families, usually over-involvement, hostility or criticism, result in higher relapse rates; patients should be discharged into such families with care and FAMILY THERAPY, treating the whole family to reduce deleterious communication, can benefit the patient.

THE PERSONAL CONSTRUCT MODEL OF SCHIZOPHRENIA

In personal construct theory, the most important empirical observation is that schizophrenics have loose construing, with many unrelated constructs; as such the construct system is similar to that of an obsessional but without the obsessional's single monolithic construct system — and it is of interest that obsessive-compulsives are at higher risk of subsequent schizophrenia. How does this system develop? As in neurosis, the driving force is anxiety resulting from invalidation and hence threatened change of the system, particularly due to SERIAL INVALIDATION, which shows similarities to Bateson's theory of the double-bind. Imagine that some person, X, is nasty to Y, the patient. X is construed by Y as 'hating'. Next time however X is nice to Y, and Y therefore changes their construction of X to 'loving'. The next occasion though X is nasty again, Y's construing changes back to 'hating'; and so on, X never behaving consistently, so that Y cannot construe them successfully, and Y's construct system is invalidated every time. There are two ways to make the system work in some degree. The relationship between constructs can be altered to produce IDIOSYNCRATIC CONSTRUING, the links between 'loving-hating' and other constructs such as 'considerate-inconsiderate' being reversed from the normal, so that, say, 'loving' and 'inconsiderate' are linked; when X is nasty they are then construed as 'loving and inconsiderate', and the system is not actually invalidated (although it predicts almost nothing, and is almost incapable of falsification). The alternative solution is LOOSE CONSTRUING, where 'loving-hating' exists in isolation from other constructs, so that X's nastiness predicts nothing else about X. Since the system predicts nothing, it also cannot be invalidated.

Loose construing is typically found in thought disordered non-paranoid schizophrenia, whereas idiosyncratic construing is typical of paranoid schizophrenia. Serial invalidation is thought to occur in childhood for the non-paranoid schizophrenic, producing an inadequate construct system that cannot cope with adult life, so that schizophrenia develops at a young age. By contrast in paranoid schizophrenia a normal childhood allows development of an adequate construct system, but serial invalidation in middle life then causes idiosyncratic construing. Serial invalidation does not produce generalized disordered construing, since schizophrenics have relatively normal construing of *physical objects*, but are especially loose at construing *people*, emphasizing the role of the social environment in causing schizophrenia.

Personal construct theory suggests therefore that schizophrenic thought is not meaningless noise but has a sense and meaning, albeit known principally to the patient themself, but which is accessible through careful analysis. Figure 30.3 summarizes diagrammatically the structures proposed by personal construct theory in neurosis and psychosis.

THE PSYCHOANALYTIC MODEL OF SCHIZOPHRENIA

Freud recognized early in his career that psychoanalytic therapy worked only with neurotics, and not with psychotics. In neurosis, psychotherapy works by the patient developing strong emotional attachments to the therapist (the TRANSFERENCE) and the therapist forming a relationship to the patient (usually attachment, but sometimes a dislike), COUNTER-TRANSFERENCE. The transference induces conflict between the patient's wishes and the analyst's wishes producing RESISTANCE and forming the TRANSFERENCE NEUROSIS, whose working through is therapeutic for the neurosis proper, for which the transference neurosis has acted as a surrogate.

Psychosis is untreatable by psychoanalysis because there is no transference, the patient being unable to form relationships. Freud said that in psychotics a breakdown in EGO-FUNCTIONS caused impaired REALITY TESTING and hence delusions and hallucinations, with loss of personal identity and failure to differentiate the internal world from the outside world: 'In a neurosis the ego . . . suppresses a piece of the id . . . whereas in a psychosis the ego, in the service of the id, withdraws from a piece of reality'. To Freud psychotic symptoms were a 'waking dream', PRIMARY PROCESS THINKING (akin to latent dream content) being unacted upon by censorship to produce SECONDARY PROCESS THINKING (the dream's manifest content), and emerging unchanged in unconsciousness producing conflicts and terrors. Freud merely described schizophrenia, but did not explain its origins, except in suggesting a failure

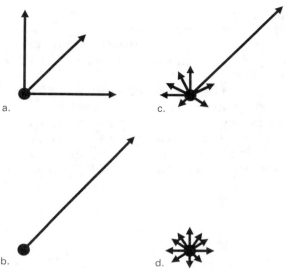

Fig. 30.3 A diagrammatic summary of the personal construct theory models of neurosis and psychosis. Each arrow represents an independent dimension in construct space (and the space can be multidimensional). The length of an arrow is proportional to the degree to which that dimension accounts for the relationships expressed in the repertory grid. In normal individuals (*a*) there are typically 3 or 4 principal dimensions underlying constructs. In individuals with phobias there is a single construct dimension (*b*), and in individuals with obsessional neurosis there is a single predominant dimension, but also a large number of small, independent dimensions (*c*). In schizophrenia there are large numbers of independent dimensions, each of which accounts for only a small proportion of the information in a repertory grid (*d*), and this looks similar to the subsidiary portion of the construct space found in obsessional neurosis.

of development early in childhood.

Melanie Klein said that schizophrenia resulted from problems at the very earliest recognizable age of psychological development, the PARANOID-SCHIZOID POSITION, early in the oral stage. Internal and external reality are not yet properly differentiated, introjection and projection meaning that the child confuses its own actions with those of objects in the world, a failure of ego differentiation. Objects therefore acquire by projection the ego's emotions, becoming perhaps loving or hating, and their properties are also introjected within the mind. Normal transition to the depressive position is helped by a mother who is neither confusing nor contradictory (the GOOD ENOUGH MOTHER in the jargon), and allows the child to develop a sense of object realities, and to dissipate the hatred developed in the paranoid-schizoid position. If this process fails then emotions are not projected onto external objects but back onto the child itself, resulting in NARCISSISM, or self-love, and the development of either MEGALOMANIA (grandiose thinking) if accompanied by positive emotions, or PARANOIA if accompanied by negative emotions.

This chapter should have made it clear that at present no complete description of schizophrenia is possible; such a description cannot be couched solely in terms of abnormal neurochemistry, although that must be a part of it, but must also explain the especial mental life, and the early infantile experiences of the schizophrenic, so that an integrated picture can help make possible adequate and humane treatments.

31

Mental retardation

- Children with mental retardation of ORGANIC origin tend to show greater intellectual impairment than those with a FAMILIAL AETI-OLOGY, who are typically of lower social class or have experienced environmental deprivation.
- Mentally retarded children are often slow at learning because of a lack of experience at learning, because of inexperience with social rewards, and because of learned helplessness.
- Retarded children can often be helped by BEHAVIOUR MODIFICATION in which a problem is IDENTIFIED, a GOAL set, BASE-LINE BEHAVIOUR measured, a specific INTERVENTION is used to modify the behaviour and its CONSEQUENCES monitored.
- Beneficial behaviours can be increased in frequency by positive reinforcement, most successfully using either TOKENS as secondary reinforcers, or by means of SOCIAL REINFORCERS.
- Successful reinforcers are CONTINGENT, IMMEDIATE, CONSISTENT and CLEAR.
- Deleterious behaviours can be decreased in frequency by a careful use of PUNISHMENT, often in the form of TIME OUT, which should be administered in small, frequent amounts.

One in forty of the population is MENTALLY RETARDED (the preferred term, which has replaced mental subnormality or deficiency which have pejorative overtones). Definition is not easy, although that of the American Association on Mental Deficiency (AAMD) is probably satisfactory:

> 'Mental retardation refers to significantly sub-average intellectual functioning resulting in or associated with impairment in adaptive behaviour and manifested during the developmental period'.

Notice the separate emphases on *intellectual functioning*, social or *adaptive behaviour*, and on the *developmental period*. In practice, retardation is often defined solely in terms of an IQ of two or more standard deviations below the mean for age (i.e. less than 70). Although apparently arbitrary, the criterion is useful in practice, broadly separating those in need of care and attention from those able to live a normal life; nevertheless, it must be emphasized that half of the retarded will marry, have jobs, and live in the community. Severity of retardation is classified as MILD (IQ 50–70), MODERATE (IQ 35–50), SEVERE (IQ 20–34) and PROFOUND (IQ less than 20). Retardation is also defined legally in many countries, and Figure 31.1 summarizes the terminology of successive Acts of Parliament in the UK. The MENTAL HEALTH ACT OF 1983 defined both 'MENTAL IMPAIRMENT' and 'SEVERE MENTAL IMPAIRMENT', the latter being:

'a state of arrested or incomplete development of mind which includes severe impairment of intelligence or social functioning *and is associated with abnormally aggressive or seriously irresponsible conduct on the part of the person concerned*' (my italics).

A key innovation of this Act is that retardation alone is not sufficient for compulsory detention in hospital, instead *impairment* is required, thereby restoring a number of civil rights to the majority of the mentally handicapped.

Mental retardation is also classified aetiologically into two major groups. Some 25 to 50% of retardates show ORGANIC aetiology, with over 200 causes being described, broadly grouped into PRENATAL (e.g. chromosomal problems, such as Down's syndrome and fragile-X syndrome, genetic defects, and teratogenic syndromes, such as intra-uterine rubella infection), PERINATAL (e.g. intrapartum cerebral anoxia), and POSTNATAL (e.g. secondary to meningitis, encephalitis, or head injury). The remaining 50 to 75% of cases are described as FAMILIAL AETIOLOGY, mostly being the tail of the normal distribution of IQ (essentially a poor deal in the lottery of polygenic inheritance) or, more rarely, environmental deprivation. The two aetiologies differ in IQ, familial retardation mainly being mild, while organic retardation is often severe (Fig. 31.2); they also differ in many other features (Fig. 31.3), the most important being that organic aetiology comes from all social classes, whereas familial aetiology arises principally in social class IV and V, where mean intelligence is lower and environmental deprivation greater.

By definition, the mentally retarded are less able to carry out intellectual tasks. The reasons are complex, and two theoretical positions can be distinguished. DEVELOPMENTAL THEORIES say that intellectual growth is simply delayed, with slower progression through the same stages as the non-retarded child, and hence a lower final level. DIFFERENCE (or DEFICIT) THEORIES say the retarded are not just quantitatively different but differ qualitatively, having specific problems with some aspects of cognition, such as language, attention, or sensory processing, and developing differently to non-retarded children. Although controversial, current consensus sees familial retardation as developmental and organic retardation as due to deficit.

Care must be taken to distinguish two possible reasons for slower

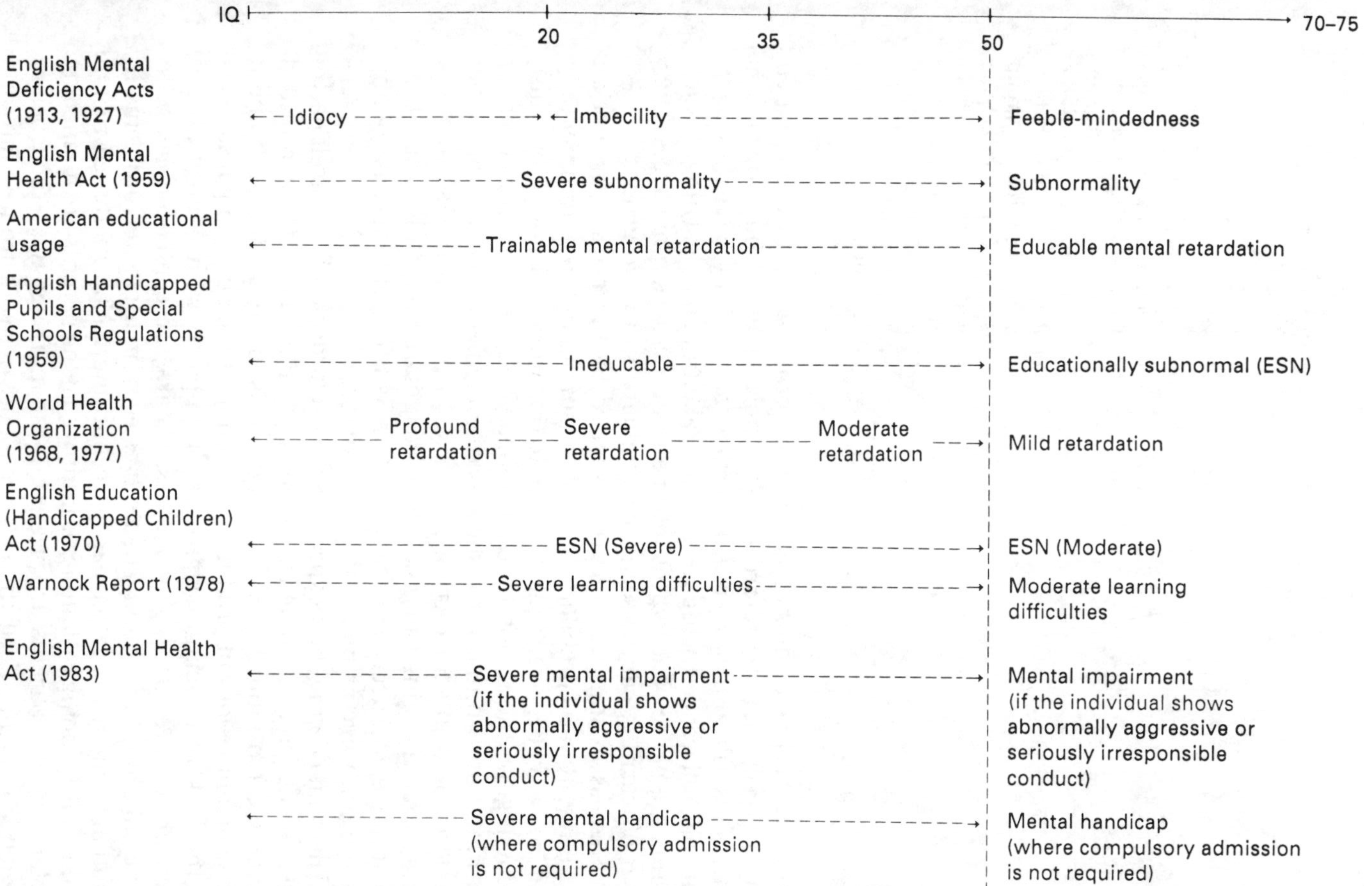

IQ |————————|————————|————————|————————|——————→ 70–75
                    20   35   50

English Mental Deficiency Acts (1913, 1927)
Idiocy ←——————————————→ Imbecility   Feeble-mindedness

English Mental Health Act (1959)
←———————— Severe subnormality ————————→   Subnormality

American educational usage
←———————— Trainable mental retardation ————————→   Educable mental retardation

English Handicapped Pupils and Special Schools Regulations (1959)
←———————— Ineducable ————————→   Educationally subnormal (ESN)

World Health Organization (1968, 1977)
Profound retardation — Severe retardation — Moderate retardation   Mild retardation

English Education (Handicapped Children) Act (1970)
←———————— ESN (Severe) ————————→   ESN (Moderate)

Warnock Report (1978)
←———————— Severe learning difficulties ————————→   Moderate learning difficulties

English Mental Health Act (1983)
←———————— Severe mental impairment (if the individual shows abnormally aggressive or seriously irresponsible conduct) ————————→   Mental impairment (if the individual shows abnormally aggressive or seriously irresponsible conduct)

Severe mental handicap (where compulsory admission is not required)   Mental handicap (where compulsory admission is not required)

Fig. 31.1 The changing terminology of degree of mental retardation in relation to IQ. Reproduced with permission from Clarke A M, Clarke A D B and Berg J M (1985). *Mental deficiency: the changing outlook*, 4th edn. London, Methuen, 40.

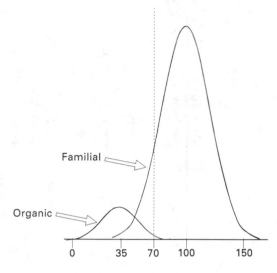

Fig. 31.2 Typical distributions of intelligence in organic and familial mental retardation, showing how the familial group forms the lower end of the population distribution, whereas the organic group forms a separate overlapping distribution. Adapted from Zigler E and Hodapp R M (1986), *Understanding mental retardation*, Cambridge, Cambridge University Press, 73.

learning. Averaged rates of learning in normal and retarded children may suggest that the retarded learn more slowly. That however is not necessarily the case. *When learning starts* it may be as fast as in controls, differences being in the time taken to start learning; if such results are plotted backwards in time from a criterion of success then rates of learning can be seen to be similar in the two groups.

Slowness in starting to learn is caused by several factors, not all cognitive. Retarded children are often surprisingly environmentally and socially deprived, partly due to institutionalization, but also occurring in those not in institutions. They are inexperienced at learning, and unused to social reinforcement, such that social reinforcement in an experimental situation often distracts attention, rather than assisting the task. Retarded children often also learn they are unable to succeed at tasks, this LEARNED HELPLESSNESS becoming greater with age as more failure is experienced.

The social deprivation experienced by retarded children itself partly reflects the child's influence upon its family. Parents of retarded children often mourn after the diagnosis is made, feeling guilt and a sense of failure for not producing a normal child, and being frustrated at the lack of educational progress. Compared with control groups the parents are more often depressed, are more preoccupied with their children, have diminished self-esteem, and greater problems in handling anger, the latter partly accounting for an increased risk of child abuse. Coping by families is improved if the parents are financially well off, if both parents are present, if the marriage was stable before the child's birth, and if there is a support network from family and friends. The material consequences of a retarded child should also not be forgotten, a retarded child typically needing seven hours care per

IQ	Organic 0–70	Familial 50–70
CLASSIFICATORY PRINCIPLE	Demonstrable organic aetiology	No demostrable organic aetiology. Parents have this same type of retardation
CORRELATES	Found at all SES levels	More prevalent at lower SES levels
	IQs most often below 50	IQs rarely below 50
	Siblings usually of normal intelligence	Siblings often at lower levels of intelligence
	Often accompanied by severe health problems	Health within normal range
	Appearance often marred by physical stigmata	Normal appearance
	Mortality rate higher (More likely to die at a younger age than the general population)	Normal mortality rate
	Often dependent on care from others throughout life	With some support can lead an independent existence as adults
	Unlikely to marry and often infertile	Likely to marry and produce children of low intelligence
	Unlikely to experience neglect in their homes	More likely to experience neglect in their homes
	High prevalence of other physical handicaps (e.g., epilepsy, cerebral palsy)	Less likely to have other physical handicaps

Fig. 31.3 Differences between mental retardates with organic and familial aetiology. Some individuals cannot reliably be placed in either of the two groups and would therefore be classed as 'Undifferentiated'. Adapted from Zigler E and Hodapp R M (1986), *Understanding mental retardation*, Cambridge, Cambridge University Press, 53.

day, and considerable financial expenditure; families with retarded children fail to show the typical social and economic upward mobility seen in parents entering middle age.

Help for the retarded takes many forms, although in general there are unlikely to be 'miracle cures' (despite occasional claims in the popular press). Prophylaxis is successful in rare cases, such as a phenylalanine free diet in phenylketonuria. Physical treatments have little role. A controversial exception is partial glossectomy to reduce the bulky protruding tongue in Down's syndrome, thus allowing the mouth to close, improving speech and language, preventing dribbling, and producing a more normal appearance which diminishes stereo-typing and discrimination by adults and children, and allows more normal social interactions.

Appropriate education for retarded children is required by law in the UK, and frequently this is a special education in institutions specializing in the needs of the retarded. Some carefully selected children (Figure 31.4) benefit from MAINSTREAMING, education in a normal school with ordinary children, a process that also benefits the normal children, by demonstrating the range of human variability, and reducing subsequent negative attitudes towards retardation.

For moderate and severe retardation much benefit is attained through programmes of specific BEHAVIOUR MODIFICATION. Although far from confined to the treatment of mental retardation, this is a convenient place to describe these important techniques in detail.

The mentally retarded present many problems of practical manage-ment for carers, be they parents, teachers or nurses. Some absent behaviours could help the child, allowing more integration and benefit from society; examples are toilet training, ability to feed or dress, and improved language use. Other behaviours that are present are deleterious, such as temper tantrums, masturbation, or faeces smear-ing, and can be life-threatening, as with compulsive desires to climb or jump, head-banging or self-mutilation. Changing these behaviours is not easy in the absence of sufficient intellectual or linguistic skills for psychotherapy or reasoning, so that the only practical techniques are BEHAVIOUR MODIFICATION or BEHAVIOUR THERAPY, using the principles of learning theory, and especially of operant conditioning. Many techniques are now available and a few will be described here, emphasizing the principles of practical behaviour change.

Engineering human behaviour is similar to other forms of engineer-ing, beginning with an objective description of the problem, and of the desired end product; a hypothesis is then proposed to explain the aberrant behaviour, and the hypothesis tested by implementing a process of change; and finally the outcome is evaluated to assess success or otherwise. Probably the key improvement over informal approaches to behaviour change (as practised by parents and teachers for generations) is the emphasis upon objective measurement of

A child should be mainstreamed	Caution should be used in considering mainstreaming
If the child is young and the problem has been identified rather early in the school year.	If the child is older and the problem has continued unimproved for some time in the regular class.
If the child's problem is mild and not readily apparent outside of the school context.	If the child's problem is severe and pervades other areas of the child's life.
If the child's problem is limited to a single area of functioning.	If the child's problems are multiple (e.g. mild retardation *and* a behaviour problem).
If remediation of the child's problem does not require complicated equipment or materials.	If the child's condition requires complicated remedial equipment or teaching methods.
If the child appears to have friends or the ability to develop supportive friendships with normal children.	If the child has had repeated difficulty in developing friendships with nonhandicapped children.
If the regular classroom contains less than 25 or 30 children.	If the regular classroom contains more than 30 or 35 children.
If the child's regular-class teacher appears knowledgeable and willing to deal with the child's problem.	If the child's teacher appears to be unwilling or grossly unable to continue working with the child.
If the child's family appear to be willing and able to deal effectively with his or her problem.	If the child's family appears to lack extensive support for dealing with his or her problem.

Fig. 31.4 Criteria for differentiating retarded children for whom mainstreaming is likely to be successful from those for whom it will probably be unsuccessful. Adapted from Forness S R (1979), *Psychology in the Schools*, **16**, 508–14.

behaviour, so that it can be seen directly whether a manipulation has worked, and if not, change it.

Programmes for behaviour modification must be tailored for each individual problem and person, there being no 'off-the-peg' solutions, although general techniques sometimes transfer, although not always successfully if applied uncritically.

The first, most important step is to IDENTIFY THE PROBLEM and SELECT A TARGET, which should be realistic, within the ability range of the child. Since problems do not exist in a vacuum but are part of a social world, the social situation may be a part or even the major cause of a problem, a behaviour occurring only in some places or with certain individuals. Identification of the problem requires MEASUREMENT, the child's behaviour being closely observed over an extended period of days or weeks, to establish a BASE-LINE level before intervention. Measurement uses many techniques, from simple checklists (e.g. Fig. 31.5), through observational methods derived from ETHOLOGY (the study of animal behaviour), assessing the timing and frequency of specific EVENTS in a SAMPLING PERIOD (e.g. the number of tantrums occurring each hour between 8 am and 6 pm), or the DURATION of behaviours (e.g. how long does the child take to get dressed?), through sophisticated methods of INTERVAL RECORDING by a trained observer who by using a pre-coded schema on a keyboard records all the behaviours occurring in each 15 second epoch.

After the base-line has been recorded a programme of intervention can be devised. Different techniques are used for initiating behaviours or preventing them, and they will be considered separately.

Mentally retarded children need to know many skills, which they do not learn by imitation or modelling, examples being teeth cleaning, hair combing and use of knife and fork, the behaviours generally being completely absent, or else poorly formed and non-functional. The LAW OF EFFECT says behaviours change in response to their consequences, and hence behaviours are increased or improved by associating them with beneficial results; they are REINFORCED. Reinforcers are divided into three groups: PRIMARY REINFORCERS, such as food, drink, and warmth, which satisfy biological needs; SECONDARY REINFORCERS such as money or tokens without intrinsic effect, but which give access to primary reinforcers; and SOCIAL REINFORCERS, such as attention, praise, cuddling, hugging or smiling, which are perceived positively, but not because of their association with biological needs. Primary reinforcers are powerful but impractical, food, for instance, being messy and inconvenient, showing satiation, and requiring time out from training for its consumption. Sweets as reinforcers ('Smarties' being very popular) also cause obesity and dental problems if overused. In general, therefore, either social reinforcers or secondary reinforcers such as tokens are used. Most children rapidly learn that a token gives access to future rewards (be they sweets, television, games, or

A. Eating skills	Cannot	Can with help	Can by self but messy	Can by self neatly
Chews adequately				
Tries to feed self with fingers				
Eats with spoon				
Eats with spoon and fork				
Eats with fork alone				
Uses fork and knife				
Uses knife as pusher				
Cuts with knife				
Spreads with knife				
Drinks from cup				

B. Social training				
Finds own place and sits				
Sits still during meals				
Waits for others to finish				
Lays table				
Pours from jug				
Serves with spoon				
Carries plate				
Passes plates				

C. Behaviour problems	Often	Sometimes	Rarely	Never
Uses fingers unnecessarily				
Tips drink over				
Throws or tips food				
Grabs other people's food				
Regurgitates food				
Faddiness about food				
Bolts food				
Excessively slow				
Eats from plate with mouth				

Fig. 31.5 Example of an assessment form used in the monitoring of behaviour and self-care during feeding. Reproduced with permission from Carr J and Wilson B (1980), in Yule W and Carr J, Eds, *Behaviour modification for the mentally handicapped*, London, Croom Helm, 116–32.

swimming), and then behaviours may be reinforced by the tokens themselves, which are clean, easy to distribute, do not satiate, and require no time for consumption. TOKEN ECONOMIES also provide social training in handling those important tokens that motivate so much normal adult behaviour, money. Tokens may also reinforce group behaviour by rewarding individuals only if the entire group has acted in a particular way. Finding a reinforcer for a particular child is usually straightforward, since usually one can ask the child what they like, look at what they like doing, or present alternatives and observe preference. Occasionally no reinforcer is obvious and problems result. A solution uses the PREMACK PRINCIPLE, in which the child is left on its own and observed; any behaviour performed frequently, even if stereotyped, such as plaiting string or clapping hands, can be presumed to be intrinsically rewarding, and access to the behaviour will act as a reinforcer. Occasionally, observation reveals an undesirable behaviour such as masturbation or head-banging; that also can sometimes be used to gain behavioural control, and then itself phased out. All the reinforcers thus far have been positive; negative reinforcers, the removal of aversive events, find little practical use in behaviour modification.

If the desired behaviour occurs spontaneously then its frequency can be increased by reinforcement, successful reinforcement having the four features of being CONTINGENT, occurring only together with the target behaviour, being IMMEDIATE, as soon as the target behaviour has occurred, being CONSISTENT, and being CLEAR, so that there is no doubt about the relation between behaviour and reward. CONTINUOUS REINFORCEMENT, when each occurrence of the behaviour is reinforced, is more successful in the early stages of training than INTERMITTENT REINFORCEMENT, but gradually transfer is made to intermittent schedules, such as the variable rate schedule (see Chapter 3), which are more resistant to extinction, and correspond more closely to the vicissitudes of the real world.

Very often a behaviour is desirable but not even occasional reasonable efforts are made at performing it. SHAPING is used, so that at first crude approximations are rewarded, and then reinforcement gradually given only for the desired components; thus a child can be taught to use a spoon, firstly by rewarding for touching the spoon, then for holding or picking it up, then for holding it the right way up, followed by rewards only if the spoon is held near the mouth or put in it; and so on. In some sense this is how all children have learnt to use a spoon, using social reinforcers from parents, coupled with imitation. Some behaviours have the additional complication that the individual components are inherently simple, but the components must be assembled in the correct sequence; there is little point in brushing your teeth without firstly putting toothpaste on the brush. CHAINING is trained by rewarding for partial sequences, with reinforcers

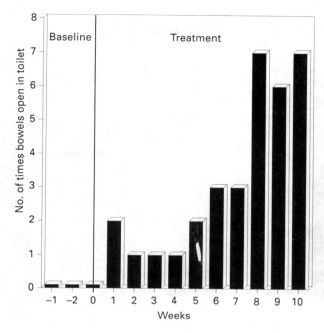

Fig. 31.6 The treatment of faecal soiling by the use of positive reinforcement with tokens in a five year old mildly mentally handicapped girl. Redrawn with permission from Wilson B (1980), in Yule W and Carr J, Eds, *Behaviour modification for the mentally handicapped*, London, Croom Helm, 135–50.

being given for longer and longer sequences. BACKWARD CHAINING, teaching the last item of the sequence first, is generally more effective than FORWARD CHAINING, when the steps are taught in their natural order. Sometimes children must be trained to GENERALIZE behaviour if, for example, toilet training is successful only at home but not at a nursery; alternatively they may need to learn DISCRIMINATION, that behaviours should only occur in response to specific stimuli, so that, for instance, food is only eaten at a dinner table at meal times, and not whenever it is seen, be it in the kitchen or the supermarket. Programmes of reinforcement usually provide such refinements with relative ease.

Figure 31.6 shows a successful behaviour modification programme for a five year old mentally retarded child who did not use a toilet for defecation (although she did use it for micturition), and instead soiled herself, ENCOPRESIS). Initially the mother taught her not to be afraid of the toilet by rewarding her with sweets whenever she sat on the toilet seat. However, she still did not defecate in the toilet, and after a baseline recording when the mother recorded where and when the child defecated (pants, floor, bed, toilet) a token system was instigated by the psychologist simply explaining to the child that each week they would visit the shops and buy an ice-cream or sweets if the child had collected enough 'stars', one star being given for each successful bowel opening. As Figure 31.6 shows, the programme was rapidly successul. However, encopresis can be particularly resistant to training, in part because the stimulus of rectal distention occurs infrequently each day;

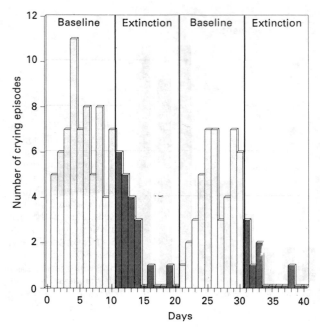

Fig. 31.7 The role of inadvertent social reinforcement in maintaining crying and tantrums in a four-year-old, and its extinction by ignoring of crying episodes. Redrawn with permission from Hart, Allen, Buell, Harris and Wolf (1964), Effects of social conditioning on operant crying, *J Exp Child Psychol*, **1**, 145–53.

that problem can be solved by administering a mild purgative. Similarly administration of oral fluids helps bladder control training by increasing the rate of bladder distention.

Decreasing a deviant or undesirable behaviour is more problematic than increasing the rate of a behaviour. Occasionally behaviours can be removed by altering the environment, by changing stimuli associated with the behaviour, or by gradually removing the reward associated with the behaviour. A child was excessively attached to a blanket that it would drag around all day, having tantrums whenever it was removed, and not taking part in more constructive educational activities; the mother was advised to cut a small portion from the blanket each night so that after a few weeks the child carried round only a tattered bundle of threads, in which it then lost interest.

Some behaviours can be removed by EXTINCTION. Behaviours must be maintained by being rewarded, so that if the reward is found and removed then the behaviour will decrease. Rewards are often social reinforcers, since behaviours attract attention or care from parents and carers. Figure 31.7 is an example of a four-year-old boy crying continuously at nursery school, as is seen in the base-line observations. Careful study showed crying to be rewarded by extra care and attention from staff, so that during extinction, staff were instructed to ignore the child, when the behaviour rapidly disappeared. In a test period, care and attention were reintroduced in response to crying and rapidly produced increased crying, after which a second extinction period eliminated the behaviour even more quickly than before. Although often successful, extinction has the problem of being slow (especially when compared with punishment), particularly when previous reinforcement has been on an intermittent schedule; there is also often an EXTINCTION BURST, which is very unpleasant for carers, and sometimes dangerous for the child with behaviours such as head-banging. It also fails if reward is intrinsic, and so cannot be dissociated from behaviour, as in masturbation. Finally, it is practically difficult to ensure all carers produce the appropriate behaviour, such as ignoring *all* tantrums; a single failure will result in continuation of the behaviour, perhaps directed specifically at the most vulnerable member of staff.

Much more successful at removing unwanted behaviours is PUNISHMENT (used in the technical sense of an action that decreases the frequency of a behaviour, rather than simply as a coercive, moral or physical force, or threats of such behaviour). Corporal punishment is actually rarely used, partly because it is not very effective (being associated with positive reinforcers unbeknown to the administrator, such as elevation of status in the eyes of peers), partly because it degrades the carers, distracting them from their role of *caring*, and partly because of ethical problems within institutions. The most used punishment is TIME OUT (strictly, 'time out from positive reinforcement'), in which a pleasant stimulus is removed. A child misbehaving at dinner table is removed for several minutes, after which they are allowed to return. Similarly, televisions or gramophones are turned off, usually for a few minutes for each transgression, small repeated applications of punishment being more successful than a single large punishment. The events removed must genuinely be positive reinforcers; a child who is frightened of other children and misbehaves to attract teacher's attention will be *rewarded* by being placed outside the classroom, and the behaviour will increase in frequency. Occasionally, restraint is used as a punishment, such as a child's arms being pinioned to its side for 20 seconds or so, by an attendant or, very rarely, by a chair with straps. The latter is counter-productive in self-mutilating children since the restraint is a positive reinforcer to such children and hence increases the rate of the behaviour. In exceptional cases which involve life-threatening self-destructive behaviours electric shocks are used with effect. The crucial thing about punishment in behaviour modification is that it is *not* being used as a moral instrument, as a form of retribution or of 'just desserts', and there is no intention of making the punishment be proportional to or seem to atone for any supposed 'crime'. Punishments are small and mild but used frequently, in ways directly contingent upon behaviour, with the express intention of decreasing those behaviours. A final method of removing undesirable behaviours is DIFFERENTIAL REINFORCEMENT OF OTHER BEHAVIOURS (DRO). Since a child can carry out only one task at a time, if more desirable behaviours are reinforced and increase in rate then it is a necessary consequence that undesirable behaviours will decrease in frequency.

Behaviour modification can dramatically improve the life-style and social skills of mentally handicapped children (and many other groups of individuals), and make life more pleasant for them and their carers; nevertheless it must be carried out systematically, and with careful monitoring by the team of carers, as an integral part of caring. Common sense and intuition are no substitutes in psychology, or elsewhere, for the careful and systematic analysis of problems and the consequences of actions.

Further reading

Further reading

In the past quarter of a century, over half a million research papers have been published in psychology, as well as countless numbers of books. Any guide to further reading must therefore be highly selective. The books cited will, it is hoped, help you to gain access to this voluminous literature, in part by giving you a single title which will then allow you to find similar volumes on nearby shelves. The best way of finding information on a particular detailed topic is to use the *Psychological Abstracts* or *Index Medicus* (both published as annual volumes and available for on-line computer access). For succinct up to date research reviews, consult the major reviewing journals, of which such series as the American *Annual Review of Psychology* and the British Psychological Society's *Psychology Survey* (published biennially) are good, or look in the index of journals such as *Psychological Review* and *Psychological Bulletin*. For direct entry to the research literature, the journals published by the British Psychological Society will provide a useful guide to current interests, with the *British Journal of Psychology* covering cognitive psychology and areas of general interest, the *British Journal of Clinical Psychology* and the *British Journal of Medical Psychology* covering topics relevant to medicine, and the *British Journal of Social Psychology* and *British Journal of Developmental Psychology* covering social and developmental topics. For clinical and particularly psychiatric aspects of psychology, look at *Psychological Medicine* and the *Journal of Psychosomatic Research*, and for the newly emergent area of health psychology look at *Psychology and Health*. Any university with a department of psychology will almost certainly have most of the above in its library. There are hundreds of other journals in addition that often cover relatively obscure areas of the subject.

Useful works for following up or reading around topics mentioned in this volume are:

On psychology in general

Colman A M (1987), *Facts, fallacies and frauds in psychology*, London, Hutchinson.

Lloyd P, Mayes A, Manstead A S R, Meudell P R and Wagner H L (1984), *Introduction to psychology: an integrated approach*, London, Fontana.

Reber A S (1988), *The Penguin dictionary of psychology*, Harmondsworth, Penguin.

Tajfel H and Fraser C (1978), Eds, *Introducing social psychology*, Harmondsworth, Penguin.

Valentine E R (1982), *Conceptual issues in psychology*, London, George Allen and Unwin.

On psychology applied to medicine in general

Brewin C (1988), *Cognitive foundations of clinical psychology*, Hove, Lawrence Erlbaum.
Fitzpatrick R, Hinton J, Newman S, Scambler G and Thompson J (1984), *The experience of illness*, London, Tavistock.
Gatchel R J, Baum A and Krantz D S (1989), *An introduction to health psychology*, 2nd edn, New York, Random House.
Kent G and Dalgleish M (1983), *Psychology and medical care*, Wokingham, Von Nostrand Reinhold.
Leigh H and Reiser M F (1980) *The patient: biological, psychological and social dimensions of medical practice*, New York, Plenum.
Rachman S (1977, 1980 and 1984), Ed, *Contributions to medical psychology*, vol 1, 2 and 3, Oxford, Pergamon.
Taylor S E (1986), *Health psychology*, New York, Random House.

Perception and sensation

Bruce V and Green P (1985), *Visual perception: physiology, psychology and ecology*, London, Lawrence Erlbaum.
Frisby J (1979), *Seeing: illusion, brain and mind*, Oxford, Oxford University Press.
Gregory R L (1966), *Eye and brain: the psychology of seeing*, London, World University Library.
McNicol D (1972), *A primer of signal detection theory*, London, George Allen and Unwin.
Osherson D N, Kosslyn S M and Hollerbach J M (1990), *An invitation to cognitive science: volume 2, Visual cognition and action*, Cambridge, MTP.
Spoehr K T and Lehmkuhle S W (1982), *Visual information processing*, San Francisco, W H Freeman.

Learning

Davey G M (1981), *Animal learning and conditioning*, London, MacMillan.
Dickinson A (1980), *Contemporary animal learning theory*, Cambridge, Cambridge University Press.
Sheldon B (1982), *Behaviour modification: theory, practice and philosophy*, London, Tavistock.

Memory

Baddeley A D (1976), *The psychology of memory*, 2nd edn, New York, Harper & Row.
Baddeley A D (1990), *Human memory: theory and practice*, Hove, Lawrence Erlbaum.

Cohen G, Eysenck M W and LeVoi M E (1986), *Memory: a cognitive approach*, Milton Keynes, Open University Press.

John E R *et al*. (1985), 'Double-labelled metabolic maps of memory', *Science*, **233**, 1167–75.

Kopelman M D (1986), 'The memory deficits in Alzheimer-type dementia: a review', *Q J Exp Psychol*, **38A**, 535–73

Luria A R (1975), *The mind of a mnemonist*, Harmondsworth, Penguin.

Squire L R (1986), 'Mechanisms of memory', *Science*, **232**, 1612–20.

Thompson R F (1986), 'The neurobiology of learning and memory', *Science*, **233**, 941–7.

Whitty C W M and Zangwill O L (1977), *Amnesia*, 2nd edn, London, Butterworths.

Cognition

Cohen G (1983), *The psychology of cognition*, 2nd edn, London, Academic.

Johnson-Laird P N and Wason P C (1977), Eds, *Thinking: readings in cognitive science*, Cambridge, Cambridge University Press.

Johnson-Laird P N (1983), *Mental models*, Cambridge, Cambridge University Press.

Kahneman D, Slovic P and Tversky A (1982), Eds, *Judgement under uncertainty: heuristics and biases*, Cambridge, Cambridge University Press.

Osherson D N and Smith E E (1990), Eds, *An invitation to cognitive science: volume 3; Thinking*, Cambridge, MIT Press.

Language

Aitchison J (1983), *The articulate mammal: an introduction to psycholinguistics*, London, Hutchinson.

Argyle M (1975), *Bodily communication*, London, Methuen.

De Villiers P A and De Villiers J G (1979), *Early language*, London, Fontana.

Miller G A (1981), *Language and speech*, San Francisco, W H Freeman.

Osherson D N and Lasnik H (1990), Eds, *An invitation to cognitive science: volume 1, Language*, Cambridge, MIT press.

Intelligence

Kaplan R M and Saccuzzo D P (1982), *Psychological testing: principles, applications and issues*, Monterey, Brooks/Cole.

Sternberg R J (1982), Ed, *Handbook of human intelligence*, Cambridge, Cambridge University Press.

Vernon P E (1979), *Intelligence: heredity and environment*, San Francisco, W H Freeman.

Zajonc R B (1983), 'Validating the confluence model', *Psychol Bull*, **93**, 457–80.

Personality

Eysenck H J (1970), *The structure of human personality*, 3rd edn, London, Methuen.

Kline P (1983), *Personality: measurement and theory*, London, Hutchinson.
Lynn R (1981), *Dimensions of personality: papers in honour of H J Eysenck*, Oxford, Pergamon.
Powell G E (1980), *Brain and personality*, Farnborough, Gower.

Emotion

Adelmann P K and Zajonc R B (1989), 'Facial efference and the experience of emotion', *Annu Rev Psychol*, **40**, 249–80.
Robins P V *et al.* (1986), 'Structural brain correlates of emotional disorder in multiple sclerosis', *Brain*, **109**, 585–97.
Strongman K T (1978), *The psychology of emotion*, 2nd edn, Chichester, John Wiley.

Child development

Bower T G R (1971), 'The object in the world of the infant', *Scientific American*, **225** (4), 30–8.
Bower T G R (1979), *Human development*, San Francisco, W H Freeman.
Fischer K W and Lazerson A (1988), *Human development: from conception through adolescence*, New York, W H Freeman.
Meadows S (1986), *Understanding child development*, London, Hutchinson.
Piaget J and Inhelder B (1969), *The psychology of the child*, London, Routledge and Kegan Paul.
Richmond P G (1970), *An introduction to Piaget*, London, Routledge and Kegan Paul.
Rutter M (1981), *Maternal deprivation reassessed*, 2nd edn, Harmondsworth, Penguin.

Freud

Appignanesi R and Zarate O (1992), *Freud for beginners*, London, Icon Books.
Brown D and Pedder J (1979), *Introduction to psychotherapy: an outline of psychodynamic principles and practice*, London, Tavistock.
Erdelyi M H (1985), *Psychoanalysis: Freud's cognitive psychology*, New York, W H Freeman.
Isbister J N (1985) *Freud: an introduction to his life and work*, Cambridge, Polity Press.
Kline P (1981), *Fact and fantasy in Freudian theory*, 2nd edn, London, Methuen.

Attitudes

Ajzen I and Fishbein M (1980), *Understanding attitudes and predicting social behaviour*, New Jersey, Prentice-Hall.
Hewstone M (1989), *Causal attribution: from cognitive processes to collective beliefs*, Oxford, Basil Blackwell.
Hewstone M, Stroebe W, Codol J-P and Stephenson G M (1988), Eds, *Introduction to social psychology*, Oxford, Basil Blackwell.

Personal construct theory

Bannister D and Fransella F (1971), *Inquiring man: the theory of personal constructs*, 2nd edn, Harmondsworth, Penguin.
Fransella F and Bannister D (1977), *A manual for repertory grid technique*, London, Academic.
Kelly G A (1955), *The psychology of personal constructs*, New York, W W Norton.

Group processes

Argyle M and Henderson M (1985), *The anatomy of relationships*, Harmondsworth, Penguin.
Cartwright D and Zander A (1968), *Group processes: research and theory*, 3rd Edn, London, Tavistock.
Gahagan J (1975), *Interpersonal and group behaviour*, London, Methuen.
Smith P B (1983), 'Social influence processes in groups', in Nicholson J and Foss B M, Eds, *Psychology survey No. 4*, Leicester, British Psychological Society, 88–108.

Doctor-patient communication

Bennett A E (1976), Ed, *Communication between doctors and patients*, London, Oxford University Press.
Byrne P S and Long B E L (1984), *Doctors talking to patients*, Exeter, Royal College of General Practitioners.
Hargie O (1986), Ed, *A handbook of communication skills*, London, Croom Helm.
Ley P (1988), *Communicating with patients: Improving communication, satisfaction and compliance*, London, Croom Helm.
Pendleton D and Hasler J (1983), *Doctor-patient communication*, London, Academic.

Diagnosis

Adams I D *et al.* (1986), 'Computer-aided diagnosis of acute abdominal pain: a multi-centre study', *Br Med J*, **293**, 800–4.
Elstein A S, Shulman L S and Sprafka S A (1978), *Medical problem solving: an analysis of clinical reasoning*, Cambridge, Harvard University Press.
Gale J and Marsden P (1983), *Medical diagnosis: from student to clinician*, Oxford, Oxford University Press.
Schwartz S and Griffin T (1986), *Medical thinking: the psychology of medical judgement and decision making*, New York, Springer-Verlag.
Taylor T R, Aitchison J and McGirr E M (1971), 'Doctors as decision makers: a computer-assisted study of diagnosis as a cognitive skill', *Br Med J*, **2**, 35–40.

Ageing

Bromley D B (1966), *The psychology of human ageing*, Harmondsworth, Penguin.

Erikson E H (1977), *Childhood and society*, London, Triad/Paladin.
Levy R and Post F (1982), Eds, *The psychiatry of late life*, Oxford, Blackwell.

Death, dying and bereavement

Anthony S (1971), *The discovery of death in childhood and after*, London, Allen Lane.
Bowlby J (1981), *Attachment and loss: vol III: Loss: sadness and depression*, Harmondsworth, Penguin.
Hinton J (1972), *Dying*, 2nd edn, Harmondsworth, Penguin.
Parkes C M (1986), *Bereavement: studies of grief in adult life*, 2nd edn, Harmondsworth, Penguin.
Worden J W (1983), *Grief counselling and grief therapy*, London, Tavistock.

Sleep

Hartmann E L (1973), *The functions of sleep*, New Haven, Yale University Press.
Horne J (1989), *Why do we sleep: the functions of sleep in humans and other mammals*, Oxford, Oxford University Press.
Mayes A (1983), Ed, *Sleep mechanisms and functions in humans and animals — an evolutionary perspective*, Wokingham, Van Nostrand Reinhold.
Mendelson W B, Gillin J C and Wyatt R J (1977), *Human sleep and its disorders*, New York, Plenum.

Pain

Melzack R and Wall P D (1982), *The challenge of pain*, Harmondsworth, Penguin.
Pearce S (1983), 'Pain', in Nicholson J and Foss B, Eds, *Psychology Survey No. 4*, Leicester, British Psychological Society, 170–202.

Drugs, placebos and addiction

Glass I B (1991), *The international handbook of addiction behaviour*, London, Routledge.
Iversen S D and Iversen L L (1981), *Behavioural pharmacology*, 2nd edn.
Stimson G V (1973), *Heroin and behaviour*, Shannon, Irish Universities Press.
Stimson G V and Oppenheimer E (1982), *Heroin addiction: treatment and control in Britain*, London, Tavistock.

Stress, anxiety and psychosomatics

Cox T (1978), *Stress*, London, MacMillan.
Gray J A (1987), *The psychology of fear and stress*, Cambridge, Cambridge University Press.
Henry J P and Stephens P M (1977), *Stress, health and the social environment*, New York, Springer-Verlag.
Johnston M and Wallace L (1990), *Stress and medical procedures*, 3rd edn, Oxford, Oxford University Press.

Levitt E E (1980), *The psychology of anxiety, 2nd edn*, Hillsdale, Lawrence Erlbaum.

Neuropsychology

Beaton A (1985), *Right side, left side: a review of laterality research*, London, Batsford.
Ellis A (1984), *Reading, writing and dyslexia: a cognitive analysis*, London, Lawrence Erlbaum.
Gardner H (1976), *The shattered mind*, New York, Vintage.
Humphreys G W and Riddoch M J (1987), *To see but not to see: a case study of visual agnosia*, London, Lawrence Erlbaum.
Kolb B and Whishaw I Q (1985), *Fundamentals of human neuropsychology*, 2nd edn, New York, W H Freeman.
McManus I C (1985), Handedness, language dominance and aphasia: a genetic model, *Psychol Med, Monograph supplement No. 8.*
Shallice T (1988), *From neuropsychology to mental structure*, Cambridge, Cambridge University Press.

Smoking

Ashton H and Stepney R (1982), *Smoking: psychology and pharmacology*, London, Tavistock.
Royal College of Physicians (1983), *Health or smoking?*, London, Pitman.
Warburton D M (1989), 'Is nicotine use an addiction?', *The Psychologist: Bulletin of the British Psychological Society*, **4**, 166–70.

Alcohol

Eastman C (1984), *Drink and drinking problems*, London, Longman.
Hore B D (1976), *Alcohol dependence*, London, Butterworths.
Robertson I and Heather N (1986), *Let's drink to your health: a self-help guide to sensible drinking*, Leicester, British Psychological Society.
Royal College of Psychiatrists (1979), *Alcohol and alcoholism*, London, Tavistock.

Eating and obesity

Garrow J S (1981), *Treat obesity seriously: a clinical manual*, Edinburgh, Churchill Livingstone.
Le Magnen J (1985), *Hunger*, Cambridge, Cambridge University Press.
Logue A W (1986), *The psychology of eating and drinking*, New York, W H Freeman.

Models of mental illness

Hare R M (1986), 'Health', *J Med Ethics*, **12**, 174–81.
Miller E and Morley S (1986), *Investigating abnormal behaviour*, London, Weidenfeld and Nicolson.

Siegler M and Osmond H (1966), 'Models of madness', *Br J Psychiatr*, **112**, 1193–1203.

Neurosis

Beech H R and Vaughan M (1978), *Behavioural treatments of obsessional states*, London, John Wiley.
Eysenck H J and Rachmann S (1965), *The causes and cures of neurosis*, London, Routledge and Kegan Paul.

Depression

Brown G and Harris T (1978), *Social origins of depression*, London, Tavistock.
Garber J G and Seligman M E P (1980), *Human helplessness: theory and applications*, New York, Academic.
Gilbert P (1984), *Depression: from psychology to brain state*, London, Lawrence Erlbaum.
Scott W C M (1948), 'A psycho-analytic concept of the origin of depression', *Br Med J*, **1**, 538.
Segal H (1979), *Klein*, London, Fontana.

Schizophrenia

Laing R D and Esterson A (1970), *Sanity, madness and the family*, Harmondsworth, Penguin.
Miller R (1984), 'Major psychosis and dopamine: controversial features and suggestions', *Psychol Med*, **14**, 779–89.
Tsuang M T and Vandermey R (1980), *Genes and the mind: inheritance of mental illness*, Oxford, Oxford University Press.
Wing J K (1978), *Schizophrenia: towards a new synthesis*, London, Academic.

Mental subnormality

Clarke A M, Clarke A D B and Berg J M (1985), *Mental deficiency: the changing outlook*, 4th edn, London, Methuen.
Lewis V (1987), *Development and handicap*, Oxford, Blackwell.
Yule W and Carr J (1980), Eds, *Behaviour modification for the mentally handicapped*, London, Croom Helm.
Zigler E and Hodapp R M (1986), *Understanding mental retardation*, Cambridge, Cambridge University Press.

Index